Principles of
Clinical
Electrocardiography

11th edition

Principles of Clinical Electrocardiography

MERVIN J. GOLDMAN, MD

Clinical Professor of Medicine
University of California School of Medicine
San Francisco

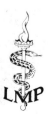

LANGE Medical Publications   Los Altos, California 94022

A Concise Medical Library for Practitioner and Student

Lithographed in USA

Table of Contents

Preface

It is the author's intention to present in this volume the basic concepts of electrocardiography and their clinical application. He realizes that material so presented must be simplified and that an exhaustive and detailed treatment of the subject matter to be covered will not be possible.

Emphasis has been placed on the unipolar leads. To one who first learned electrocardiography by memorizing patterns in the bipolar standard leads and later followed the development of unipolar electrocardiography, the latter offers a more logical approach to the subject material. Vector analysis of the ECG offers an intelligent means of understanding the electrical potentials generated from the heart. There should be no major disagreement between vector and unipolar electrocardiographic analysis. Both are descriptive of the same phenomena, the former offering an evaluation of the electrical potentials as oriented in space and the latter as reflected in the resulting electrocardiographic pattern.

A knowledge of basic electrophysiologic principles is essential in the understanding of the ECG. These are emphasized throughout the text. Such information permits a more logical and meaningful appreciation of electrocardiography.

The author cannot too strongly emphasize the fact that the ECG is a laboratory test only. Like all laboratory findings, an abnormal electrocardiographic tracing is significant only when interpreted in the light of clinical findings. Ideally, the person best qualified to interpret the ECG is the physician caring for the patient.

The chapter on spatial vectorcardiography and corrected orthogonal lead systems is intended to give the reader an insight into this relatively new field and not as a comprehensive discussion of the subject.

For the eleventh edition, new concepts pertaining to the differential diagnosis of transmural versus nontransmural myocardial infarction have been introduced; a section has been added on left anterior conduction delay; and a third appendix describes the application of statistics to the interpretation of the ECG. The section on electrical pacing has been expanded, and 44 new ECGs have been added.

We are most gratified with the acceptance this Review has received among students and physicians both here and abroad. Spanish, Italian, Japanese, Polish, Portuguese, French, and Greek translations are now available; German and Turkish translations are in preparation.

The many letters received are hereby acknowledged and are most welcome.

Mervin J. Goldman, MD

San Francisco
August, 1982

Introduction to Electrocardiography | 1

The electrocardiogram (ECG) is a graphic recording of the electrical potentials produced in association with the heartbeat. The heart is unique among the muscles of the body in that it possesses the property of automatic rhythmic contraction. The impulses that precede contraction arise in the conduction system of the heart. These impulses result in excitation of the muscle fibers throughout the myocardium. Impulse formation and conduction produce weak electrical currents that spread through the entire body. By applying electrodes to various positions on the body and connecting these electrodes to an electrocardiographic apparatus, the ECG is recorded. The connections of the apparatus are such that an upright deflection indicates positive potential and a downward deflection indicates negative potential.

USEFULNESS OF THE ELECTROCARDIOGRAM

With advances in electrocardiography, the accuracy of electrocardiographic diagnosis has been greatly increased. The ECG is of particular value in the following clinical conditions:

(1) Atrial and ventricular hypertrophy.

(2) Myocardial ischemia and infarction: Multiple leads, vectorcardiograms, and modern exercise testing have increased the accuracy of diagnosis and of estimates of extent of disease.

(3) Arrhythmias: Not only can more exact diagnoses be made, but unipolar and intracardiac electrocardiography have also contributed substantially to our basic understanding of the origin and conduction of abnormal rhythms.

(4) Pericarditis.

(5) Systemic diseases that affect the heart.

(6) Effect of cardiac drugs, especially digitalis and quinidine.

(7) Disturbances in electrolyte metabolism, especially potassium abnormalities.

Caution to the Beginner

The ECG is a laboratory test only and is not a sine qua non of heart disease diagnosis. A patient with an organic heart disorder may have a normal ECG, and a perfectly normal individual may show nonspecific electrocardiographic abnormalities. All too often a patient is relegated to the status of a cardiac invalid solely on the basis of some electrocardiographic abnormality. On the other hand, a patient may be given unwarranted assurance of the absence of heart disease solely on the basis of a normal ECG. The ECG must always be interpreted in conjunction with the clinical findings. In general, the person best qualified to interpret the ECG is the physician caring for the patient.

ELECTROCARDIOGRAPHIC APPARATUS

In modern electrocardiography, 2 types of apparatus are used: the string galvanometer and the radio amplifier. The former records its pattern on photographic paper which must then be developed. It requires more experience to operate, and caution must be taken to prevent damage to the valuable string. The radio amplifier has been combined with a direct writer; it is a compact, light, and mobile unit which is very simple to operate, and there is much less chance of damaging the machine by technical errors of operation. It has the additional advantage of producing an instantaneous recording, thus making the record immediately available for interpretation. Many modern machines record multiple (3 or 6) leads simultaneously.

Oscilloscopic viewing of the ECG is commonly used in clinical medicine. This produces a constant electrocardiographic pattern on a fluorescent screen, and permanent records can be obtained by connecting the machine to a direct-writing apparatus. Such pieces of equipment are now routine in coronary and intensive care units and in surgery.

Small electrocardiographic tape recorders can be attached to a patient and continuous recordings obtained while the patient is ambulatory (or at rest) for 24-hour periods. The tape is then reviewed by the physician. This is of special value in the study of patients with arrhythmias and myocardial ischemia.

ECGs can be transmitted via telemetry or telephone lines, thus permitting constant or temporary

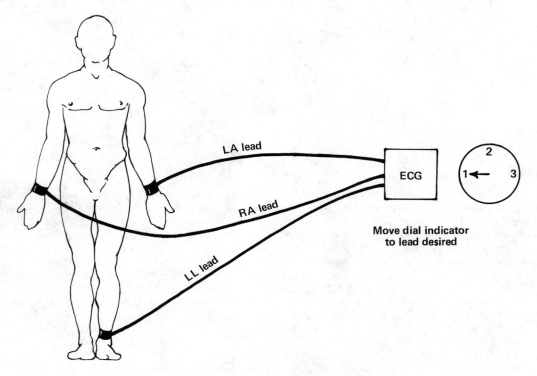

Figure 1–1. Standard leads.

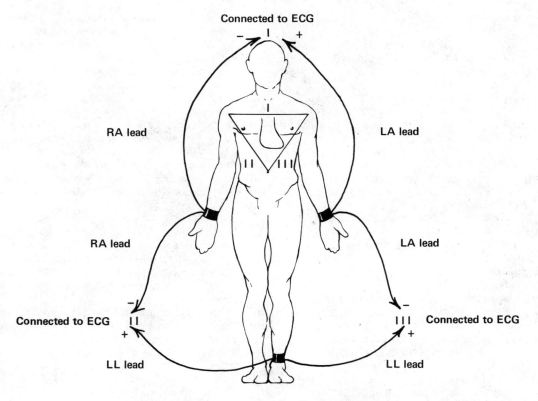

Figure 1–2. Connections for bipolar standard leads I, II, and III.

monitoring and interpretation by a physician many miles from the patient. Memory loops are available to record events prior to the onset of an arrhythmia. Computer facilities are available not only for electrocardiographic interpretation but for the recognition and quantitation of arrhythmias.

BIPOLAR STANDARD LEADS

The bipolar standard leads (I, II, and III) are the original leads selected by Einthoven to record the electrical potentials in the frontal plane. Electrodes are applied to the left arm, right arm, and left leg. Proper skin contact must be made by rubbing electrode paste on the skin. The LA (left arm), RA (right arm), and LL (left leg) leads are then attached to their respective electrodes. By turning the selector dial to 1, 2, and 3, the 3 standard leads (I, II, and III) are taken.

All electrocardiographic machines also have a right leg electrode and lead. This acts as a ground wire and plays no role in the production of the ECG. In areas where there is electrical interference, it may be necessary to run a ground wire from the bed or the machine to an appropriate ground (water pipe or steam pipe).

Electrical Potential

The bipolar leads represent a difference of electrical potential between 2 selected sites.

Lead I = Difference of potential between the left arm and the right arm (LA − RA).

Lead II = Difference of potential between the left leg and the right arm (LL − RA).

Lead III = Difference of potential between the left leg and the left arm (LL − LA).

The relation between the 3 leads is expressed algebraically by Einthoven's equation: lead II = lead I + lead III. This is based on Kirchoff's law, which states that the algebraic sum of all the potential differences in a closed circuit equals zero. If Einthoven had reversed the polarity of lead II (ie, RA − LL), the 3 bipolar lead axes would result in a closed circuit (Fig 1–17), and leads I + II + III would equal zero. However, since Einthoven did make this alteration in the polarity of the lead II axis, the equation becomes: I − II + III = 0. Hence II = I + III.

The electrical potential as recorded from any one extremity will be the same no matter where the electrode is placed on the extremity. The electrodes are usually applied just above the wrists and ankles. If an extremity has been amputated, the electrode can be applied to the stump. In a patient with an uncontrollable tremor, a more satisfactory record may be obtained by applying the electrodes to the upper portions of the limbs.

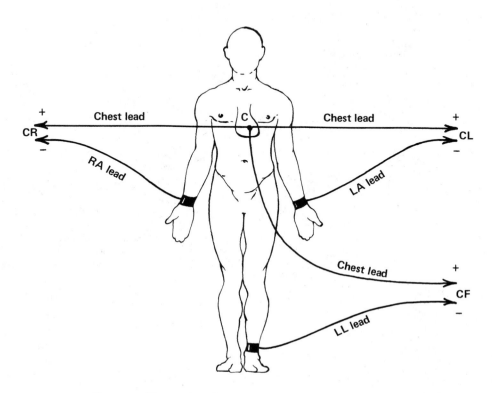

Figure 1–3. Connections for bipolar chest leads CR, CL, and CF.

BIPOLAR CHEST LEADS

Bipolar chest leads record differences of potential between any given position on the chest (C) and one extremity. Before unipolar electrocardiography was introduced, the left leg (F) was used as the "indifferent" electrode, and the leads were called CF leads. Less commonly, the right arm (CR leads) or the left arm (CL leads) was used. It was assumed that the left leg (or right or left arm) was so remote from the heart that it would act as an "indifferent" electrode and not interfere with the chest potential. However, it is now realized that the potentials in the extremities can appreciably alter the pattern of the chest lead. For this reason CF, CR, and CL leads are not frequently used today.

A special bipolar chest lead (Lewis lead) is of value in amplifying the waves of atrial activity and thereby clarifying the mechanism of an atrial arrhythmia. The right arm electrode is placed in the second intercostal space to the right of the sternum. The left arm electrode is placed in the fourth intercostal space to the right of the sternum. The tracing is then recorded on lead I. The above 2 electrodes may be interchanged (RA and LA). This will reverse the polarity of all the complexes, but it will not alter the interpretation since the basic purpose is to identify atrial activity.

UNIPOLAR LEADS
(Extremity Leads, Precordial [Chest] Leads, Esophageal Leads)

Unipolar leads (VR, VL, VF, multiple chest leads "V," and esophageal leads "E") were introduced into clinical electrocardiography by Wilson in 1932. The frontal plane unipolar leads (VR, VL, VF) bear a definite mathematical relationship to the standard (I, II, III) bipolar leads (see p 13). The precordial (V) leads record potentials in the horizontal plane without being influenced by actual potentials from an "indifferent" electrode used in recording bipolar chest leads. One concept must be clearly understood: A unipolar precordial (or esophageal) lead does not record only the electrical potential from a small area of the underlying myocardium; it records all of the electrical events of the entire cardiac cycle as viewed from the selected lead site.

All modern electrocardiographic machines are constructed so that augmented extremity leads can be taken with the same hookup as used for standard leads by turning the selector dial to aVR, aVL, and aVF. Unipolar chest leads are taken by applying the chest lead and its electrode to any desired position on the chest and turning the selector dial to the V position. Multiple chest leads are taken by changing the position

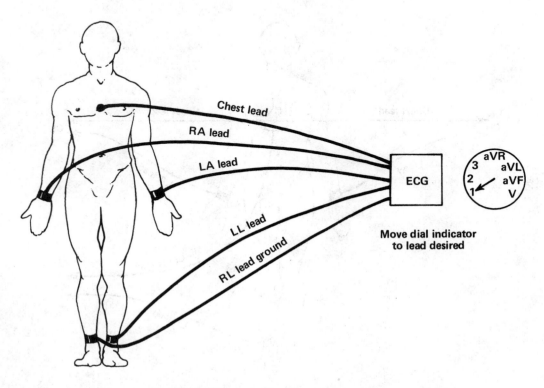

Figure 1–4. Unipolar leads with modern equipment.

of the chest electrode (Fig 1–9). Unipolar esophageal leads are taken by attaching the esophageal lead to the chest lead and turning the selector dial to the V position (Fig 1–14).

A universal lead selector is available for a 3-lead electrocardiographic apparatus. With this unit attached, the standard, unipolar extremity, and chest leads can be taken by simply rotating the selector dial as is done with all modern electrocardiographic machines.

IMPROVISED UNIPOLAR LEADS USING AN INDIFFERENT ELECTRODE

If a modern electrocardiographic machine or universal lead selector is not available, an electrocardiograph that can record standard leads I, II, and III can be used to obtain perfectly satisfactory unipolar leads. To do so, one first constructs an indifferent electrode. This is easily made by fastening 3 separate lengths of insulated copper wire (each about 4 feet long) together at one end with a battery clip. This end becomes the central terminal (T). The 3 free ends are connected to the LA, RA, and LL electrodes. The central terminal is connected to the RA lead of the electrocardiograph. The LA lead becomes the exploring electrode for any desired unipolar lead. All such leads are taken with the selector dial on lead I.

arm is recorded. Although it is technically a bipolar lead, it represents a unipolar lead since one of the potentials is zero. This is designated as VR (vector of right arm). The left arm (VL) and left leg (VF) potentials are obtained in the same way. The selector dial is set on lead I (Fig 1–6).

(1) To take VR, the LA lead of the machine is attached to an electrode placed on the right arm at a different site from the RA electrode connected to the central terminal.

(2) To take VL, the LA lead of the machine is attached to an electrode on the left arm.

(3) To take VF, the LA lead of the machine is attached to an electrode on the left leg.

Augmented Extremity Leads aVR, aVL, aVF

By a slight change in technique from above (this is automatically accomplished by all modern electrocardiographic machines), the amplitude of the deflections of VR, VL, and VF can be increased by about 50%.* These leads are called augmented unipolar extremity leads and are designated as aVR, aVL, and aVF. It must be emphasized that the only difference between leads VR, VL, and VF and leads aVR, aVL, and aVF is this difference in amplitude. In routine electrocardiographic practice, the augmented leads have replaced the nonaugmented unipolar extremity leads because they are easier to read. (Hereafter in this text, the term "extremity leads" will refer to the augmented leads.)

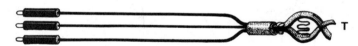

Figure 1–5. Indifferent electrode.

In principle, the unipolar leads attempt to represent potentials in a given lead axis and not differences in potential. Since it is generally accepted that the sum of the potentials of the 3 extremity leads is zero (RA + LA + LL = 0), the connection of these 3 extremity leads (the central terminal) will for all clinical purposes result in a zero potential.

UNIPOLAR EXTREMITY LEADS

Unipolar Nonaugmented Extremity Leads VR, VL, VF

These have been replaced by the augmented extremity leads aVR, aVL, and aVF and are not commonly taken.

Using the indifferent electrode (RA + LA + LL) as one terminal and placing another electrode on the right arm, a bipolar lead can be taken. This represents the difference between the potential of the right arm and the zero potential of the central terminal (RA − 0 = RA). Therefore, the "actual" potential of the right

*Using lead aVR as an example, this can be shown as follows. Since aVR represents a difference of potential between the right arm (RA or VR) and the average of the potential of the left leg and left arm, the following equation (1) can be established:

$$(1) \quad aVR = RA - \left[\frac{LL + LA}{2}\right]$$

By changing signs in (1):

$$(2) \quad aVR = RA + \left[-\frac{LL + LA}{2}\right]$$

From Einthoven's equation it is known that:

$$(3) \quad RA + LA + LL = 0$$

By subtracting LA + LL from both sides of (3):

$$(4) \quad RA = -(LA + LL)$$

By substituting equation (4) in (2):

$$(5) \quad aVR = RA + \left[\frac{RA}{2}\right] = 3/2 \text{ RA (or 3/2 VR)}$$

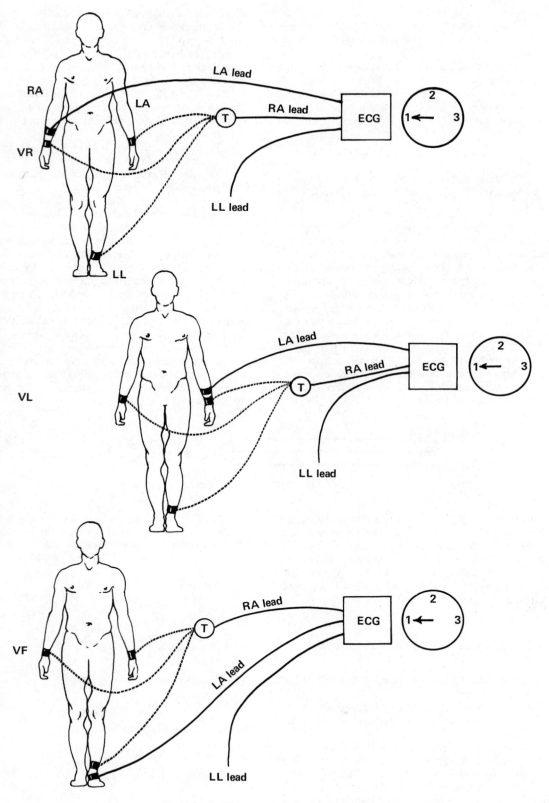

Figure 1–6. Nonaugmented extremity leads.

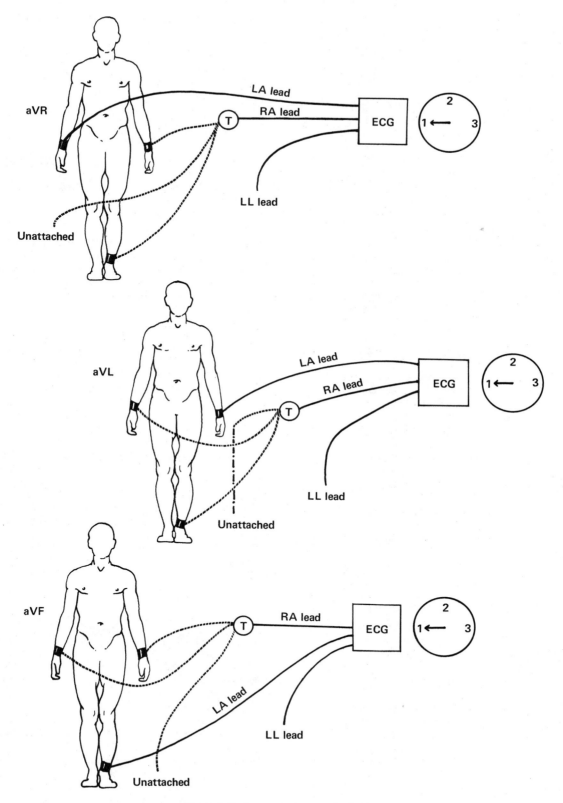

Figure 1–7. Augmented extremity leads.

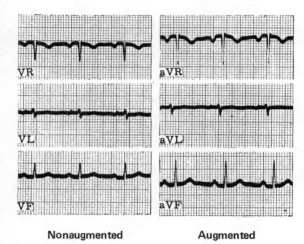

| Nonaugmented | Augmented |

Figure 1–8. Comparison of nonaugmented and augmented extremity leads. All of the above leads are taken on the same individual. Note that the pattern in comparable leads is the same; the only difference is that the augmented extremity leads are of greater voltage (approximately 3/2).

V_1: Fourth intercostal space at the right sternal border.

V_2: Fourth intercostal space at the left sternal border.

V_3: Equidistant between V_2 and V_4.

V_4: Fifth intercostal space in the left midclavicular line. All subsequent leads (V_{5-9}) are taken in the same horizontal plane as V_4.

V_5: Anterior axillary line.

V_6: Midaxillary line.

V_7: Posterior axillary line.

V_8: Posterior scapular line.

V_9: Left border of the spine.

V_{3R-9R}: Taken on the right side of the chest in the same location as the left-sided leads V_{3-9}. V_{2R} is therefore the same as V_1.

$3V_{1-9}$: Taken one interspace higher than V_{1-9}; these are the third interspace leads. The same terminology can be applied to leads taken in other interspaces, eg, $2V_{1-9}$, $6V_{1-9}$, etc.

V_{3R-9R}: Right precordial leads taken one interspace higher than V_{3R-9R}.

VE: Taken over the ensiform cartilage.

The usual routine ECG consists of 12 leads: I, II, III; aVR, aVL, aVF; and V_{1-6}.

As in the nonaugmented leads, the 3 wires of the indifferent electrode are connected to the 3 extremities (LA, RA, and LL); the central terminal is connected to the RA lead of the machine; the LA lead of the machine becomes the exploring electrode; and the selector dial is set on lead I. (See Fig 1–7.)

(1) To take aVR, the indifferent lead to the right arm is removed and left unattached, and the LA lead of the machine is attached to the RA electrode.

(2) To take aVL, the indifferent lead to the left arm is removed and left unattached, and the LA lead of the machine is attached to the LA electrode. (Of course, the indifferent electrode removed from the right arm in taking aVR has been replaced.)

(3) To take aVF, the indifferent lead to the left leg is removed and left unattached, and the LA lead of the machine is attached to the LL electrode.

UNIPOLAR PRECORDIAL (CHEST) LEADS

These are obtained by turning the selector to V on the dial or, in the older machines, by using the following directions:

The indifferent electrode leads remain connected to the 3 extremities. The central terminal is attached to the RA lead of the machine. The selector dial is set on lead I. The LA lead of the machine is attached to an electrode that can be applied to the desired chest positions, producing multiple unipolar chest leads. (See Fig 1–11.) This results in a V lead. The common precordial positions used (as recommended by the American Heart Association) are as follows:

MONITOR LEADS

Although it is possible to use any lead (or multiple simultaneous leads if equipment is available) in a specialized area such as a coronary care unit, it is more common to use a modified bipolar chest lead. The positive electrode is placed in the usual V_1 position and the negative electrode near the left shoulder. A third electrode is placed at a more remote area of the chest and serves as a ground. The recording will be similar to V_1 (a modified CL_1). This lead is of major value in rhythm evaluation. However, if it is deemed necessary to monitor the patient for ST–T changes due to ischemia or potassium abnormalities, it is advisable to place the positive electrode in the V_4 or V_5 position.

UNIPOLAR ESOPHAGEAL LEADS

Esophageal leads can be taken by attaching an esophageal lead to the V (chest) lead of the modern machine or the left arm lead of the improvised machine, using the indifferent electrode.

Esophageal leads are taken from within the esophagus. A nasal catheter through which is threaded a wire with an electrode attached to its tip can be passed through the nares into the esophagus. Using this as one terminal and the zero potential as the other terminal, a unipolar esophageal lead can be obtained. This is designated an E lead. The nomenclature of the lead is derived from the distance in centimeters from the tip of

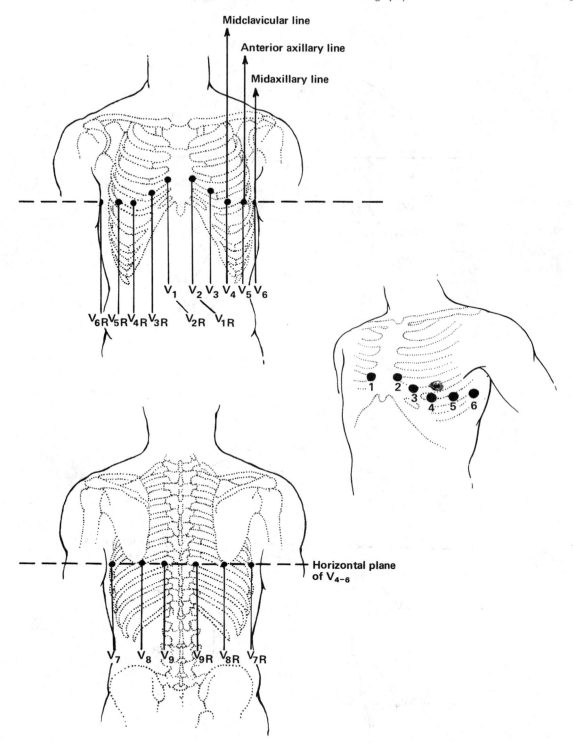

Figure 1–9. Locations of unipolar precordial leads.

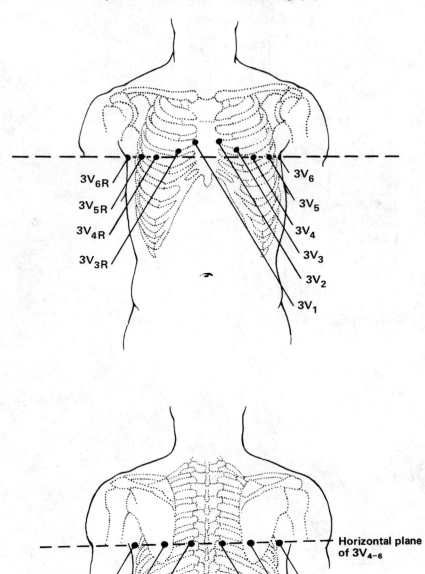

Figure 1–10. Third interspace leads.

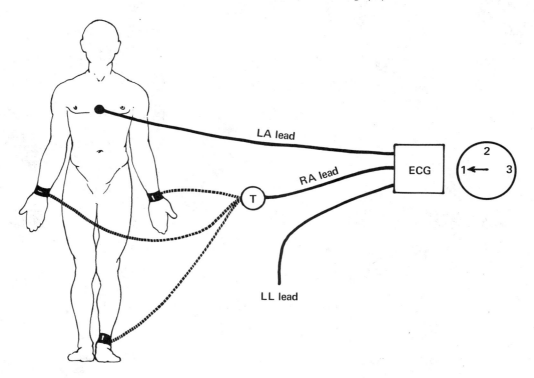

Figure 1–11. Unipolar chest leads.

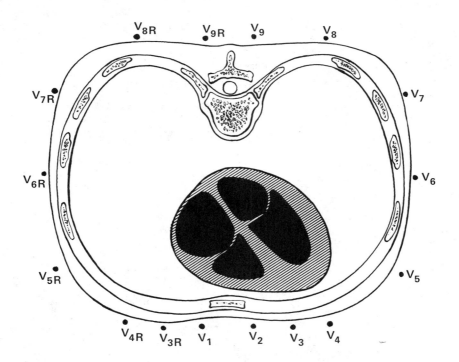

Figure 1–12. Transverse section of thorax illustrating position of the unipolar chest leads.

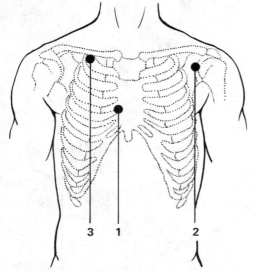

Figure 1–13. Modified CL$_1$ lead system for monitoring. (1) Positive electrode in V$_1$ position. (2) Negative electrode near left shoulder. (3) Ground electrode.

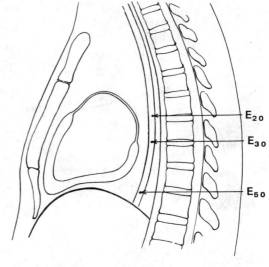

Figure 1–14. Sagittal view of thorax illustrating position of the unipolar esophageal leads.

the nares to the electrode. Thus, E$_{50}$ represents a unipolar esophageal lead at a distance of 50 cm from the nares. Leads E$_{40-50}$ usually reflect the posterior surface of the left ventricle; leads E$_{15-25}$, the atrial area; and leads E$_{25-35}$, the region of the atrioventricular groove. Since these positions vary tremendously with individual differences in body size and shape and heart position, no interpretation should be made from a single esophageal lead; an entire series of low to high esophageal levels must be studied for proper evaluation. For more accurate localization of the position of the esophageal electrode, fluoroscopy may be used.

Esophageal leads are especially useful in recording the atrial complexes, which are greatly magnified at this location, and in exploring the posterior surface of the left ventricle.

UNIPOLAR INTRACARDIAC LEADS

An electrode contained in a cardiac catheter is attached to the V (chest) lead. Unipolar ECGs can then be recorded from various intracardiac chambers, such as the right atrium and right ventricle, depending upon the position of the catheter tip. This technique is of clinical value in (1) clarification of an arrhythmia by amplification of the waves of atrial activity and (2) localization of the catheter tip when a "floating" pacemaker is inserted without fluoroscopic guidance. The nature of the P waves and QRS complexes will identify the location of the catheter tip.

With appropriate catheter electrodes inserted under fluoroscopic vision, recordings can be made of bundle of His potentials. This technique, although

limited to the cardiac laboratory, has resulted in major advances in the understanding and interpretation of arrhythmias and atrioventricular conduction. Multiple intracardiac recordings in association with appropriate electrical stimulation can be performed in specialized electrophysiology laboratories. They are of value in determination of the site of ectopic activity, the induction of arrhythmias by programmed stimulation and the efficacy of specific drug therapy, and the identification of accessory pathways.

Attachment of the V lead to a pericardiocentesis needle, under sterile precautions, permits electrocardiographic recording during this procedure. When the needle strikes the epicardium, ST elevation will be recorded and is an indication for withdrawal of the needle.

In all situations in which an actual or potential electrode is in direct contact with the myocardium, proper electrical grounding is essential. Currents as low as 10 μA can induce ventricular fibrillation.

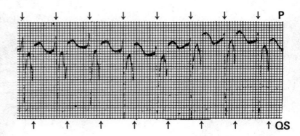

Figure 1–15. Unipolar ECG recorded with a catheter electrode in the right atrium. The very large diphasic complexes are P waves which are followed by QS complexes of ventricular activation.

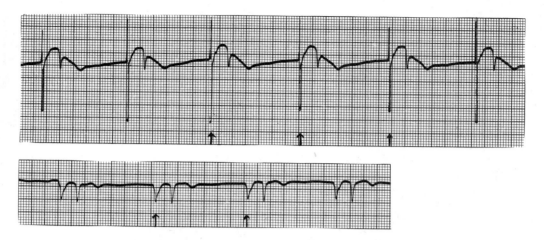

Figure 1–16. Intra-atrial electrogram. Unipolar electrograms recorded from an electrode within the right atrium. In the top recording, the very large, slender diphasic complexes (indicated by arrows) are the P waves. Note the elevation of the PR segment. This is the result of the electrode touching the endocardial surface of the right atrium and producing an acute current of injury (see p 140). In the bottom strip, the electrode is free in the upper portion of the right atrium and records an inverted P wave. The PR segment is isoelectric.

RELATIONSHIP BETWEEN UNIPOLAR EXTREMITY LEADS & STANDARD BIPOLAR LEADS

Leads I, II, III, aVR, aVL, and aVF all represent frontal plane vectors (see p 29). As stated on p 3: $I = VL - VR (LA - RA)$, $II = VF - VR (LL - RA)$, and $III = VF - VL (LL - LA)$.

Since the augmented extremity leads are 3/2 the nonaugmented extremity leads, the equations are changed to: $I = 2/3 (aVL - aVR)$, $II = 2/3 (aVF - aVR)$, and $III = 2/3 (aVF - aVL)$.

The relationship of the extremity leads to the standard leads is derived from Einthoven's formula:

(1) $VR + VL + VF = 0$

(2) $VR = - VL - VF$

(3) Adding 2VR to equation (2),

$$3VR = - VL - VF + 2VR$$

(4) $VR = \dfrac{- VL - VF + 2VR}{3}$

(5) $VR = \dfrac{- VL + VR - VF + VR}{3}$

(6) $VR = - \dfrac{(VL - VR) + (VF - VR)}{3}$

(7) $VR = - \dfrac{I + II}{3}$

In the same manner, the relationships of the extremity leads to the standard leads can be derived. The nonaugmented leads are multiplied by 3/2 to give the other augmented leads.

$$VR = - \dfrac{I + II}{3}$$

$$aVR = - \dfrac{I + II}{3} \times \dfrac{3}{2} = - \dfrac{I + II}{2}$$

$$VL = \dfrac{I - III}{3}$$

$$aVL = \dfrac{I - III}{3} \times \dfrac{3}{2} = \dfrac{I - III}{2}$$

$$VF = \dfrac{II + III}{3}$$

$$aVF = \dfrac{II + III}{3} \times \dfrac{3}{2} = \dfrac{II + III}{2}$$

Bipolar and unipolar leads are not of equal lead strength. A nonaugmented unipolar lead is 58% of the lead strength of a bipolar lead. An augmented unipolar lead is 87% (ie, $3/2 \times 58\%$) of the lead strength of a bipolar lead. Therefore, the above equations must be corrected by these factors. When the strength (voltage) of an augmented unipolar lead is determined from bipolar lead values, the latter is corrected by multiplying the result by 0.87. When the strength of a bipolar lead is determined from augmented unipolar lead values, the latter is corrected by multiplying by 1.15 (100/87). An example is shown in Fig 1–17.

The measured voltages of the individual R waves in the 6 leads are as follows (method of measurement is

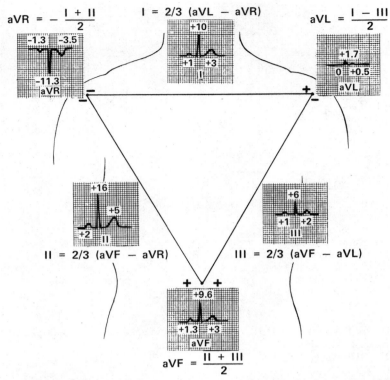

Figure 1–17. Illustration of the relationship of unipolar limb and standard leads. In order for the determinations to be accurate, the leads should be taken simultaneously.

given on p 28): I: R = +10, II: R = +16, III: R = +6, aVR: R = −11.3, aVL: R = +1.7, and aVF: R = +9.6.

To determine the voltage in augmented extremity leads from the actual measurements of the standard leads (only R will be calculated, but the same method is to be used for P and T):

$$aVR = -\frac{I + II}{2}(0.87) = -\left[\frac{10 + 16}{2}\right](0.87) = -11.3$$

$$aVL = \frac{I - III}{2}(0.87) = \left[\frac{10 - 6}{2}\right](0.87) = +1.7$$

$$aVF = \frac{II + III}{2}(0.87) = \left[\frac{16 + 6}{2}\right](0.87) = +9.6$$

To determine the voltage in standard leads from the actual measurement of the augmented extremity leads (again calculating only the R wave):

I = 2/3 (aVL − aVR) (1.15) =
    2/3 (1.7 + 11.3) (1.15) = +10

II = 2/3 (aVF − aVR) (1.15) =
    2/3 (9.6 + 11.3) (1.15) = +16

III = 2/3 (aVF − aVL) (1.15) =
    2/3 (9.6 − 1.7) (1.15) = +6

TECHNICAL DIFFICULTIES AFFECTING THE ELECTROCARDIOGRAM

Attention to the following details will ensure against artifacts and poor technical records:

(1) The examination should be conducted on a comfortable bed or table large enough to support the patient's entire body, and the patient must be completely relaxed in order to ensure a satisfactory tracing. It is best to explain the procedure in advance to an apprehensive patient in order to allay any fears or anxieties. Any muscular motions or twitchings by the patient can alter the record.

(2) Be certain there is good contact between the skin and the electrode. A poor contact can result in a poor record.

(3) The machine must be properly standardized so that 1 mV will produce a deflection of 1 cm. Incorrect standardization will produce inaccurate voltage of the complexes and can lead to faulty interpretation.

(4) The patient and the machine must be properly grounded to avoid alternating current interference.

(5) Any electronic equipment that comes in contact with the patient can produce artifacts in the ECG—eg, an electrically regulated intravenous infusion pump.

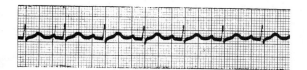

Figure 1–18. A technically good tracing.

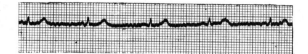

Figure 1–19. Effect of muscle twitchings.

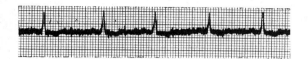

Figure 1–20. Effect of poor contact.

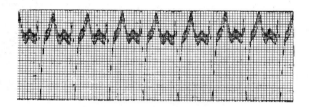

Figure 1–21. Effect of alternating current interference.

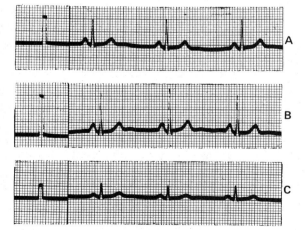

Figure 1–22. Effect of standardization. *A:* Proper standardization: 1 cm deflection. *B:* Overstandardization: 1.4 cm deflection. This increases the voltage of the complexes. *C:* Understandardization: 0.5 cm deflection. This decreases the voltage of the complexes.

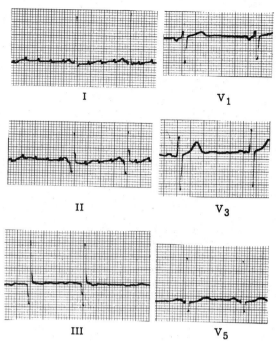

I   V₁

II   V₃

III   V₅

Figure 1–23. Regular deflections at a rate of 300 are recorded in leads I and II, which could result in an interpretation of atrial flutter (see p 225). However, lead III and all precordial leads indicate sinus rhythm. The above was due to artifact from an intravenous infusion pump unit inserted into a right forearm vein. In addition, there is evidence of inferior myocardial infarction (see p 169).

POTENTIAL ERROR OF THE INDIFFERENT ELECTRODE

The indifferent electrode in the unipolar lead system has zero potential because the sum of the potentials of RA + LA + LL = 0. On rare occasions this is not true, and the sum of RA + LA + LL has a finite potential. This can lead to an erroneous interpretation of the ECG. *Example:* A V_1 lead in a normal individual records an rS complex with r voltage = 0.2 mV and S = −0.6 mV, resulting in a mean of −0.4 mV. Let us assume that the central terminal (indifferent electrode) has a potential of −0.8 mV instead of zero. Therefore, V_1 would record the true forces in V_1 (−0.4 mV) minus −0.8 mV (instead of zero) = +4 mV. This would result in an abnormally tall R wave that could lead to incorrect interpretation (eg, right ventricular hypertrophy).

2 | Electrophysiology of the Heart

The following factors are involved in the genesis of the ECG: (1) initiation of impulse formation in the primary pacemaker (sinus node), (2) transmission of the impulse through the specialized conduction system of the heart, (3) activation (depolarization) of the atrial and ventricular myocardium, and (4) recovery (repolarization) of all the above areas. In order for one to have an understanding of the ECG, it is necessary to have a basic knowledge of intracellular and surface potentials.

INTRACELLULAR POTENTIALS

If one electrode is placed on the surface of a resting muscle cell and a second indifferent electrode is placed in a remote location, no electrical potential (ie, zero potential) will be recorded because of the high impedance of the cell membrane. However, if the cell membrane is penetrated by a capillary electrode, a negative potential of about 90 millivolts (mV) will be recorded. This is known as the membrane resting potential (MRP). The major factor that determines the MRP is the gradient of the potassium ions (K^+) across the cell membrane. The intracellular concentration of K^+ is approximately 150 mEq/L, and the extracellular concentration is approximately 5 mEq/L. This K^+ gradient of 30:1 is sufficient to explain the recorded MRP (−90 mV). On the other hand, an opposite gradient exists for the sodium ions (Na^+). There is a relatively high extracellular Na^+ concentration in relation to intracellular Na^+ concentration. This Na^+ gradient, opposite in polarity to that of the K^+ gradient, does not appreciably alter the MRP because the cell membrane is considerably less permeable to Na^+ than to K^+. It is estimated that the cell membrane in the resting state is 30 times more permeable to K^+ than to Na^+.

At the onset of depolarization of a cardiac muscle cell (eg, a ventricular muscle cell), there is an abrupt change in permeability of the cell membrane to sodium. Sodium ions (and calcium ions to a lesser degree) enter the cell and result in a sharp rise of intracellular potential to positivity (approximately 20 mV). This is designated as phase 0 and represents the fast inward current typical of normal myocardial cells and Purkinje fibers. Pacemaker cells of the SA node

and cells in the proximal region of the AV node are depolarized by a slow inward current of calcium. Under abnormal conditions, cells whose fast inward current via sodium channels is inhibited can be depolarized by the slow inward current via calcium channels.

Following depolarization, there is a relatively slow and gradual return of intracellular potential to the MRP (phase 4). This is repolarization and is divided into 3 phases: *Phase 1:* An initial rapid return of intracellular potential to 0 mV. This is largely the result of abrupt closing of the sodium channels. It has been suggested that chloride ions entering the cell may contribute to phase 1. *Phase 2:* A plateau phase of repolarization owing to the slow entrance of calcium ions into the cell. These are the same channels that can result in the slow inward type of depolarization. *Phase 3:* This represents the slow, gradual return of the intracellular potential to MRP. It results from extrusion of potassium ions out of the cell, which reestablishes the normal negative resting potential. However, the cell is left with an excess of sodium ions and a deficit of potassium ions. To restore the original ion concentration, a cell membrane sodium-potassium pump mechanism becomes effective. The energy required for this pump is derived from conversion of ATP to ADP. This pump removes sodium from the cell and permits potassium influx.

The summation of all phase 0 potentials of atrial myocardial cells results in the P wave of the ECG. All phase 0 potentials of ventricular muscle cells produce the QRS complex. Phase 2 correlates with the ST segment and phase 3 with the T wave of the ECG.

The entire curve of intracellular potential, as illustrated in Fig 2–1, is the monophasic action potential. The duration of this curve from the onset of depolarization to the termination of repolarization is the duration of action potential.

The monophasic action potential curve of an atrial muscle cell is different from that of a ventricular muscle cell. Phase 4 (MRP) and phase 0 (depolarization) are similar, but the duration of repolarization, and hence the duration of action potential, is shorter in an atrial muscle cell. This is largely due to a shortening and steepening of the slope in phase 2.

The monophasic action potential curve of a cell in the sinoatrial (SA) node is markedly different from the above:

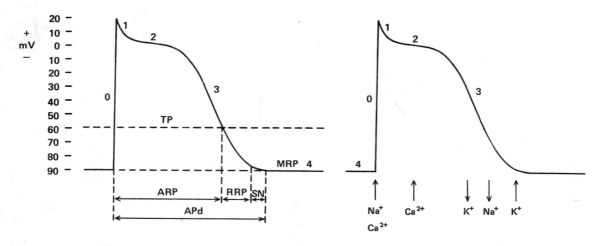

Figure 2–1. Diagrams of the action potential of a ventricular muscle cell. MRP = membrane resting potential; 0 = depolarization; 1, 2, 3 = phases of repolarization; 4 = diastolic phase = MRP; APd = duration of action potential; TP = threshold potential; ARP = absolute refractory period; RRP = relative refractory period; SN = supernormal period. *Phase 4:* Membrane resting potential = −90 mV. *Phase 0:* Rapid depolarization due to Na⁺ and Ca²⁺ influx. *Phase 1:* Initial phase of repolarization. *Phase 2:* Plateau phase of repolarization in which there is a slow influx of Ca²⁺. *Phase 3:* Efflux of K⁺ resulting in slow return of intracellular potential to −90 mV. At the termination of phase 3 the active transport system extrudes Na⁺ from the cell and pumps K⁺ into the cell. (Diagram on right reproduced, with permission, from Medical Staff Conference, University of California, San Francisco: The significance and treatment of long-term ventricular arrhythmias. *West J Med* 1977; **126:**209.)

(1) There is a lower MRP (−60 to −70 mV) at the onset of diastole.

(2) A prepotential is present in diastole (phase 4). Instead of the MRP remaining at a constant level during diastole, as is typical of ventricular and atrial muscle cells, there is a gradual rise of the MRP during diastole. It is this prepotential that explains the automatic function of the sinus pacemaker.

(3) Depolarization is slower and does not reach sufficient positive potential to be recorded on a surface electrogram.

(4) The peak of the action potential is rounded, and repolarization is a single slow curve in which phases 1, 2, and 3 cannot be defined.

The major portion of the AV node does not have the property of prepotential. The configuration of the action potential of cells in the bundle of His and the Purkinje fibers is similar to that of a ventricular muscle cell except that some degree of prepotential is present which allows these centers to assume pacemaker activity under appropriate conditions. The duration of action potential is longer in a Purkinje fiber than in any other site. This is due to prolongation of phases 2 and 3 and results in the U wave of the ECG.

Conduction Velocity

The speed at which the electrical potential spreads through the heart varies considerably depending upon the inherent properties of different portions of the specialized conduction system and the myocardium. Velocity is most rapid in Purkinje fibers and slowest in the midportion of the AV node. The following figures are averages of many experiments done on various animal species: SA node, 0.05 m/s; atrial muscle, 0.8–1 m/s; AV node, 0.05 m/s; bundle of His, 0.8–1 m/s; Purkinje fiber, 4 m/s; and ventricular muscle, 0.9–1 m/s.

Excitation & Threshold Potential

Excitation of cardiac muscle occurs when the stimulus reduces the transmembrane potential to a certain critical level: the threshold potential. This is approximately −60 mV in atrial and ventricular muscle cells. Thus, excitation will result from a relatively weak stimulus if the MRP is lowered and therefore closer to the level of threshold potential (providing other factors such as membrane resistance are constant). Conversely, excitation will require a stronger stimulus if the MRP is increased and therefore farther removed from the level of threshold potential.

Refractoriness of Heart Muscle

That period of time in the action potential curve during which no stimulus will propagate another action potential is known as the absolute refractory period. This period includes phases 0, 1, 2, and part of phase 3. Following this, there is a period during which a strong stimulus can evoke a response. This is the relative (or effective) refractory period. It begins when the transmembrane potential in phase 3 reaches the threshold potential level (about −60 mV) and ends just before the termination of phase 3. This is followed by a period of supernormal excitability (terminal part of phase 3 and beginning of phase 4), during which time a relatively weak stimulus can evoke a response.

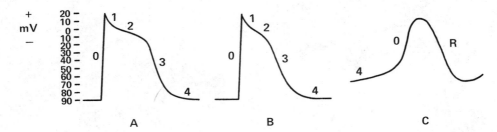

Figure 2–2. Diagrams of action potential curves. *A:* Ventricular muscle cell. *B:* Atrial muscle cell. *C:* SA node. R = repolarization phase of SA node, not divisible into phases 1, 2, and 3.

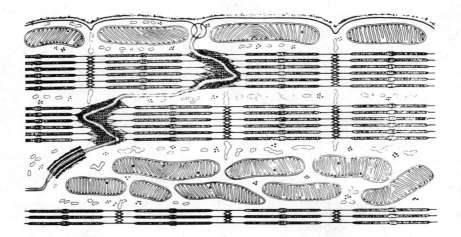

Figure 2–3. Diagrammatic reconstruction of mammalian cardiac muscle based on electron microscopic findings. The ovoid structures are mitochondria; the parallel bars are muscle filaments. An intercalated disk is shown coursing downward and to the left from the top of the picture. It has a low resistance membrane which facilitates electrical cell-to-cell transmission. (Reproduced, with permission, from Sjöstrand FS et al: *J Ultrastruct Res* 1958;1:271.)

Cell-to-Cell Conduction

It had been assumed that cell-to-cell conduction and impulse transmission occurred through "intracellular bridges" between muscle cells. However, with electron microscopy it was shown that cells are bounded on all sides by membranes, and no "bridges" are present. The membrane of the cell has a high resistance that should make electrical conduction impossible; for this reason, chemical transmission was postulated. However, it is now known that, although the cells have a true membrane along their longitudinal axes, the intercalated disks that cross the short axes of the cells are low resistance membranes. These disks have a resistance of 1/1000 of cell membrane and thereby readily permit electrical transmission from cell to cell.

ELECTRICAL POTENTIALS PRODUCED BY NORMAL CARDIAC MUSCLE

One can arrive at a basic understanding of the principles involved in electrocardiographic interpretation by an examination of the physiologic and electrical events that occur in isolated muscle strip experiments.

As stated above, if an electrode (E) is placed on the surface of a resting muscle strip and connected to a galvanometer, no deflection occurs since the entire surface of the muscle strip has zero potential because of the high impedance of cell membranes.

When an isolated muscle strip is stimulated (S), the surface of the stimulated portion becomes electrically negative. As the impulse traverses the muscle strip, there is a progressively advancing negative charge, whereas the portion of the muscle that has not as yet received the stimulus is electrically positive.

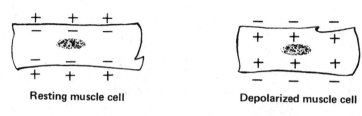

Resting muscle cell   Depolarized muscle cell

Figure 2–4. Potential of resting and depolarized muscle.

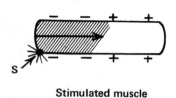

Resting muscle; no deflection

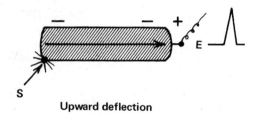

Stimulated muscle

Figure 2–5. Electrical potential of resting and stimulated muscle.

THE ELECTROGRAM

A tracing (electrogram) of the electrical potentials of a stimulated muscle strip is analogous to a unipolar ECG. There are 2 parts to the electrogram: (1) that produced during the passage of the stimulus (depolarization) and (2) that produced when the muscle returns to a resting state (repolarization).

Depolarization

The initial spread of the stimulus through the muscle is known as depolarization. The direction in which a stimulus spreads through the muscle and the position of the electrode in relation to the spread of the stimulus determine the deflection of the tracing.

A. In a Single Muscle Strip:

1. Upward deflection–The deflection will be upward if the stimulus spreads toward the electrode that is at the positively charged end of the muscle strip.

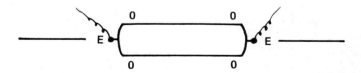

Upward deflection

2. Downward deflection–The deflection will be downward if the stimulus spreads away from the electrode that is at the negatively charged end of the muscle strip.

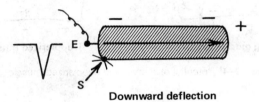

Downward deflection

3. Diphasic deflection–The deflection will be diphasic if the electrode overlies the midportion of the muscle strip. The initial deflection will be upward as a result of the advancing positive charge; the second deflection will be downward from the effect of the passing negative charge.

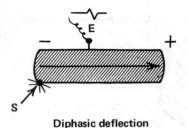

Diphasic deflection

B. In a Double Muscle Strip:

1. Muscles of equal size–If 2 muscle strips of approximately equal size are stimulated at a central point, a positive deflection (of depolarization) of equal magnitude will occur at either end.

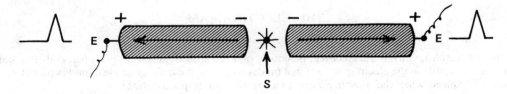

Two muscle strips of equal size

2. Muscles of unequal size–If 2 muscle masses of markedly different sizes (analogous to the right and left ventricles) are stimulated at a central point, a large positive deflection will result over the larger muscle mass, and a small positive deflection followed by a deep negative deflection (or an entirely negative deflection) will result over the smaller muscle mass.

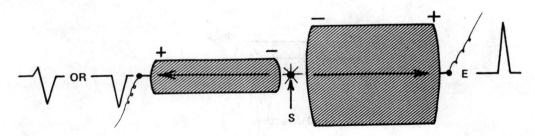

Two muscle strips of markedly different sizes

Intrinsic Deflection (Ventricular Activation Time, VAT)

The time required for the spread of the impulse from the stimulated end to the opposite end of the muscle strip can be correlated with the electrogram by measuring the interval from the onset to the peak of the depolarization wave. In clinical electrocardiography, this has been termed the intrinsic (or intrinsicoid) deflection, the ventricular activation time (VAT), or the R-peak time.

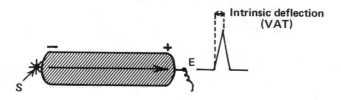

Repolarization

The return of the stimulated muscle to the resting state is known as repolarization.

A. Right to Left: If repolarization occurs in a direction opposite that of depolarization, the deflection will be in the same direction as that produced by depolarization. Repolarization from right to left is illustrated in the following 3 diagrams:

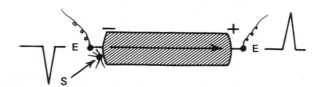

Depolarization from left to right

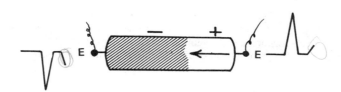

Repolarization beginning from right to left

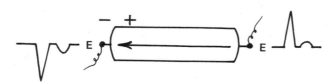

Repolarization completed

B. Left to Right: If repolarization occurs in the same direction as that of depolarization, the deflection will be opposite that of depolarization. Repolarization from left to right is illustrated in the following 3 diagrams:

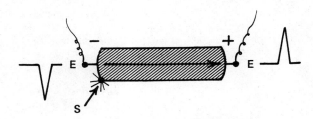

Depolarization from left to right

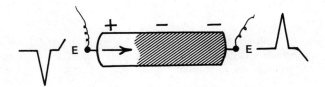

Repolarization beginning from left to right

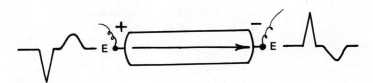

Repolarization completed

In isolated muscle strip experiments, the wave of repolarization is opposite to that of depolarization, indicating that repolarization has occurred in the same direction as depolarization. However, this finding does not prove that a similar direction of repolarization occurs in the intact human heart.

Definitions of Electrocardiographic Configurations | 3

The Electrocardiographic Grid

Electrocardiographic paper is a graph in which horizontal and vertical lines are present at 1 mm intervals. A heavier line is present every 5 mm. Time is measured along the horizontal lines: 1 mm = 0.04 s; 5 mm = 0.2 s. Voltage is measured along the vertical lines and is expressed as mm (10 mm = 1 mV). In routine electrocardiographic practice, the recording speed is 25 mm/s. The usual calibration is a 1 mV signal which produces a 10 mm deflection.

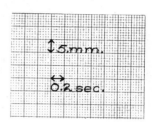

(The above and all subsequent electrocardiographic illustrations are 70% of actual size.)

NORMAL ELECTROCARDIOGRAPHIC COMPLEXES

Capital letters (Q, R, S) refer to relatively large waves (over 5 mm); small letters (q, r, s) refer to relatively small waves (under 5 mm).

P wave: The deflection produced by atrial depolarization.

T$_a$ (or P$_t$) wave: The deflection produced by atrial repolarization. This deflection is usually not seen in the average 12-lead ECG.

Q (q) wave: The initial negative deflection resulting from ventricular depolarization. It precedes the first positive deflection (R).

R (r) wave: The first positive deflection during ventricular depolarization.

S (s) wave: The first negative deflection of ventricular depolarization that follows the first positive deflection (R).

R' (r') wave: The second positive deflection, ie, the first positive deflection during ventricular depolarization that follows the S wave. The negative deflection following the r' is termed the s'.

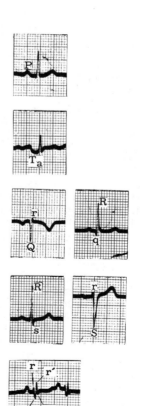

T wave: The deflection produced by ventricular repolarization.

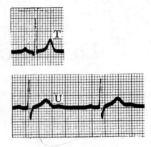

U wave: A deflection (usually positive) seen following the T wave and preceding the next P wave. The exact cause of this wave is unknown. It is currently thought to be the result of the slow repolarization of the intraventricular (Purkinje) conduction system (see p 17).

NORMAL INTERVAL VALUES

R–R interval: The R–R interval is the distance between 2 successive R waves. If the ventricular rhythm is regular, the interval in seconds (or fractions of a second) between the peaks of 2 successive R waves divided into 60 (seconds) will give the heart rate per minute. This is more easily determined by consulting Table 3–1. If the ventricular rhythm is irregular, the number of R waves in a given period of time (eg, 10 seconds) should be counted and the results converted into the number per minute. For example, if 20 R waves are counted in a 10-second interval, the ventricular rate is counted as 120 per minute.

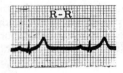

P–P interval: In regular sinus rhythm (Fig 12–5), the P–P interval will be the same as the R–R interval. However, when the ventricular rhythm is irregular or when atrial and ventricular rates are different but regular, the P–P interval should be measured from the same point on 2 successive P waves and the atrial rate per minute computed in the same manner as the ventricular rate.

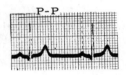

P–R interval: This measures the AV conduction time. It includes the time required for (1) atrial depolarization, (2) the normal conduction delay in the AV node (approximately 0.07 s), and (3) the passage of the impulse through the bundle of His and bundle branches to the onset of ventricular depolarization. It is measured from the onset of the P wave to the beginning of the QRS complex. Although the term P–R is in common use, P–Q would be more accurate. The normal value is in the range of 0.12–0.20 s (possibly up to 0.22 s). This must be correlated with the heart rate; normally, the slower the heart rate, the longer the P–R interval. A P–R interval of 0.2 s may be of no clinical significance with a heart rate of 60 but may well be significant with a heart rate of 100. The values vary also with age and body build (Table 3–2).

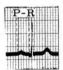

QRS interval: This is the measurement of total ventricular depolarization time. It is measured from the onset of the Q wave (or R if no Q is visible) to the termination of the S wave. The upper limit of normal is 0.1 s in frontal plane leads. Occasionally in precordial leads V_2 or V_3 this interval may be 0.11 s.

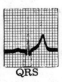

Ventricular activation time (VAT): The time it takes an impulse to traverse the myocardium from the endocardial to the epicardial surface is assumed to be reflected in a measurement from the beginning of the Q wave to the peak of the R wave. Such a measurement is accurate only when recorded directly from the surface of the heart (intrinsic deflection), preferably with closely placed bipolar electrodes. The accuracy and significance of this measurement diminishes with body surface unipolar recordings (intrinsicoid deflection). The VAT should not exceed 0.03 s in V_{1-2} and 0.05 s in V_{5-6}.

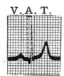

V. A. T.

Q–T interval: This is measured from the onset of the Q wave to the end of the T wave. It measures the duration of electrical systole. The Q–T interval varies with the heart rate and must be corrected (Q–T_c). This is easily done by use of the nomogram in Fig 3–1, which gives the Q–T_c for a heart rate of 60. The normal Q–T_c should not exceed 0.42 s in men and 0.43 s in women.

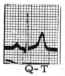

Q-T

Q–U interval: This measures the interval from the beginning of the Q wave to the end of the U wave. It measures total ventricular repolarization, including Purkinje fibers.

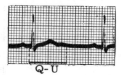

Q-U

S–T interval: The duration of the RS–T segment (see below).

NORMAL SEGMENTS & JUNCTIONS

PR segment: That portion of the electrocardiographic tracing from the end of the P wave to the onset of the QRS complex. It is normally isoelectric.

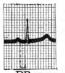

PR segment

RS–T junction (J): The point at which the QRS complex ends and the RS–T segment begins.

RS–T segment (usually called the ST segment): That portion of the tracing from the J to the onset of the T wave. This segment is usually isoelectric but may vary from −0.5 to +2 mm in precordial leads (see p 82). It is elevated or depressed in comparison with that portion of the base line between the termination of the T wave and the beginning of the P wave (T–P segment) or when related to the level of the PR segment.

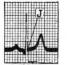

ST segment

Table 3—1. Determination of heart rate.*

To find the heart rate, select the figure in column L that represents the cycle duration in seconds measured on the ECG. The corresponding number in column R gives the rate per minute. Thus, if the interval between P waves (or R waves) of 2 consecutive beats is 0.60, the heart rate is 100. Accurate values are obtained only if rhythm is regular.

L†	R‡	L	R	L	R	L	R	L	R	L	R
0.10	600	0.33	182	0.57	105	0.80	75	1.07	56	1.82	33
0.11	550	0.34	177	0.58	103	0.81	74	1.09	55	1.86	32
0.12	510	0.35	173	0.59	101	0.82	73	1.11	54	1.92	31
0.13	470	0.36	168	0.60	100	0.83	72	1.13	53	2.00	30
0.14	430	0.37	164	0.61	98	0.84	71	1.15	52	2.06	29
0.15	400	0.38	158	0.62	96	0.85		1.17	51	2.15	28
0.16	375	0.39	155	0.63	95	0.86	70	1.20	50	2.22	27
0.17	350	0.40	150	0.64	93	0.87	69	1.23	49	2.30	26
0.18	335	0.41	145	0.65	92	0.88	68	1.25	48	2.40	25
0.19	315	0.42	142	0.66	91	0.89	67	1.27	47	2.50	24
0.20	300	0.43	138	0.67	90	0.90		1.29	46	2.60	23
0.21	284	0.44	136	0.68	89	0.91	66	1.33	45	2.70	22
0.22	270	0.45	133	0.69	87	0.92	65	1.36	44	2.84	21
0.23	260	0.46	129	0.70	85	0.93	64	1.38	43	3.00	20
0.24	250	0.47	127	0.71	84	0.94	63	1.42	42	3.15	19
0.25	240	0.48	125	0.72	83	0.95		1.45	41	3.35	18
0.26	230	0.49	123	0.73	82	0.96	62	1.50	40	3.50	17
0.27	222	0.50	120	0.74	81	0.97	61	1.55	39	3.75	16
0.28	215	0.51	117	0.75	80	0.98		1.58	38	4.00	15
0.29	206	0.52	115	0.76	79	0.99	60	1.64	37	4.30	14
0.30	200	0.53	113	0.77	78	1.00		1.68	36	4.70	13
0.31	192	0.54	111	0.78	77	1.01	59	1.73	35	5.10	12
0.32	186	0.55	109	0.79	76	1.03	58	1.77	34	5.50	11
		0.56	107			1.05	57			6.00	10

*Modified and reproduced, with permission, from Ashman R, Hull E: *Essentials of Electrocardiography*, 2nd ed. Macmillan, 1941.
†L = heart cycle duration in seconds.
‡R = heart rate per minute.

Table 3—2. Upper limits of the normal P—R intervals.*
(Intervals measured in fractions of a second.)

Rate	Below 70	71—90	91—110	111—130	Above 130
Large adults	0.21	0.20	0.19	0.18	0.17
Small adults	0.20	0.19	0.18	0.17	0.16
Children, ages 14—17	0.19	0.18	0.17	0.16	0.15
Children, ages 7—13	0.18	0.17	0.16	0.15	0.14
Children, ages 1½—6	0.17	0.165	0.155	0.145	0.135
Children, ages 0—1½	0.16	0.15	0.145	0.135	0.125

*Reproduced, with permission, from Ashman R, Hull E: *Essentials of Electrocardiography*. Macmillan, 1937.

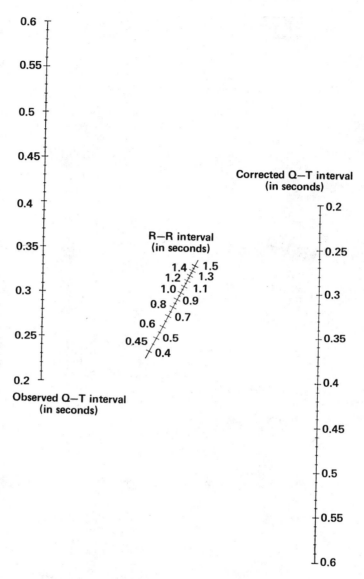

Figure 3–1. Nomogram for rate correction of Q–T interval. Measure the observed Q–T interval and the R–R interval. Mark these values in the respective columns of the chart (left and middle). Place a ruler across these 2 points. The point at which the extension of this line crosses the third column is read as the corrected Q–T interval (Q–Tc). (Reproduced, with permission, from Kissin et al: *Am Heart J* 1948;**35**:990.)

VOLTAGE MEASUREMENTS

The voltage of upright deflections (upright P, R, upright T) is measured from the upper portion of the base line to the peak of the wave.

The voltage of negative deflections (inverted P, Q, S, inverted T) is measured from the lower portion of the base line to the nadir of the wave.

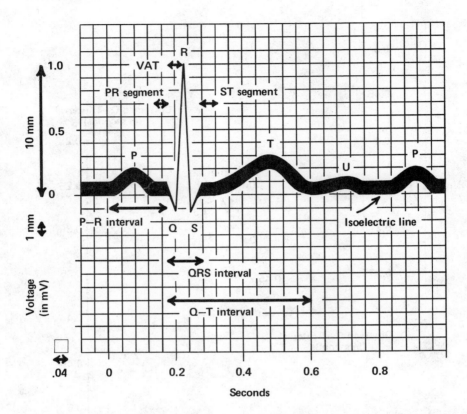

Figure 3–2. Diagram of electrocardiographic complexes, intervals, and segments.

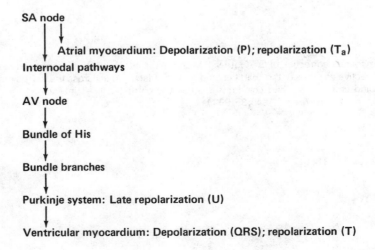

Figure 3–3. Summary of conduction and excitation.

The term *cardiac vector* designates all of the electromotive forces of the heart cycle. It has known magnitude, direction, and polarity. It must be appreciated that at any given instant during depolarization and repolarization, electrical potentials are being propagated in many directions in space. Over 80% of these potentials are canceled out by opposing forces, and only the net is recorded. The *instantaneous vector* represents the net electrical force at a given instant. A *mean vector* of any given portion of the heart cycle (eg, QRS) represents the mean magnitude, direction, and polarity for that period (eg, the mean QRS vector).

The mathematical symbol of a vector is an arrow pointing in the direction of the net potential (positive or negative); the length of the arrow indicates the magnitude of the electrical force.

A vector can be drawn for atrial depolarization (P), ventricular depolarization (QRS), and ventricular repolarization (T). Each vector is constantly changing: starting at a central point, spreading through the heart, and then returning to the starting point. It therefore forms a 3-dimensional loop, ie, the spatial vectorcardiogram or VCG (see Chapter 20). Cathode ray oscilloscopes are now available that can record the vectorcardiogram in 3 planes—frontal, horizontal, and sagittal—and also record the 3 orthogonal scalar leads X, Y, and Z (see Chapter 20). This method of recording is gaining popularity in many medical centers throughout the world.

FRONTAL PLANE VECTORS

The result of the electrical potentials of the entire cardiac cycle as reflected in the frontal plane of the body is the frontal plane vector. The Einthoven triangle diagrammatically illustrates the bipolar standard leads (Fig 4–1).

Einthoven devised this equilateral triangle on the following assumptions:

(1) The "dipolar hypothesis." It is believed that each instantaneous vector is the result of an electrical potential which acts as a dipole, as illustrated in Fig 4–2.

(2) The center of electrical activity of the heart is located in the anatomic center of the chest.

(3) Leads I, II, and III are all equidistant from the center of electrical activity.

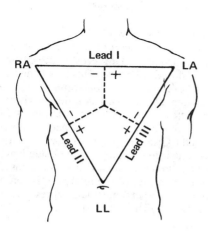

Figure 4–1. Frontal plane leads. If a perpendicular is dropped from the center of each lead axis, the intersection of these will theoretically represent the center of electrical activity.

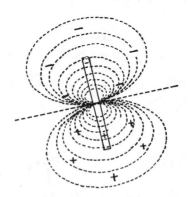

Figure 4–2. Dipolar hypothesis. One half of the dipole is positive, and the opposite half is negative. One half of the electrical field is positive, the other half negative. The greatest electrical potential, either positive or negative, will be along a line parallel with the dipole. Electrical potential along a line perpendicular to the dipole at its electrical center will be practically nil.

(4) The human torso can be assumed to be spherical in shape.

(5) All body tissues and fluids can be assumed to be equally good conductors of electrical potential.

However, it is now recognized that assumptions (2), (3), (4), and (5) above are unwarranted, and even the dipolar hypothesis is still the subject of considerable controversy. Although for mathematical accuracy it is necessary to correct for these errors, the purposes of clarification will be best served by a simplified presentation of the concept of vector analysis; the more complicated but more correct analysis will be discussed later (see Chapter 20) in relation to corrected orthogonal leads.

If the Einthoven triangle is modified so that the leads intersect at a central point, the lead axes are seen to be placed as shown in Fig 4–3. (This does not alter the mathematical relationship of the leads.)

The frontal plane unipolar leads can be diagrammed as shown in Fig 4–4.

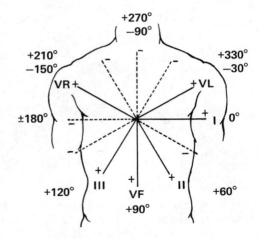

Figure 4–5. Frontal plane leads.

If Figs 4–3 and 4–4 are superimposed, a hexaxial reference system can be drawn that illustrates all 6 leads of the frontal plane (Fig 4–5).

By convention, the positive pole of lead I is designated as 0 degrees, the negative pole of lead I as ±180 degrees, the positive pole of VF as +90 degrees, the negative pole of VF as +270 degrees or −90 degrees, the positive pole of lead II as +60 degrees, the positive pole of lead III as +120 degrees, the positive pole of VR as +210 degrees or −150 degrees, and the positive pole of VL as +330 degrees or −30 degrees.

Polarity of Individual Frontal Plane Lead Axes

If a perpendicular is drawn through the center of a given lead axis, any electrical force (ie, vector) oriented in the positive half of the electrical field will record an upright deflection in that lead; any force oriented in the negative half of the electrical field will record a downward deflection. (See Fig 4–6.)

Direction of Mean Frontal Plane Axis

The mean QRS vector in the frontal plane can be approximated from standard leads by use of the reference system described above. This is only an approximation, however, since it is determined by measurement of magnitude (ie, voltage) alone, whereas the true mean QRS vector must be determined from 2 factors: magnitude and time. The net amplitude and direction of the QRS complex in any 2 of the 3 standard leads are plotted along the axes of the 2 standard leads. Perpendicular lines are drawn at these locations. A line drawn from the center of the reference system to the intersection of the perpendiculars represents the approximate mean QRS vector. Its angle is the frontal plane axis.

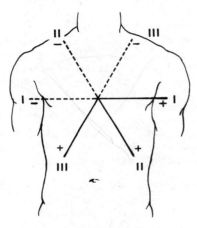

Figure 4–3. Frontal plane bipolar leads.

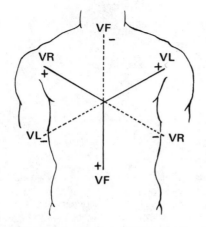

Figure 4–4. Frontal plane unipolar leads.

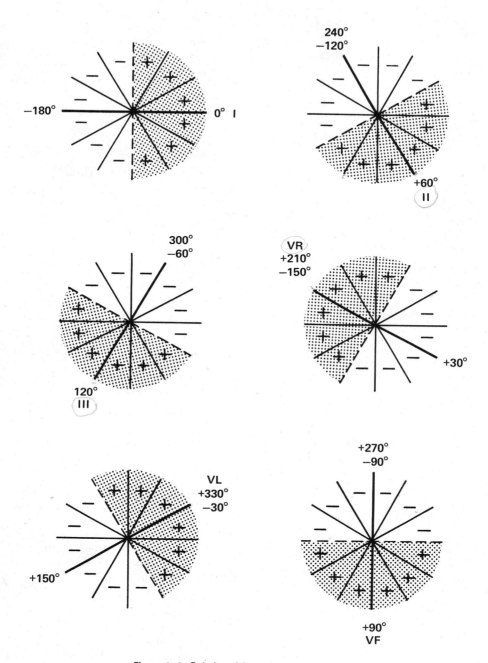

Figure 4–6. Polarity of frontal plane lead axes.

Example: (See also Fig 4–7.)

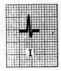
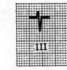

I: R = +6 mm,   III: R = +2 mm,
   S = −2 mm   S = −5 mm

The algebraic sum of R + S in I and III is determined

$$I = +6 \; -2 = +4$$
$$III = +2 \; -5 = -3$$

The values +4 and −3 are plotted on the respective lead axes. Perpendiculars are drawn from each lead axis at these points. The resultant vector is oriented at an angle of −15 degrees; its magnitude is approximately 4.1 units (See Fig 4–7.)

Another simple means of approximating the mean frontal plane QRS axis is as follows: If any one lead of the 6 frontal plane leads has a net QRS magnitude of zero, the mean QRS vector will be perpendicular to that lead axis. Inspection of another lead (I or aVF) will tell in which half of this perpendicular the mean vector is.

Example: Lead II shows a QRS complex whose net is zero. The lead II axis is +60 degrees. Therefore, the mean QRS vector in the frontal plane is perpendicular to +60 degrees, which is −30 degrees or +150 degrees. If the net QRS in lead I is positive, the mean vector is −30 degrees. If the net QRS in lead I is negative, the mean vector is +150 degrees.

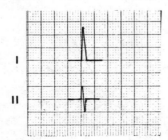

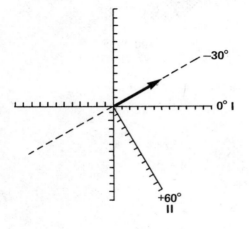

Example: Lead I shows a QRS complex whose net is zero. The lead I axis is 0 degrees. Therefore, the mean QRS vector in the frontal plane is perpendicular to 0 degrees, which is +90 degrees or −90 degrees. If the net QRS in lead aVF is positive, the mean vector is +90 degrees. If the net QRS in lead aVF is negative, the mean vector is −90 degrees.

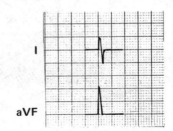

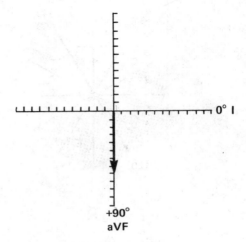

If no one frontal plane lead has a net QRS of zero, one can interpolate and estimate the mean vector by inspection of several frontal plane leads.

By the same method, the mean frontal plane axis of the P and the T can be determined.

Frontal plane QRS–T angle: Knowing the mean QRS angle and the mean T angle in the frontal plane, the QRS–T angle can be determined. Normally, this is less than 50 degrees. *Example:* The mean QRS angle = −10 degrees, and the mean T angle = 30 degrees. The QRS–T angle = 40 degrees.

Thus, if one knows the direction and magnitude of a cardiac vector, one can derive its direction and magnitude in any of the frontal plane leads.

On p 33 is illustrated a cardiac vector (A) whose angle in the frontal plane is +45 degrees. The magnitude is indicated by the length of the arrow. On the scale used in this diagram, the vector has an arbitrary magnitude of 8.6 units. If one draws a perpendicular from the tip of the arrow to each of the standard lead axes, the polarity (positive or negative) and magnitude for each lead can be determined. Thus, I = +6 units, II = +8 units, and III = +2.7 units.

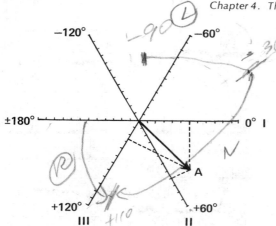

Axis Deviation

The angle of the mean frontal QRS vector determines its frontal plane axis. In the earlier days of electrocardiography, the normal axis was considered to be 0 to +90 degrees, right axis deviation +90 to +180 degrees, and left axis deviation 0 to −90 degrees. However, in order to facilitate the differentiation of normal and abnormal ECGs, the following criterion is now accepted: The normal axis lies between −30 and +110 degrees; therefore, left axis deviation between −30 and −90 degrees, and right axis deviation between +110 and ±180 degrees, are abnormal. Within the range of normal (−30 to +110

degrees), left axis deviation (0 to −30 degrees) represents a normal horizontal heart position in unipolar terminology; and right axis deviation (+75 to +110 degrees) represents a normal vertical heart position (Figs 6–3 and 6–4).* See also Fig 4–7.

HORIZONTAL PLANE VECTORS

The unipolar precordial leads represent approximations of the electrical potentials (ie, the vector forces) in the horizontal plane. This can be diagrammed as shown in Fig 4–9.

As has been illustrated for the frontal plane, a perpendicular can be drawn through the zero point of any unipolar precordial lead axis. Any electrical force oriented in the positive half of the electrical field will record a positive (upright) deflection in that lead; any force oriented in the negative half of the electrical field will record a negative (downward) deflection in that lead.

Examples are shown in Fig 4–10.

*Although the term left axis is traditional, a more accurate term would be superior axis. Any force of unchanging magnitude that is oriented between −30 degrees and −90 degrees will be more superior than leftward. The greatest leftward magnitude will be represented on the 0 degree axis (lead I).

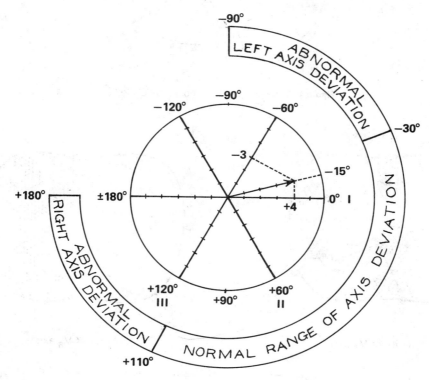

Figure 4–7. Determination of axis deviation.

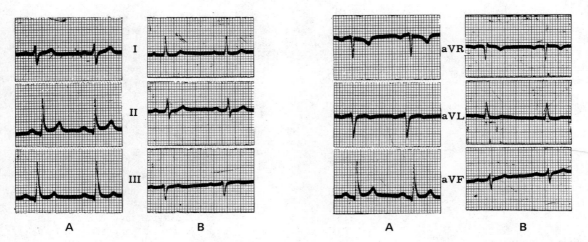

Figure 4–8. Examples of variations in frontal plane QRS axis. *A:* Frontal plane QRS axis = +96 degrees, T axis = +60 degrees; QRS–T angle = 36 degrees; vertical heart position. *B:* Frontal plane QRS axis = −10 degrees, T axis = +40 degrees; QRS–T angle = 50 degrees; horizontal heart position.

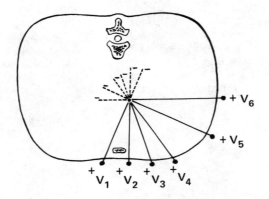

Figure 4–9. Lead axes in the horizontal plane.

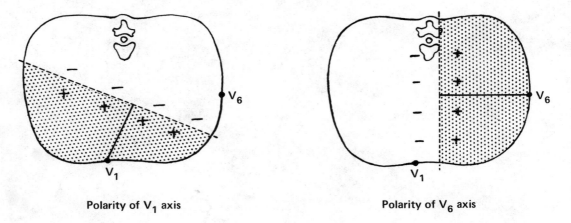

Polarity of V_1 axis   Polarity of V_6 axis

Figure 4–10. Polarity of V_1 and V_6 axes.

SAGITTAL PLANE VECTORS

The unipolar esophageal leads approximate the electrical potentials in the sagittal plane. Following the principles as outlined above, a diagram can be drawn for the sagittal plane (Fig 4–11).

VALUE OF VECTOR ANALYSIS

Vector analysis of the ECG (vector electrocardiography) serves its most useful purpose in the teaching and understanding of the propagation of the electrical events of the cardiac cycle. It is the author's opinion that the details and interpretation of these phenomena can best be learned from the study of spatial vectorcardiography. For this reason, in Chapters 5 through 19, only brief mention will be made of vector analysis of the normal and abnormal electrocardiographic patterns. A more detailed and accurate concept of vector analysis will be deferred to the chapter on spatial vectorcardiography (Chapter 20).

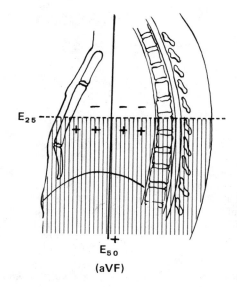

Figure 4–11. Polarity of the long axis.

5 | Normal Electrocardiographic Complexes

Anatomy & Physiology of the Conduction System

The heart possesses the property of automatic and rhythmic contraction. It has the inherent ability to initiate and conduct impulses which stimulate muscular contraction. This ability is located in the specialized neuromuscular tissue known as the conduction system. The conduction system consists of (1) the sinoatrial (SA) node, (2) the internodal atrial pathways, (3) the atrioventricular (AV) node, (4) the bundle of His, (5) the right and left bundle branches, and (6) the Purkinje system.

SA Node

The heartbeat is normally controlled by rhythmic impulses which arise in the SA node, and the latter is therefore the cardiac pacemaker. It consists of a bundle of specialized neuromuscular tissue measuring approximately 5 × 20 mm which lies on the endocardial surface of the right atrium at the junction of the superior vena cava and the right atrial appendage. The impulse then spreads through both atria, producing the P wave.

Internodal Atrial Pathways

Conduction through the atria occurs through 3 bundles of myocardium which contain Purkinje type fibers: (1) The anterior internodal tract (Bachmann) leaves the SA node in a forward direction and curves about the superior vena cava and anterior wall of the right atrium. There it divides into 2 bundles of fibers,

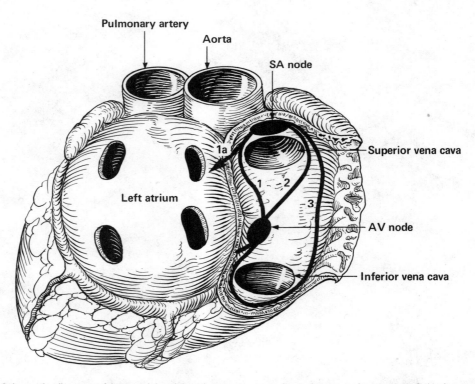

Figure 5–1. Schematic diagram of internodal atrial pathways as seen from the posterior aspect of the heart with the posterior wall of the right atrium removed. (1) Anterior internodal tract. (1a) Branch of anterior internodal tract to left atrium. (2) Middle internodal tract. (3) Posterior internodal tract.

one entering the left atrium and the other coursing over the anterior portion of the interatrial septum and descending obliquely behind the root of the aorta to enter the anterior-superior margin of the AV node. (2) The middle internodal tract (Wenckebach) leaves the posterior margin of the SA node, curves behind the superior vena cava, and courses along the posterior portion of the interatrial septum to enter the superior margin of the AV node. (3) The posterior internodal tract (Thorel) leaves the posterior margin of the SA node and follows the course of the crista terminalis and eustachian ridge to enter the posterior margin of the AV node. Lateral extensions from this tract arborize over the dorsum of the right atrium. Between all 3 tracts there are interconnecting fibers that merge just above the AV node. Some of these fibers do not enter the AV node but bypass it; they can reenter the conducting system at a place distal to the AV node.

AV Node

This bundle of specialized neuromuscular tissue measures 2 × 5 mm. It is located on the endocardial surface of the right side of the interatrial septum just inferior to the opening of the coronary sinus. The impulse which has spread through both atria enters the AV node and is normally delayed for approximately 0.07 s.

Bundle of His

The bundle of His is in direct continuity with the lower portion of the AV node. It is approximately 20 mm long and is located on the endocardial surface of the right side of the interatrial septum, immediately superior to the interventricular septum. The bundle of His is not a homogeneous mass of conducting tissue but consists of multiple individual longitudinal tracts. It is likely that specific tracts continue into specific bundle branches.

Bundle Branches

The right bundle branch arises from the bundle of His and traverses the endocardial surface of the right side of the interventricular septum. Distally, the right bundle divides into 3 divisions (anterior, lateral, and posterior). Purkinje fibers arborize from these and spread over the endocardial surface of the right ventricle and the distal portion of the interventricular septum.

On the left side of the septum, 3 fascicular radiations arise from the bundle of His. The more proximal is the left posterior fascicle, which spreads as a broad band of fibers over the posterior and inferior endocardial surfaces of the left ventricle. Immediately distal to the origin of the posterior fascicle is the left anterior fascicle, which spreads as a narrower band of fibers over the anterior and superior endocardial surfaces of the left ventricle. Separate fibers arise from the proxi-

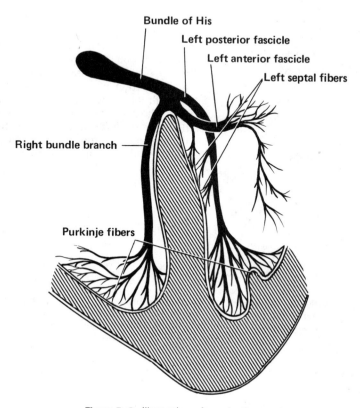

Figure 5–2. Illustration of conduction system.

mal portions of the left anterior and posterior fascicles and cover the endocardial surface of the left side of the interventricular septum. This is the septal fascicle. Those from the anterior fascicle enter the anterior and superior surfaces of the septum, and those from the posterior fascicle enter the posterior and inferior portions of the septum. Thus, the bundle branch system consists of 4 fascicles: (1) a right bundle branch, (2) a left posterior fascicle, (3) a left anterior fascicle, and (4) a left septal fascicle.

The midportion of the interventricular septum is normally activated from left to right. Purkinje fibers arise more proximally from the divisions of the left bundle than from the right bundle branch and enter the left side of the septum, which they activate initially. This wave of excitation from left to right produces the initial negativity of the left ventricular cavity and the initial positivity of the right ventricular cavity. (See p 42 and Fig 5–18.) It results in a force oriented to the right and anteriorly.

Purkinje System

After traversing the right bundle branch and the left fascicular bundle branches, the impulse passes into the multiple ramifications of the Purkinje system which cover the subendocardial surfaces of both ventricles. The impulse then travels perpendicularly from the endocardial to the epicardial surface of the myocardium. It is the propagation of the impulses through the Purkinje system into the ventricular

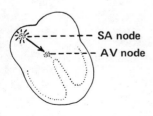

Figure 5–3. Atrial activation.

myocardium which produces the remainder of the QRS complex (after activation of the interventricular septum from left to right). (See Figs 5–19 to 5–21.)

The anteroseptal region of the right ventricle is the earliest site of free wall ventricular activation. The posterobasal region of the left ventricle, the pulmonary conus, and the uppermost portion of the interventricular septum are activated last.

ELECTRICAL CONDUCTION THROUGH THE HEART

The initial impulse in the cardiac cycle begins in the SA node.

Atrial Activation

The impulse traverses the internodal pathways to depolarize the atria, producing the P wave, and then reaches the AV node. Normally the impulse is "delayed" in the AV node for 0.07 s before passing on to the bundle of His, the right and left bundles, the ramifications of the Purkinje system, and then into the ventricles. Conduction through this electrical pathway is much more rapid than through ordinary heart muscle.

Ventricular Activation

Initial intraventricular activation occurs in the midportion of the interventricular septum in a left-to-right direction. The anteroseptal region of the ventricular myocardium is the next site of activation. The major portion of ventricular activation then occurs through the myocardium of the left and right ventricles. The last parts to be activated are the posterobasal region of the left ventricle, the pulmonary conus, and the uppermost portion of the interventricular septum. The spread of excitation through the myocardium is

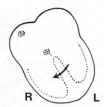

Septal activation from left to right

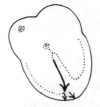

Activation of anteroseptal region of the ventricular myocardium

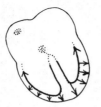

Activation of major portion of ventricular myocardium from endocardial to epicardial surfaces

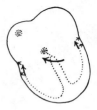

Late activation of posterobasal portion of the left ventricle, the pulmonary conus, and the uppermost portion of the interventricular septum

Figure 5–4. Ventricular activation.

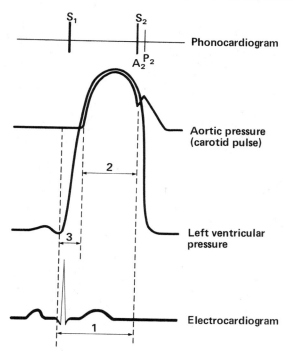

Figure 5–5. Relation between electrical and mechanical events in the cardiac cycle. The phonocardiogram, aortic pressure curve (as recorded from the carotid artery), left ventricular pressure curve, and ECG are diagrammed simultaneously. (1) Q–S_2: The total electromechanical systole, measured from the onset of the Q wave to the aortic second sound. (2) LVET: Left ventricular ejection time, measured from the upstroke to the dicrotic notch of the carotid pulse. (3) PEP: Preejection period, derived by subtracting the LVET from the Q–S_2.

from the endocardial to the epicardial surface. Thus evolves the QRS complex.

Relation Between Electrical Conduction & Contraction

The passage of the electrical impulse through any given portion of the heart precedes the resulting contraction of that portion of the myocardium. Fig 5–5 illustrates these time relationships.

ATRIAL COMPLEXES

The normal P wave in standard, extremity, and precordial leads is not over 0.11 s in duration or over 2.5 mm in height. Since the spread of excitation from the SA node to the AV node is in a leftward and head-to-foot direction, the P is normally upright in leads I, II, aVF, and V_{3-6}. The P is normally inverted in aVR and frequently in V_1 (and at times in V_2). The P

may be upright, diphasic, flat, or inverted in leads III and aVL. Thus, the normal P vector is oriented inferiorly, to the left, and slightly anteriorly. (See Fig 5–6.)

Esophageal leads will show P waves which are of greater amplitude than in any lead of the conventional 12-lead ECG. Since the P vector is directed inferiorly, the P will be inverted in high esophageal levels (E_{10-25}), ie, above the AV groove, and will be upright in low esophageal leads (E_{35-50}). In the region of the AV groove (E_{25-35}), the P wave will be a large, sharply peaked diphasic complex, simulating an RS complex of ventricular depolarization. (See Fig 5–7.)

VENTRICULAR COMPLEXES
(See Figs 5–8 to 5–12.)

UNIPOLAR ELECTROCARDIOGRAMS ON THE EXPOSED VENTRICLE

Our knowledge of unipolar electrocardiography on the exposed heart is derived from animal work and direct electrocardiography performed during operations in which the human heart is exposed. It again must be emphasized that any such unipolar lead records all of the electrical events of the cardiac cycle (ie, all the vector forces) and not merely those reflecting a small area of the underlying myocardium.

LEFT VENTRICULAR EPICARDIAL COMPLEX

Such a complex is recorded by placing an electrode directly over the left ventricle of the exposed heart. It records all of the electrical events of the cardiac cycle as viewed from this electrode site. The P wave is upright. The initial spread of excitation across the septum from left to right in a direction away from the exploring electrode (producing initial negativity of the left side of the septum which is transmitted through the left ventricular cavity and left myocardium) results in an initial downward deflection, the q wave. The spread of excitation through the large muscle mass of the left ventricle in the direction of the electrode produces a tall upright deflection, the R wave. If the electrode is so situated that the spread of excitation is directed away from the electrode to activate the remaining (posterobasal) portion of the left ventricle, a second small negative deflection will result, the s

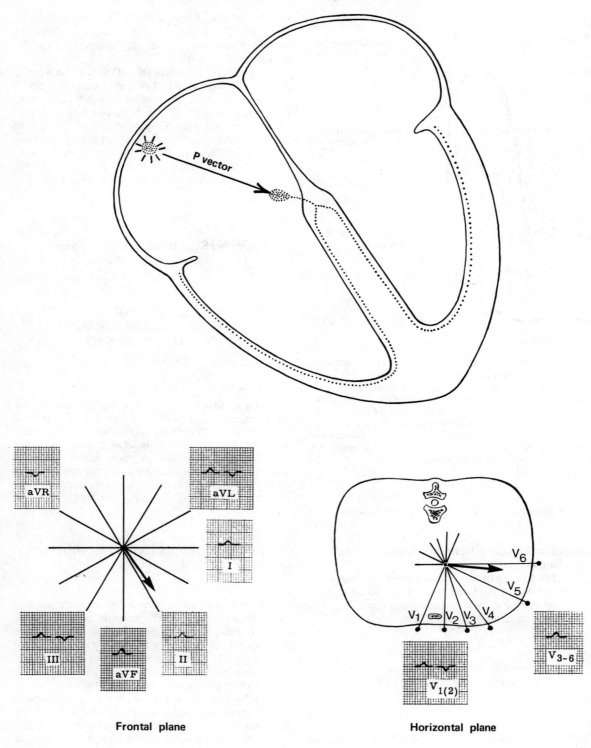

Figure 5–6. Direction of the normal frontal and horizontal plane P vectors with resulting P wave in the 12-lead ECG. The normal P vector in the frontal plane is between 0 degrees and +90 degrees. A P vector between 0 degrees and +30 degrees will produce an inverted P wave in lead III. A P vector past +60 degrees will produce an inverted P wave in lead aVL. The amount of anterior orientation in the horizontal plane will determine whether the P wave is upright or inverted in lead V₁.

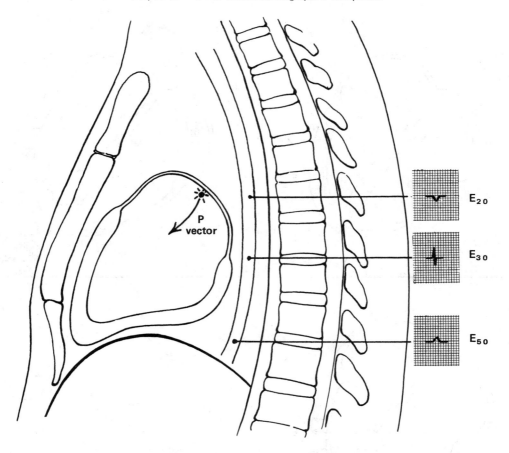

Figure 5–7. Direction of the normal P wave in esophageal leads.

wave. Thus, the typical pattern of a left ventricular epicardial lead is a qRs complex. The VAT is not over 0.04–0.05 s.

Following depolarization, the complex usually returns to the isoelectric line, producing an isoelectric ST segment.

Repolarization results in an upright T wave which is asymmetric, the upstroke being of longer duration than the downstroke. The T wave should be at least one-tenth as high as the R in the same complex.

RIGHT VENTRICULAR EPICARDIAL COMPLEX

This complex is recorded by placing an electrode directly over the right ventricle of an exposed heart. It records all of the electrical events of the cardiac cycle as viewed from this electrode site. The P wave may be upright, diphasic, or inverted. The spread of excitation through the interventricular septum from left to right in the direction of the exploring electrode (producing an initial positivity of the right side of the septum which is transmitted through the right ventricular cavity and right myocardium) produces an initial positive deflection, the r wave. Contributing to this initial upright deflection is the early activation of the right ventricular myocardium. The VAT is not over 0.02–0.03 s. Following this, the major wave of excitation is spreading away from the exploring electrode into the large muscle mass of the left ventricle, which far exceeds the spread through the smaller mass of the right ventricle, resulting in a large downward deflection. Thus, an rS complex is one typical form of right ventricular epicardial complex.

At times the initial r wave is not recorded, resulting in a completely negative deflection, or QS complex.

Occasionally (5%), the late activation of the posterobasal surface of the left ventricle and the region of the pulmonary conus, occurring in the direction of the exploring electrode, produces a second small upright deflection, an r' wave. Thus an rSr' complex or a Qr complex can occur.

The ST segment may be isoelectric or normally may be elevated 1–2 mm.

The T wave may be upright, flat, or inverted in the above complexes.

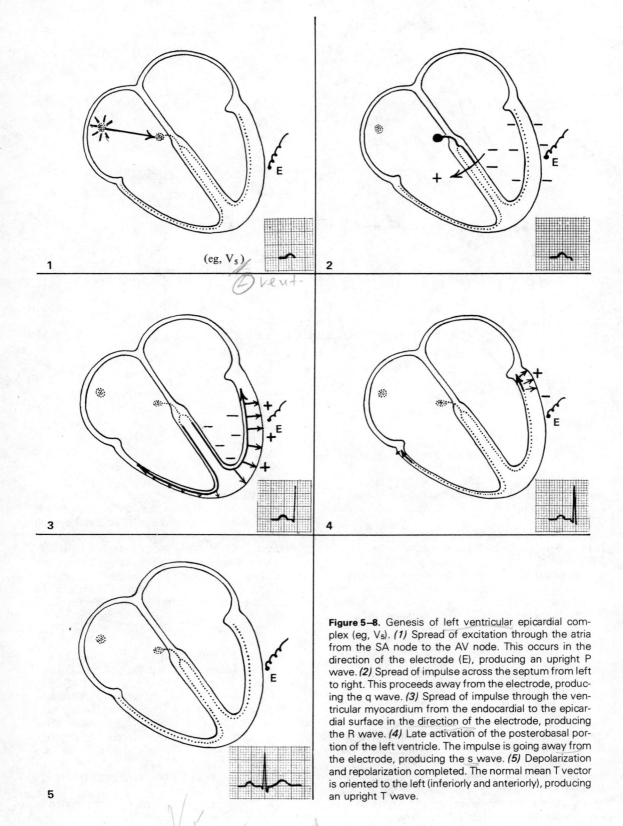

(eg, V₅)

Figure 5–8. Genesis of left ventricular epicardial complex (eg, V₅). *(1)* Spread of excitation through the atria from the SA node to the AV node. This occurs in the direction of the electrode (E), producing an upright P wave. *(2)* Spread of impulse across the septum from left to right. This proceeds away from the electrode, producing the q wave. *(3)* Spread of impulse through the ventricular myocardium from the endocardial to the epicardial surface in the direction of the electrode, producing the R wave. *(4)* Late activation of the posterobasal portion of the left ventricle. The impulse is going away from the electrode, producing the s wave. *(5)* Depolarization and repolarization completed. The normal mean T vector is oriented to the left (inferiorly and anteriorly), producing an upright T wave.

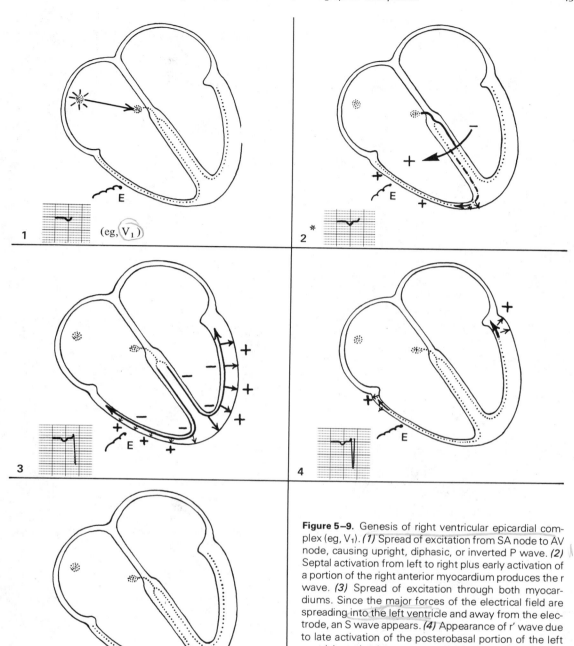

1   (eg, V₁)

2 *

3

4

5

(R. vent.)

Figure 5–9. Genesis of right ventricular epicardial complex (eg, V₁). *(1)* Spread of excitation from SA node to AV node, causing upright, diphasic, or inverted P wave. *(2)* Septal activation from left to right plus early activation of a portion of the right anterior myocardium produces the r wave. *(3)* Spread of excitation through both myocardiums. Since the major forces of the electrical field are spreading into the left ventricle and away from the electrode, an S wave appears. *(4)* Appearance of r' wave due to late activation of the posterobasal portion of the left ventricle and pulmonary conus. *(5)* Repolarization completed. This produces an upright, diphasic, or inverted T wave. ¶There may be 4 variations of the QRS pattern in a right ventricular epicardial complex†: (1) rS, (2) QS, (3) rSr' (as illustrated in sequences), and (4) Qr. ¶In any of the above, either the P wave or the T wave may be upright, diphasic, or inverted.

*The early activation of the right anterior myocardium is illustrated only in this sequence diagram. It will be omitted in all other sequence illustrations since it contributes only to the production of a part of the r wave in a right ventricular epicardial complex.

†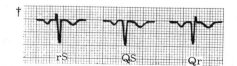

rS   QS   Qr

TRANSITIONAL ZONE VENTRICULAR EPICARDIAL COMPLEX

This complex is recorded by placing an electrode on the epicardial surface of the exposed heart overlying the interventricular septum. It records all the electrical events of the cardiac cycle as viewed from this electrical site. Since in many instances the direction of this vector force is perpendicular to the mean QRS vector, its magnitude (voltage) will be small and diphasic, resulting in an rs complex. The ST segment is isoelectric and the T wave upright.

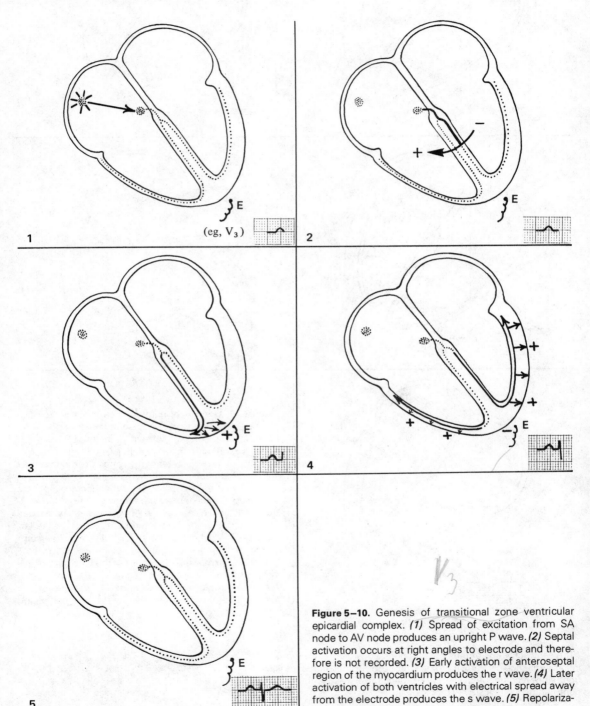

(eg, V₃)

Figure 5–10. Genesis of transitional zone ventricular epicardial complex. *(1)* Spread of excitation from SA node to AV node produces an upright P wave. *(2)* Septal activation occurs at right angles to electrode and therefore is not recorded. *(3)* Early activation of anteroseptal region of the myocardium produces the r wave. *(4)* Later activation of both ventricles with electrical spread away from the electrode produces the s wave. *(5)* Repolarization complete. This produces an upright T wave.

LEFT VENTRICULAR CAVITY COMPLEX

This complex is recorded by actually inserting an electrode within the left ventricular cavity. The P wave is inverted if the electrode is above the AV groove and upright if below. The initial septal activation as well as all subsequent myocardial activation is traveling away from the exploring electrode. Therefore, the entire ventricular depolarization complex will be a downward deflection, a QS complex. The ST segment is isoelectric, and the T wave is normally inverted.

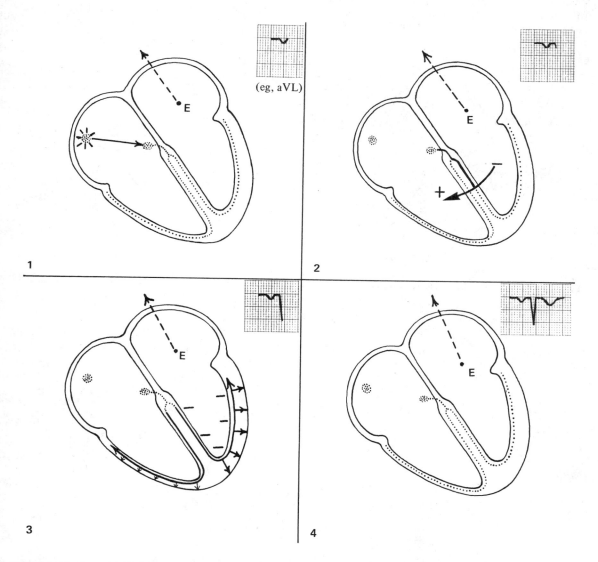

Figure 5–11. Genesis of left ventricular cavity complex (eg, aVL in a vertical heart). *(1)* Spread of excitation from SA node to AV node. Since the electrode in this diagram is above the AV groove, the P wave is inverted. *(2)* Septal activation from left to right produces the first portion of the QS complex. *(3)* Activation of the left ventricular myocardium from endocardial to epicardial surfaces renders the left ventricular cavity negative and produces the remainder of the QS complex. *(4)* Repolarization complete. This produces an inverted T wave.

RIGHT VENTRICULAR CAVITY COMPLEX

This complex is recorded by actually placing an electrode within the right ventricular cavity. The P wave is inverted, diphasic, or upright. As a result of septal activation from left to right, an initial small r wave may be registered. Actually this occurs only if the electrode is in close proximity to the septum. As the excitation wave passes through the right myocardium from endocardial to epicardial surfaces and passes into the left ventricle, all impulses will be spreading away from the electrode, producing a deep negative deflection, the S wave. For the reason given above (see p 41), a late r′ may be recorded. Thus the complexes may be (1) rS (as shown in sequence), (2) QS, (3) rSr′, or (4) Qr.* The ST segment is isoelectric and the T wave inverted.

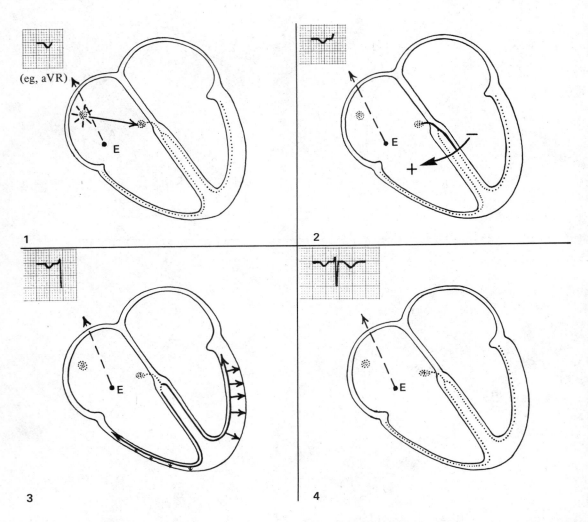

Figure 5–12. Genesis of right ventricular cavity complex (eg, aVR). *(1)* Spread of excitation from SA node to AV node. The electrode is above the level of the AV groove, resulting in an inverted P wave. *(2)* Septal activation from left to right produces initial positivity of the right ventricular cavity and hence the r wave. *(3)* Spread of excitation from the endocardial to the epicardial surface of the right and left myocardiums produces negativity of the cavity and therefore the S wave. *(4)* Repolarization complete. This produces an inverted T wave.

*The complexes not shown in the sequence are shown at the right. (Left, QS; center, rSr′; right, Qr.)

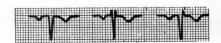

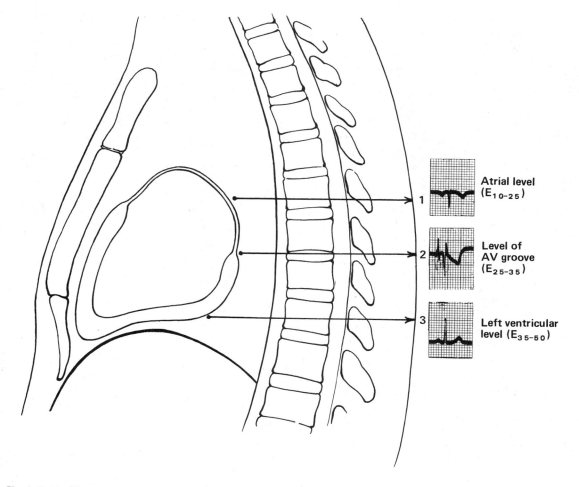

Figure 5–13. Diagram of back-of-the-heart patterns. *(1)* Atrial level. *(2)* Level of AV groove. *(3)* Left ventricular level (as recorded from esophageal electrodes, E).

"BACK–OF–THE–HEART" COMPLEXES

These are recorded by placing an exploring electrode directly on the exposed epicardial surface of the posterior aspect of the heart at varying locations.

An electrode overlying the atrial level will reflect cavity potential, thus recording an inverted P, a QS complex, and an inverted T.

An electrode placed over or just inferior to the AV groove will record a summation of cavity and left ventricular epicardial potentials: a large diphasic P, a QR complex, and an inverted T. This is the typical "back-of-the-heart" complex.

An electrode overlying the posterior aspect of the left ventricle will show a typical left ventricular epicardial complex.

In clinical practice, such recordings are obtained from an esophageal electrode.

APPLICATION OF THE COMPLEXES DESCRIBED ABOVE TO CLINICAL ELECTROCARDIOGRAPHY

The complexes described above have been obtained by actually applying the electrode to the surfaces or within the cavities of the heart. However, in clinical electrocardiography it must be remembered that all the electrodes, being on the surface of the body, are at varying distances from the heart. In unipolar electrocardiographic analysis the electrocardiographic patterns derived from body surface leads are correlated with the patterns developed from direct heart surface and cavity leads. Unipolar precordial and esophageal leads are much closer to the heart than unipolar extremity leads. The proximity of the former leads results in the major disagreement between the vector analysts and the unipolar lead analysts. The former believe that proximity leads offer no more information than can be obtained by a corrected lead system using remote leads. The unipolar lead analysts believe there may be local potentials recorded in proximity leads which are not evident in remote leads and that these may yield valuable clinical information.

Standard leads I, II, and III and unipolar extremity leads aVR, aVL, and aVF record the electrocardiographic pattern in the frontal plane. The pattern will vary depending upon the heart position.

Unipolar precordial leads V_{1-6}, etc record the electrocardiographic pattern (ie, the cardiac vector) in the horizontal plane. An individual chest lead does not represent the electrical potentials of a localized area of underlying heart muscle but records all of the electrical events of the heart cycle as viewed from that particular lead site. However, owing to the proximity of the precordial lead to the surface of the heart, those electrical potentials that are being generated in the underlying heart muscle will be magnified whereas those potentials arising from more distant locations will be of lesser magnitude (amplitude).

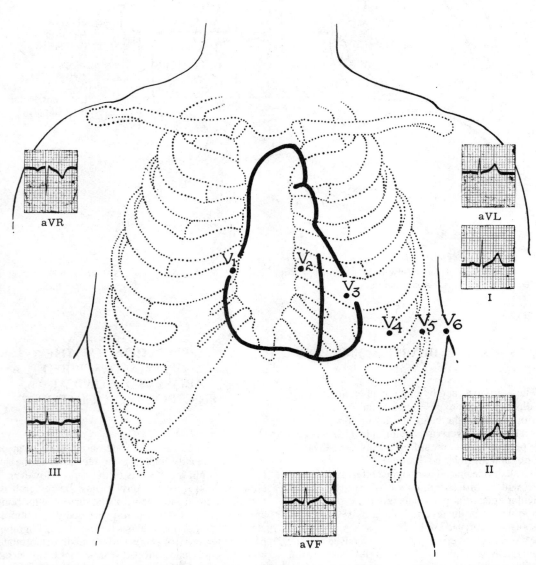

Figure 5–14. Frontal plane electrocardiographic patterns. Standard leads I, II, and III; augmented unipolar extremity leads, aVR, aVL, and aVF. Frontal plane QRS axis = +30 degrees (intermediate heart position); T axis = +15 degrees; QRS–T angle = 15 degrees.

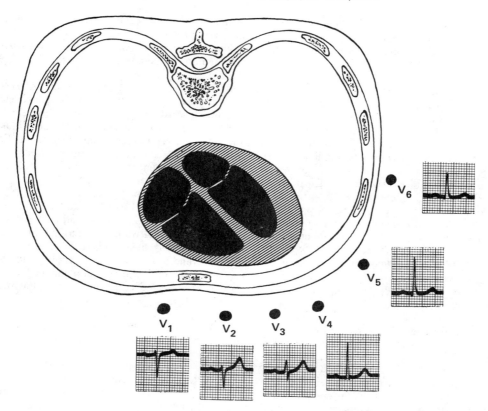

Figure 5–15. Horizontal plane electrocardiographic patterns. As the electrode is advanced from V_{1-6}, right ventricular epicardial complexes (V_{1-2}) change into left ventricular epicardial complexes (V_{4-6}). A transitional zone pattern is seen in V_3.

SUMMARY OF THE ELECTROPHYSIOLOGY OF THE NORMAL HEART & THE PRODUCTION OF THE NORMAL ELECTROCARDIOGRAM

As the electrical impulse passes through the conduction system and activates the myocardium, there is a constant changing of electrical potential which is reflected in the production of the ECG.

The pattern in any one lead of the normal ECG will depend on the relationship of its lead axis to the cardiac vector. The patterns will therefore vary with heart position (see Chapter 6). To illustrate the sequence of events in a conventional 12-lead ECG, a vertical heart position (frontal plane QRS axis = +75 degrees) will be used.

Atrial Complex

The P wave represents atrial depolarization. The P vector is directed leftward, inferiorly, and slightly anteriorly. The polarity of the P wave in any given lead will therefore depend on its relation to the direction of this vector.

A. Unipolar Extremity Leads:

1. aVR–The pattern of right arm potential is the same as the potential at the right shoulder, the arm merely acting as a conductor from the latter site. The impulse is therefore traveling away from this electrode and will result in a negative deflection, ie, an inverted P wave.

2. aVL–This lead reflecting left shoulder potential is so situated that the impulse is traveling away from it, and therefore the P wave is inverted.

3. aVF–The impulse is traveling toward the left foot electrode, and the P wave is therefore upright.

B. Standard Leads: The pattern in these leads is a further reflection of the frontal plane vector. In a normal vertical heart, the P wave is upright in all 3 leads.

C. Precordial Leads: The P wave in V_1 may be upright, diphasic, or inverted. The P wave may be inverted in V_2, but this is rare. The P wave is upright in leads V_{3-6}. (See Fig 5–16.)

D. Vector Analysis: Since the P vector is oriented to the left, inferiorly, and anteriorly, the P wave will be upright in I, II, III, and aVF, inverted in aVR and aVL, variable in V_{1-2}, and upright in V_{3-6}. (See Fig 5–6.)

After the impulse reaches the AV node, it is normally delayed for 0.07 s before the impulse passes on to the bundle of His. This produces an isoelectric PR segment in all leads. (See Fig 5–17.)

Ventricular Complex (Initial)

The initial impulse transmission in the ventricle is across the midportion of the interventricular septum from left to right. This produces initial positivity of the right ventricular cavity which is transmitted through the right ventricular myocardium and initial negativity of the left ventricular cavity which is transmitted through the left ventricular myocardium. The duration of this force is approximately 0.01 s.

A. Unipolar Extremity Leads:

1. aVR–This lead reflects right cavity potential and may record an initial small positive deflection, an r wave.

2. aVL–This lead reflects left cavity potential and will record a small negative deflection, a q wave.

3. aVF–This lead reflects left ventricular epicardial potential and will record an initial small negative deflection, a q wave.

B. Standard Leads: These reflect the pattern in extremity leads. A small q wave may be seen in leads I, II, and III.

C. Precordial Leads: Those leads reflecting right ventricular epicardial potential (V_{1-2}) will show an initial small positive deflection, the r wave. Those leads reflecting left ventricular epicardial potential (V_{4-6}) will show an initial small negative deflection, the q wave. (See Fig 5–18.)

D. Vector Analysis: The initial QRS vector is oriented to the right, anteriorly, and usually superiorly. Therefore, in the frontal plane this vector (directed to the right and superiorly) results in a small negative deflection (q) in leads I, II, III, aVL, and aVF and an upright deflection (r) in aVR. In the horizontal plane this vector (directed to the right and anteriorly) results in a small positive deflection (r) in V_{1-2} and a small negative deflection (q) in V_{4-6}.

Ventricular Complex (Major)

After activation of the midportion of the interventricular septum, the impulse passes down the right and left bundle branches into the Purkinje system, thereby activating the right and left ventricles. The impulses traverse the ventricular myocardium from the endocardial to the epicardial surface.

(1) The first portion of the ventricular myocardium to be activated is the anteroseptal region of the right ventricle. This contributes to the r wave in right precordial leads (V_{1-2}) and the q wave in I, V_5, and V_6. Its duration is approximately 0.01 s. (See Fig 5–19.)

(2) The major muscle mass of both the right and left ventricles is then activated. Since the impulse is spreading from the endocardium to the epicardium, both ventricular cavities will have a negative potential at this time. This will produce a negative wave in aVR which is an S wave since it is preceded by a positive deflection, the r wave, and hence an rS complex. It will similarly produce a negative wave in aVL. Since the initial deflection of septal activation was also negative, this completely negative wave is termed a QS complex.

Since the left ventricular muscle mass is much greater than the right, there will be greater electrical potential spreading through the left ventricle than the right. This is analogous to the muscle strip illustration on p 20. Left ventricular epicardial leads (aVF, V_{4-6}) will therefore record a tall upright deflection, the R wave, and right ventricular epicardial leads (V_{1-2}) will record deep S waves (Fig 5–20). The duration of this force is 0.03–0.05 s.

(3) Vector analysis: The major QRS vector is directed to the left, inferiorly, and posteriorly. In the frontal plane the leftward and inferiorly directed vector produces an upright deflection (R) in leads I, II, III, and aVF and a downward deflection (s) in aVR and (QS) in aVL. In the horizontal plane the leftward and posteriorly directed vector produces a downward deflection (S) in V_{1-2} and an upright deflection (R) in V_{4-6}.

(4) The last portions of the ventricular muscle mass to be activated are the posterobasal portion of the left ventricle, the region of the pulmonary conus, and the uppermost portion of the interventricular septum. This vector force is oriented to the right and superiorly. This produces a second small negative deflection in a left ventricular epicardial lead (aVF, V_{4-6}), an s wave, and, if oriented anteriorly, may produce a small second positive deflection, an r′ wave, in leads aVR and V_1 (Fig 5–21). Its duration is 0.01–0.02 s.

Repolarization

The sequences discussed above reflect ventricular depolarization. Following this, ventricular repolarization occurs. The sequence of events involved in ventricular repolarization are so complex that they cannot be illustrated. It is known that both the right and left ventricular cavities are negative during ventricular repolarization. The epicardial surface of the left ventricle is positive; that of the right ventricle may be positive or negative.

The ST segment will be isoelectric in all leads with the minor exceptions discussed on pp 25 and 82.

The T wave will be inverted in aVR and aVL (right and left cavity potential), upright in aVF and left precordial leads V_{3-6}, may be upright or inverted in V_1, and is rarely inverted in V_2. (See Fig 5–22.) The mean T vector is oriented to the left, inferiorly, and anteriorly.

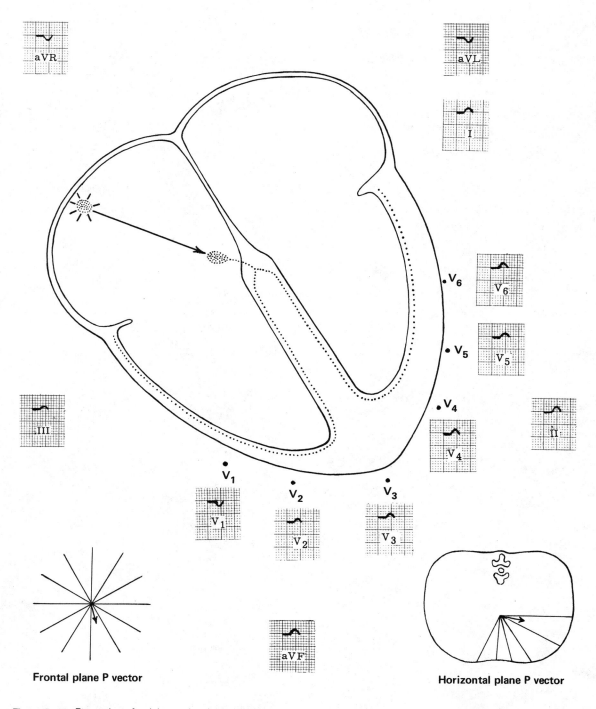

Frontal plane P vector

Horizontal plane P vector

Figure 5–16. Formation of atrial complex. In this illustration, the mean frontal plane P vector is +75 degrees. This results in upright P waves in leads I, II, III, and aVF and inverted P waves in leads aVR and aVL. The P vector in the horizontal plane is in the negative half of the V₁ axis, and the P wave is therefore inverted in lead V₁.

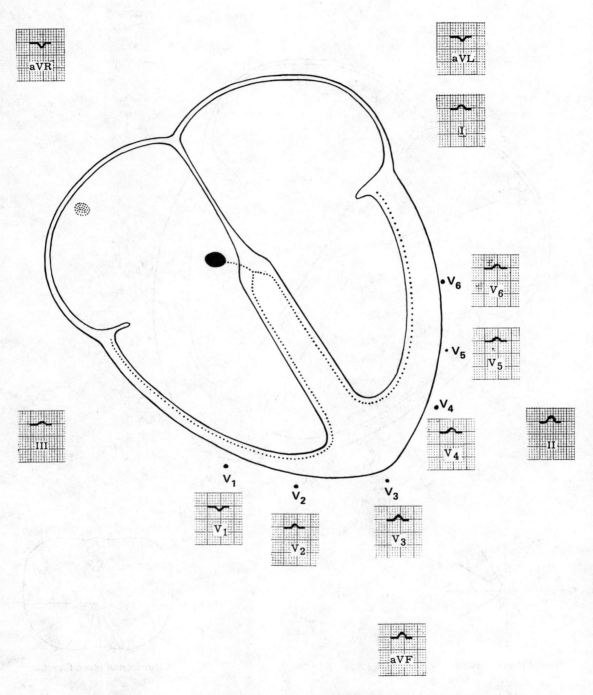

Figure 5–17. Completion of atrial complex and delay of impulse at AV node.

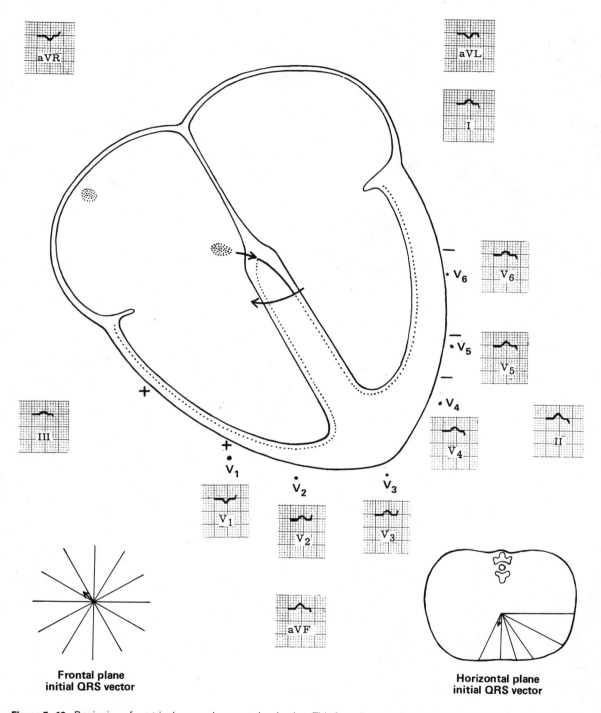

**Frontal plane
initial QRS vector**

**Horizontal plane
initial QRS vector**

Figure 5–18. Beginning of ventricular complex: septal activation. This force is normally oriented to the right and anteriorly. It may be directed superiorly (as in this illustration) or inferiorly.

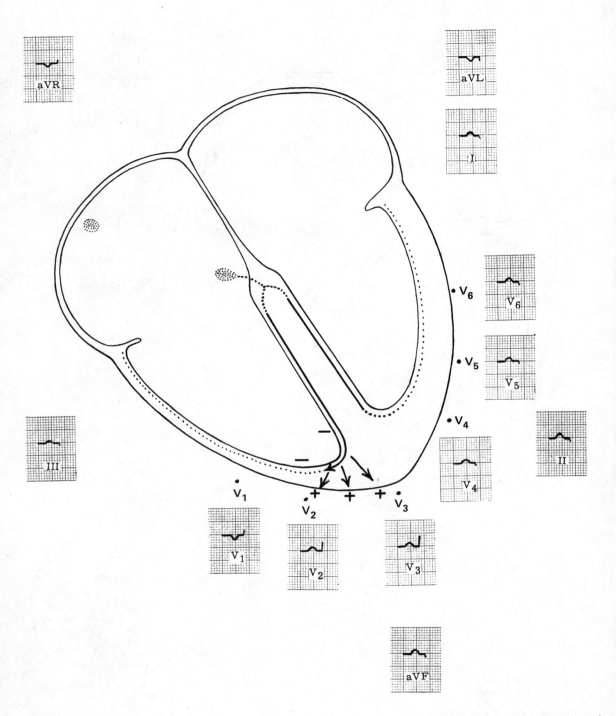

Figure 5–19. Early activation of anteroseptal region of myocardium. This produces a mean force oriented to the right and anteriorly.

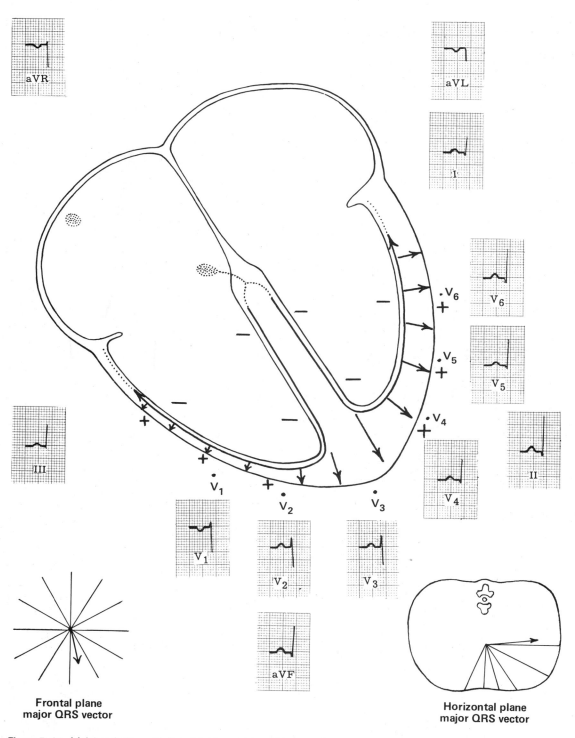

Figure 5–20. Major activation of left and right ventricles. This mean force is oriented to the left, inferiorly, and posteriorly.

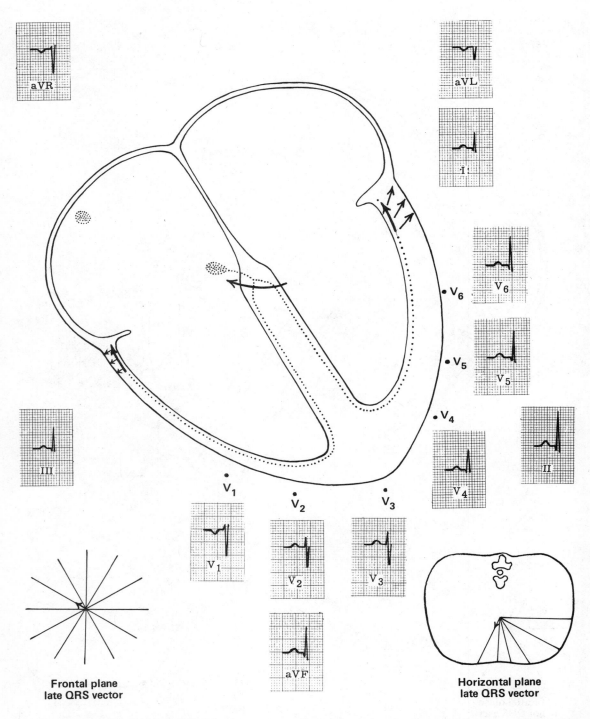

Figure 5–21. Activation of posterobasal portion of left ventricle, pulmonary conus, and uppermost portion of interventricular septum. In this illustration the mean force is oriented rightward, superiorly, and anteriorly.

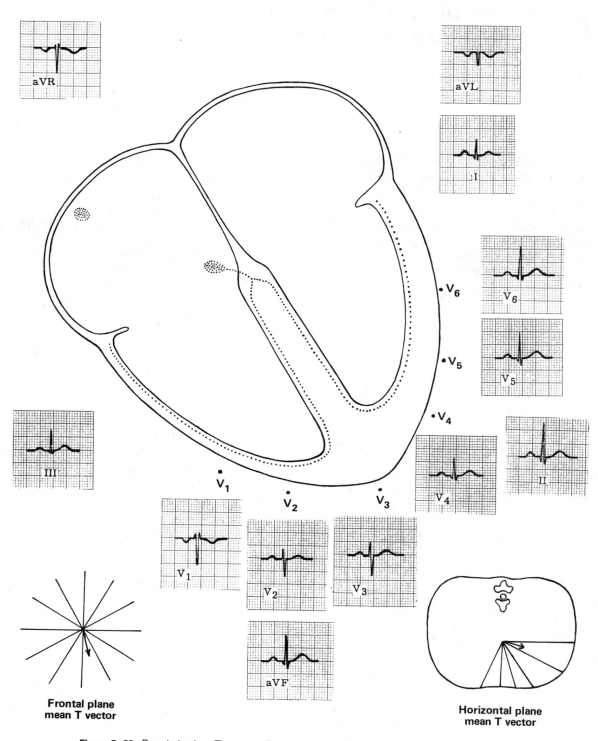

Figure 5–22. Repolarization. The mean T vector is oriented leftward, inferiorly, and anteriorly.

6 | Effect of Heart Position on the Electrocardiogram

It must be understood that when one speaks of heart position as interpreted electrocardiographically, one refers to a pattern resulting from electrical spread of excitation.

The electrical axis is not synonymous with the anatomic position of the heart. For simplicity, ECGs will be explained on the basis of the anatomic heart position, but it must be appreciated that there is not a high degree of correlation between these 2 phenomena.

In the interpretation of the ECG one should routinely determine the electrical axes along with the determination of the heart rate and rhythm. One then studies the tracing for evidence of abnormalities which are indicative of disturbances in the myocardium.

Rotation of the heart may occur on either the anteroposterior axis (frontal plane)—vertical, horizontal, intermediate, semivertical, semihorizontal—or the long axis (horizontal plane)—clockwise or counterclockwise.

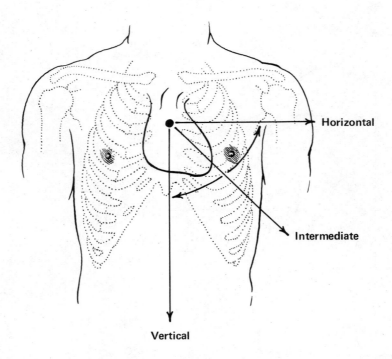

Figure 6–1. Rotation on the anteroposterior axis.

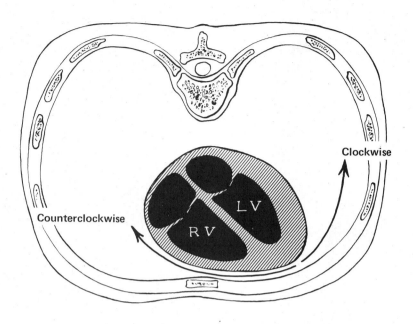

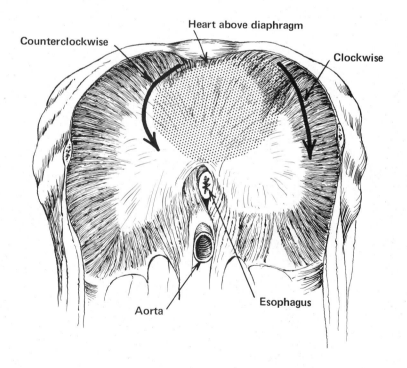

Figure 6–2. Rotation on the long axis as viewed from below the diaphragm.

ROTATION ON THE ANTEROPOSTERIOR AXIS
(Frontal Plane Axis)

Electrocardiographically, this is the more significant of the rotational patterns. The frontal plane QRS axis can be expressed in degrees (see p 30) or by the patterns in unipolar extremity leads and their resemblance to the patterns in V_1 and V_6. Both yield the same information. The latter subdivides the frontal plane axes into the following: vertical (greater than +75 degrees), semivertical (approximately +60 de-grees), intermediate (+30 degrees), semihorizontal (approximately 0 degrees), and horizontal (0 degrees to −30 degrees).

Vertical Rotation

The heart is so situated that a left ventricular epicardial complex will be recorded in aVF, a right ventricular cavity complex in aVR, and a left or right ventricular cavity complex or right ventricular epicardial complex in aVL. Thus, aVF will resemble V_6, and aVL will resemble V_1. The mean frontal plane QRS axis is +75 degrees or more.

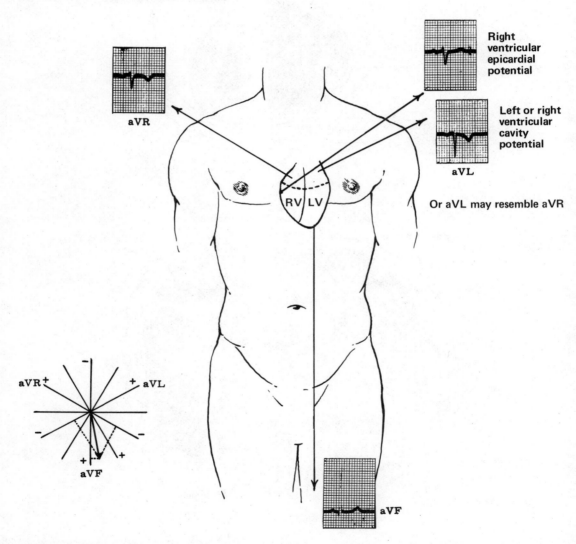

Right ventricular epicardial potential

Left or right ventricular cavity potential

aVL

Or aVL may resemble aVR

aVR

RV LV

aVR⁺   ⁺aVL

aVF

aVF

Figure 6–3. Vertical heart showing vectors. The mean QRS vector is oriented to the left and inferiorly, between +75 degrees and +110 degrees, resulting in an upright major QRS deflection in aVF and a downward major QRS deflection in aVL and aVR.

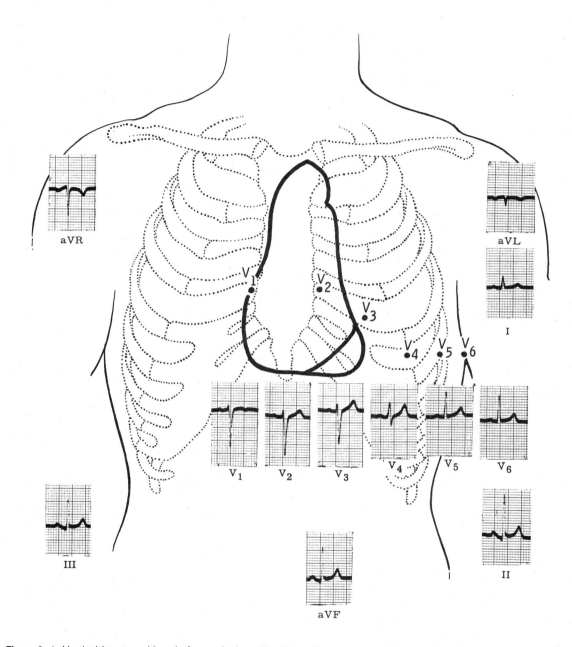

Figure 6–4. Vertical heart position. Left ventricular epicardial complex (upright P, qR, upright T) is seen in aVF, which resembles V₆; right cavity complex (inverted P, rS, inverted T) is seen in aVR; left cavity complex (inverted P, QS, inverted T) is seen in aVL. The frontal plane axis is +75 degrees.

Horizontal Rotation

A left ventricular epicardial complex is recorded in aVL (resembling V_6), either a right or left ventricular cavity complex in aVR, and a right ventricular epicardial complex in aVF (resembling V_1). This pattern is more commonly seen in heavy-set, broad-chested individuals. The mean frontal plane QRS axis is between O degrees and −30 degrees.

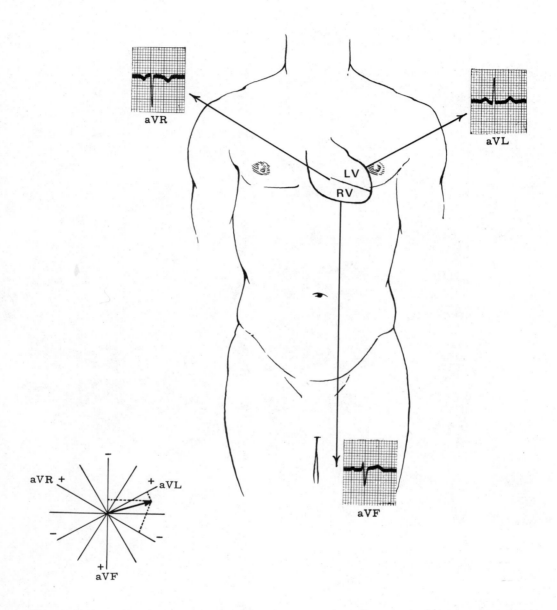

Figure 6–5. Horizontal heart showing vectors. The mean QRS vector is oriented to the left and superiorly, between 0 degrees and −30 degrees, resulting in an upright major QRS deflection in aVL and a downward major QRS deflection in aVR and aVF.

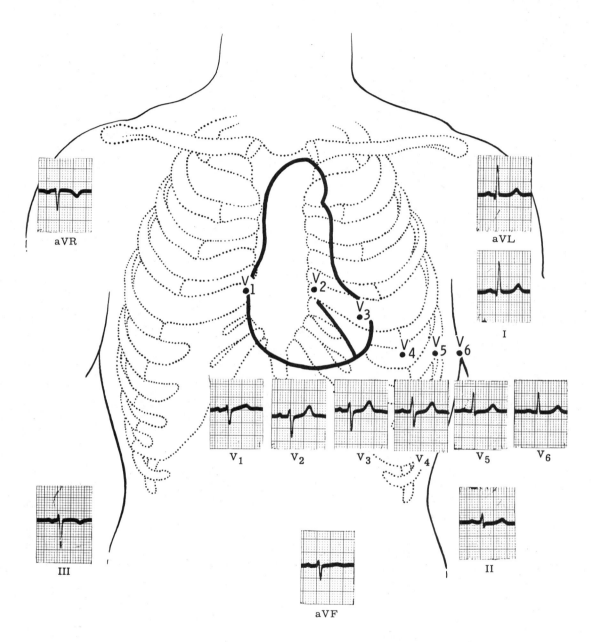

Figure 6–6. Horizontal heart position. Left ventricular epicardial complex (upright P, qR, upright T) is seen in aVL, which resembles V_6; right ventricular epicardial complex (upright P, rS, upright T) is seen in aVF, which resembles V_1; right cavity complex (inverted P, rS, inverted T) is seen in aVR. The frontal plane axis is −20 degrees.

Intermediate Rotation

This is a midway position between vertical and horizontal. A left ventricular epicardial complex is recorded in both aVL and aVF (both resembling V_6).

Either a right or left ventricular cavity complex is recorded in aVR. The mean frontal plane QRS axis is approximately +30 degrees.

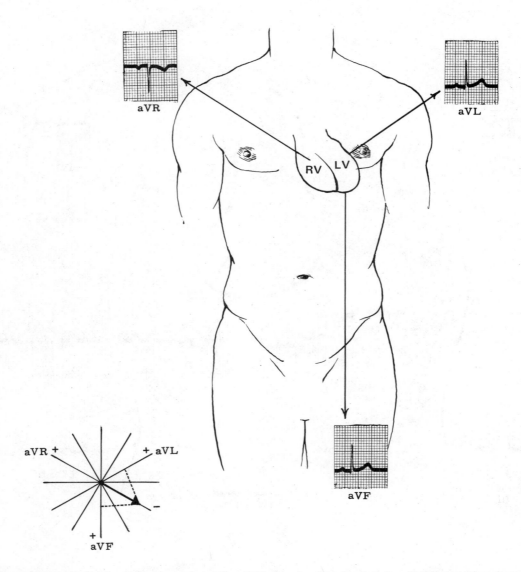

Figure 6–7. Intermediate heart showing vectors. Mean QRS vector is oriented to the left and inferiorly, halfway between the positive axes of aVF (+90 degrees) and aVL (−30 degrees). This results in an average frontal plane axis of +30 degrees with a range of +15 degrees to +45 degrees. At +30 degrees a positive QRS deflection of equal magnitude will be seen in aVL and aVF. Since the +30 degree axis is along the negative axis of aVR, the QRS deflection will be downward in aVR.

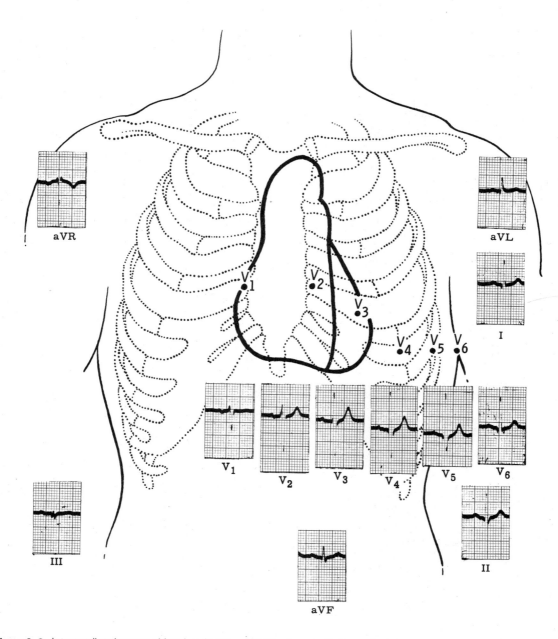

Figure 6–8. Intermediate heart position. Leads aVL and aVF both record left ventricular epicardial complex (upright P, qR in aVL, qRs in aVF; upright T) and resemble V₆; aVR records a right cavity complex (inverted P, rSr', inverted T). The frontal plane axis is +27 degrees.

Semivertical Rotation

This is a position midway between vertical and intermediate. Leads aVR and aVF are the same as in a vertical heart, but aVL consists of a small complex. The mean frontal plane QRS axis is approximately +60 degrees.

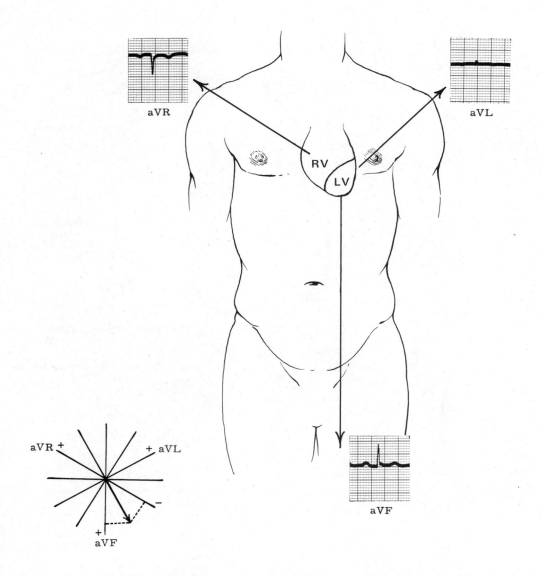

Figure 6–9. Semivertical heart showing vectors. The mean QRS vector is oriented to the left and inferiorly. Since the QRS complex in aVL is very small, the major QRS vector is pointed 90 degrees from the aVL axis (−30 degrees), or +60 degrees. This results in an upright QRS deflection in aVF and a downward deflection in aVR.

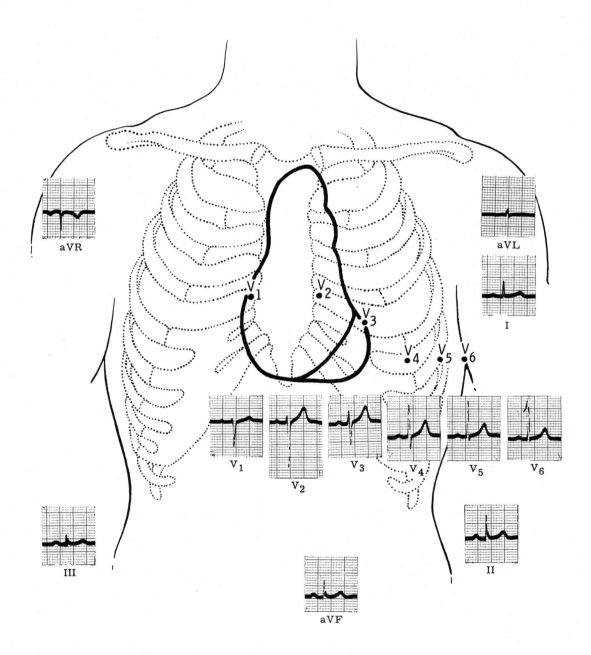

Figure 6–10. Semivertical heart position. Leads aVR and aVF are the same as in a vertical heart; however, lead aVL reveals a small complex. The frontal plane axis is +54 degrees.

Semihorizontal Rotation

This is a position midway between horizontal and intermediate. Leads aVR and aVL are the same as in a horizontal heart, but aVF consists of a small complex. The mean frontal plane QRS axis is approximately 0 degrees.

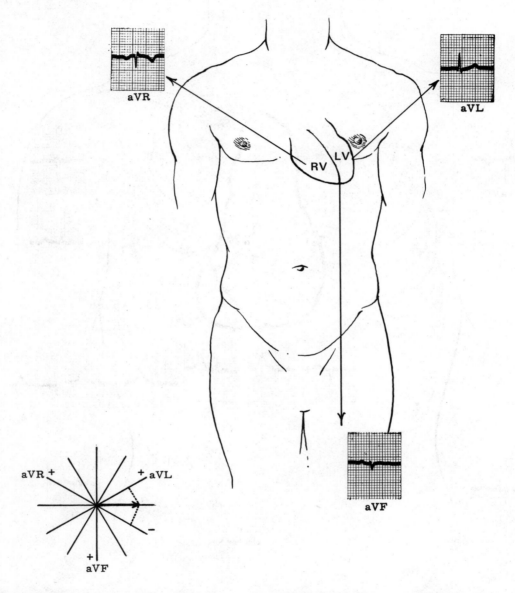

Figure 6–11. Semihorizontal heart showing vectors. The mean QRS vector is oriented to the left. Since aVF has a very small complex, the QRS vector is oriented 90 degrees from the axis of aVF (+90 degrees), or 0 degrees. This results in an upright QRS in aVL and a downward QRS in aVR.

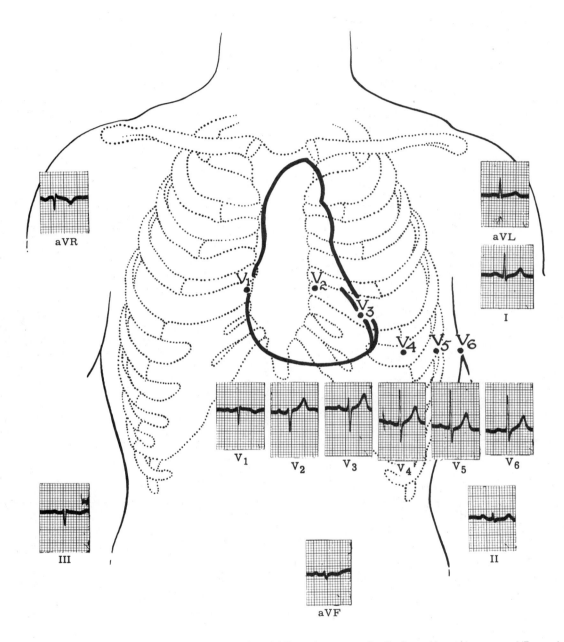

Figure 6–12. Semihorizontal heart position. Leads aVL and aVR are the same as in a horizontal heart; however, aVF reveals a small complex. The frontal plane axis is 0 degrees.

Table 6–1. Variation in patterns in unipolar extremity leads
due to rotation on the anteroposterior axis.

Frontal Plane Axis	aVR	aVL	aVF	V_1*	V_6*
Vertical	(a) Right cavity complex†	(b) Left or right cavity or right vent. epicardial complex‡	(c) Left vent. epicardial complex	(d) Right vent. epicardial complex§	(e) Left vent. epicardial complex
Semivertical	(f) Right cavity complex	(g) Small complex	(h) Left vent. epicardial complex	(i) Right vent. epicardial complex	(j) Left vent. epicardial complex
Intermediate	(k) Left or right cavity complex**	(l) Left vent. epicardial complex	(m) Left vent. epicardial complex	(n) Right vent. epicardial complex	(o) Left vent. epicardial complex
Semihorizontal	(p) Left or right cavity complex	(q) Left vent. epicardial complex	(r) Small complex	(s) Right vent. epicardial complex	(t) Left vent. epicardial complex
Horizontal	(u) Left or right cavity complex**	(v) Left vent. epicardial complex	(w) Right vent. epicardial complex	(x) Right vent. epicardial complex	(y) Left vent. epicardial complex

*Assuming no unusual rotation on the long axis.
†See ECG in Fig 5–12 for variations.
‡Or (a) or (d).
§See ECG in Fig 5–9 for variations.
**Or (a).
In (g) and (r) mean QRS = 0.

ROTATION ON THE LONG AXIS

Rotation on this axis may be clockwise or counterclockwise. The direction of rotation is defined by its appearance as viewed from the inferior surface of the heart looking upward from below the diaphragm. This rotational pattern is diagnosed by the appearance of the precordial leads. In an average case, the transitional zone is in the neighborhood of V_4.

The clinical significance of this rotation has been overemphasized in the past. Its major value is in relation to true anatomic rotation or displacement of the heart owing to congenital (eg, dextroversion, see p 78)

or acquired conditions (eg, pleural effusion, pneumothorax, atelectasis, pneumonectomy).

Clockwise Rotation

With clockwise rotation the transitional zone is displaced to the left, so the typical left ventricular epicardial pattern does not appear until V_{7-9}.

The term clockwise rotation is defined by persisting S waves in V_5 and V_6. This indicates that the terminal portion of the QRS is in the negative half of the V_5 and V_6 lead axes. This terminal force could be directed (1) rightward, in which case an S will be seen in lead I; (2) superiorly, in which case S waves will be seen in II, III, and aVF (ie, left or superior axis); or (3) posteriorly, in which case frontal plane leads are normal.

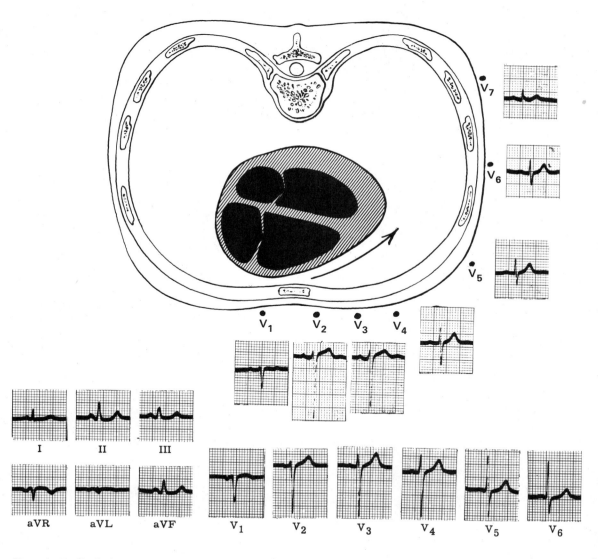

Figure 6–13. Clockwise rotation. *Extremity leads:* Semivertical heart position (frontal plane QRS axis = +60 degrees). *Precordial leads:* An RS complex is present in V_6, indicating that a left ventricular epicardial complex has not as yet been recorded.

Counterclockwise Rotation

In counterclockwise rotation the transitional zone is displaced to the right, resulting in left ventricular epicardial complexes as early as V_2. The mean QRS vector is oriented more anteriorly. ST segment elevation in V_{2-4} is a common accompaniment of counterclockwise rotation.

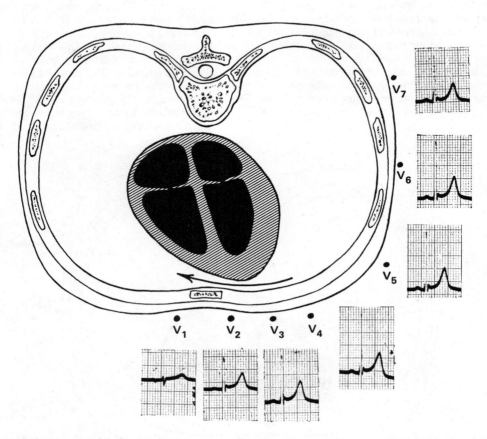

Figure 6–14. Counterclockwise rotation. A left ventricular epicardial complex is seen in V_2, indicating a transitional zone between V_1 and V_2. The ST segments are elevated in V_{2-3}, a common accompaniment of counterclockwise rotation.

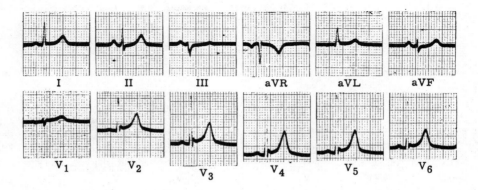

Figure 6–15. Counterclockwise rotation. *Standard leads:* Mean QRS axis = 0 degrees. *Extremity leads:* Semihorizontal heart position. *Precordial leads:* A left ventricular epicardial complex is seen in V_2, indicating counterclockwise rotation. There is associated ST segment elevation from V_{2-6}.

True Anatomic Rotation

As mentioned above, the clinical significance of this electrocardiographic description of rotation on the long axis is very limited. However, in situations in which there is true anatomic cardiac rotation or displacement, the ECG may reflect this. In the absence of clinical correlation, such ECGs can be interpreted incorrectly as other serious abnormalities. This again emphasizes the absolute necessity of correlating clinical data with the ECG. (See Figs 6–16 and 6–17.)

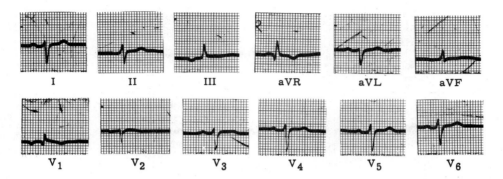

Figure 6–16. Anatomic clockwise rotation. This ECG was recorded on a 50-year-old healthy man. The frontal plane QRS axis = +150 degrees; a QR is present in V₁, and deep S waves persist through V₆. The above is consistent with right ventricular hypertrophy. There was no clinical evidence of hypertrophy, however, and cardiac catheterization revealed normal findings. The clinical diagnosis was congenital absence of the left pericardium. This anomaly permits the heart to be displaced to the left and rotated clockwise, resulting in the major QRS forces being oriented rightward and posteriorly.

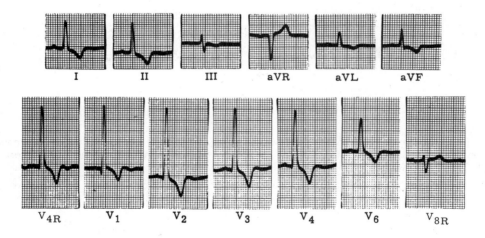

Figure 6–17. Anatomic counterclockwise rotation. The mean frontal plane QRS axis = +30 degrees. There is ST depression and T wave inversion in leads I, II, aVL, and aVF. Very tall R waves with ST depression and T wave inversion are seen in leads V₄R through V₅. Such pronounced changes could be interpreted as right ventricular hypertrophy or biventricular hypertrophy. This ECG was recorded on a 65-year-old man with hypertensive cardiovascular disease. In addition, he had congenital dextroversion. This results in true counterclockwise rotation, so that the left ventricle becomes an anterior ventricle and the pattern of left ventricular hypertrophy is reflected in the right and anterior precordial leads (see p 78).

EFFECT OF DEEP RESPIRATION ON THE ROTATIONAL PATTERNS

Deep inspiration and expiration can appreciably alter the appearance of the individual electrocardiographic leads. With deep inspiration the heart position becomes more vertical, and there is greater clockwise rotation. With deep expiration the heart becomes more horizontal, and there is greater counterclockwise rotation. Variations in right and left heart stroke volume during inspiration and expiration also play a role in these electrocardiographic changes.

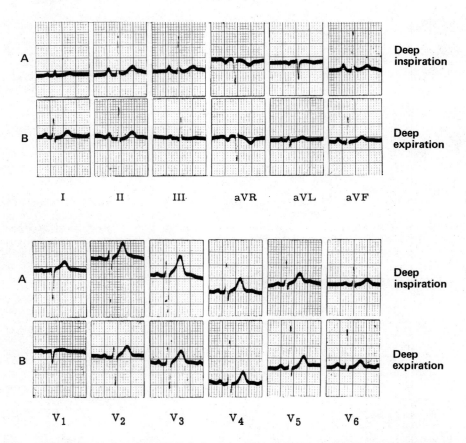

Figure 6–18. Effect of deep respiration on the ECG. *A:* Deep inspiration. *B:* Deep expiration. In deep inspiration the frontal heart position is vertical (+85 degrees); this becomes semivertical (+65 degrees) in deep expiration. In the latter phase the voltage increases in I and V_{4-6} and decreases in aVF.

The Electrocardiogram in Infants & Children; Normal Variants of the Adult Electrocardiogram | 7

FETAL ELECTROCARDIOGRAPHY

By using a standard electrocardiograph equipped with a preamplifier capable of amplifying an input signal 50 times and recording in a frequency range of 12–20 cps, it is possible to record maternal and fetal QRS complexes. After voiding, the patient lies down. One electrode of a bipolar lead is placed in the midline of the abdomen at the level of the uterine fundus; the other is placed just above the symphysis pubica.

Fetal electrocardiography is of value (1) in determining fetal life during the second and third trimesters of pregnancy; (2) in the early diagnosis of multiple pregnancy; (3) in detecting fetal arrhythmia; (4) in monitoring the fetal heart rate during labor; and (5) in determining fetal position (Fig 7–1). If the mother's QRS vector is normal (inferiorly directed, and therefore giving an upright QRS complex), the fetal QRS vector in a vertex presentation will be directed superiorly, producing an inverted QRS complex. In a breech presentation, the fetal QRS vector will be directed inferiorly, producing an upright QRS complex.

NORMAL ELECTROCARDIOGRAPHIC PATTERNS IN INFANTS & CHILDREN

Normal ECG in Infants (See Fig 7–2.)

In the fetus, the right ventricle performs more work than the left ventricle. Therefore, at birth or in infancy, there is a relative hypertrophy of the right ventricle. This will result in an electrocardiographic pattern that will simulate that of right ventricular hypertrophy in the adult, ie, tall R waves in the right precordial leads and right axis deviation. However, an initial q wave will never be seen in V_1, and the VAT is

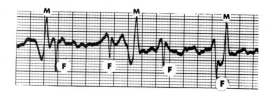
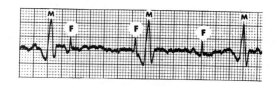

Figure 7–1. Comparison of vertex and breech presentations. Upper tracing is a vertex presentation showing the fetal QRS in opposite direction from the maternal. Lower tracing is a breech showing the fetal QRS in same direction as the maternal. (Reproduced, with permission, from Buxton TM et al: Fetal electrocardiography. *JAMA* 1963;**185**:441.)

not prolonged (Fig 8–18). Within the first 2–4 days of life, the T waves are upright in leads V_{2-6} and may be upright or inverted in V_1. After this time, the T waves normally become inverted in leads V_{1-4}.

Normal ECG in Children (See Fig 7–3.)

The tall R waves in right precordial leads usually disappear after age 5, but inverted T waves in the right precordial leads frequently persist into the second decade of life. The frontal plane QRS axis gradually shifts to the left.

Juvenile Pattern (See Fig 7–4.)

In blacks, this "juvenile pattern" of T wave inversion (as in the child) in precordial leads V_{1-4} may persist into the third decade of life.

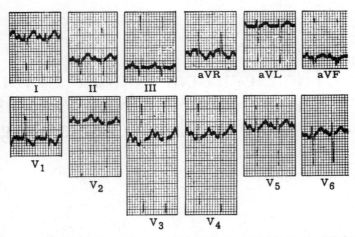

Figure 7–2. Normal ECG in an infant (age 3 days). *Standard leads:* Right axis deviation (+130 degrees). *Extremity leads:* Vertical heart position; tall R in aVR. *Precordial leads:* A tall R is present in V_1; VAT in V_1 = 0.02 s. The T waves are upright in leads V_{2-6}.

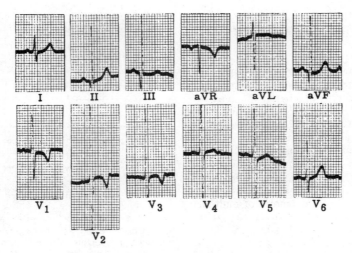

Figure 7–3. Normal ECG in an 8-year-old child. The T waves are inverted in V_{1-3}. This would be abnormal in an adult white person but is the normal pattern in a child.

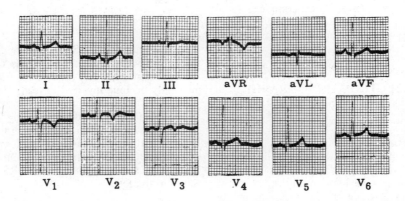

Figure 7–4. Black man, age 24, with no clinical evidence of heart disease. *Standard leads:* QRS axis = +75 degrees. *Extremity leads:* Vertical heart position. *Precordial leads:* The T waves are deeply inverted in V_{1-3}. This would be abnormal in an adult white person but can be normal in a young black. The cardiac diagnosis must depend on the result of the clinical examination. If no other abnormalities exist, this tracing can be considered to be within normal limits.

DEXTROCARDIA & DEXTROVERSION

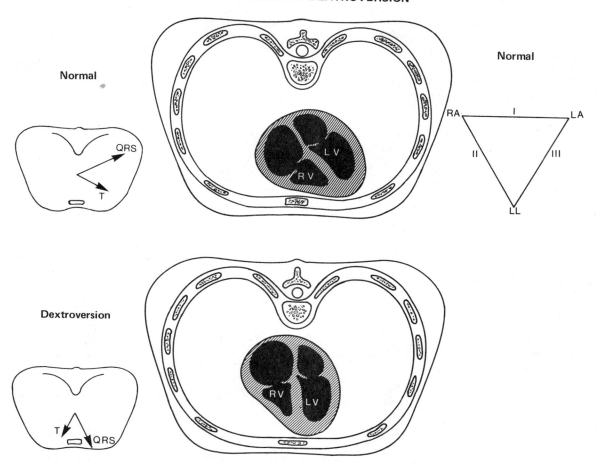

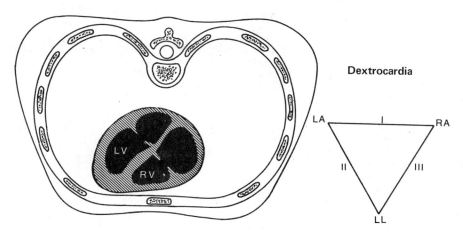

Figure 7–5a. The angle between QRS and T is the same in dextroversion as in the normal.

Figure 7–5b. RA-LA = −I, thus, P, QRS, and T are inverted; LL-LA = II (normal III); LL-RA = III (normal II); aVL and aVR are reversed.

DEXTROVERSION

Dextroversion is a congenital anomaly in which the heart is displaced to the right, and the ventricles are rotated in a counterclockwise rotation. The ventricles and atria are not transposed, the left ventricle facing to the left and the right ventricle to the right. The aorta is in a normal position. The P vector remains normal.

The mean QRS vector is oriented more anteriorly (counterclockwise rotation). The mean T vector may be oriented to the right and thus result in a negative T wave in lead I, which in this instance is not abnormal. Even though the mean QRS vector is directed anteriorly, the normal angle between the QRS and T vectors in the horizontal plane remains normal, so that the T vector is oriented rightward and anteriorly (Fig 7–5a).

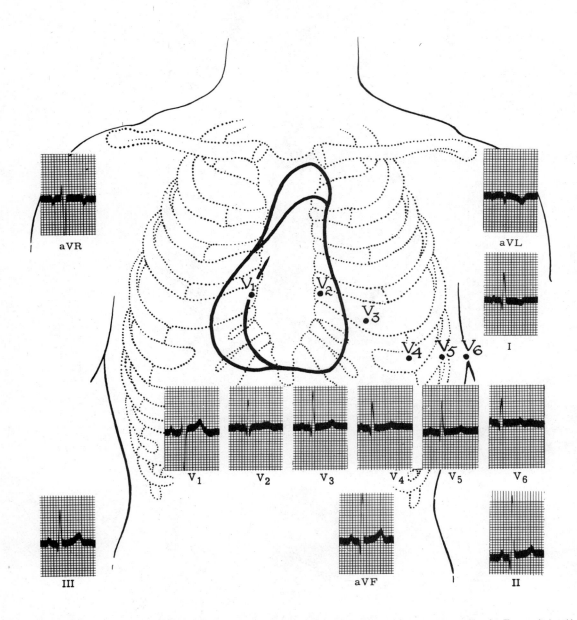

Figure 7–6. Dextroversion. The pattern in precordial leads is that of counterclockwise rotation. Note that the T wave in lead I is inverted. *Clinical findings:* Heart displaced to the right; bronchiectasis; sinusitis.

TRUE DEXTROCARDIA

This is a congenital anomaly in which there is complete transposition of both ventricles and atria. The aortic knob is also to the right. Electrically, the only abnormality is a reversal of the polarity of the L–R (I) axis. Thus, the P vector is oriented to the *right*, inferiorly, and anteriorly, producing an inverted P wave in lead I and an upright P wave in aVR. The mean QRS vector is directed to the *right*, inferiorly, and slightly posteriorly. The T vector is also oriented to the *right*, inferiorly, and anteriorly. This alters the ECG in the following fashion (Fig 7–5b):

	Normal	Dextrocardia
LA-RA	I	−I*
LL-RA	II	III
LL-LA	III	II
	aVR	aVL
	aVL	aVR
	aVF	aVF

Precordial leads V_{1-6} will reflect right ventricular epicardial and "back-of-the-heart" complexes. However, if the precordial leads are taken over the right chest, left ventricular epicardial patterns will result.

*Thus, P, QRS, and T are inverted.

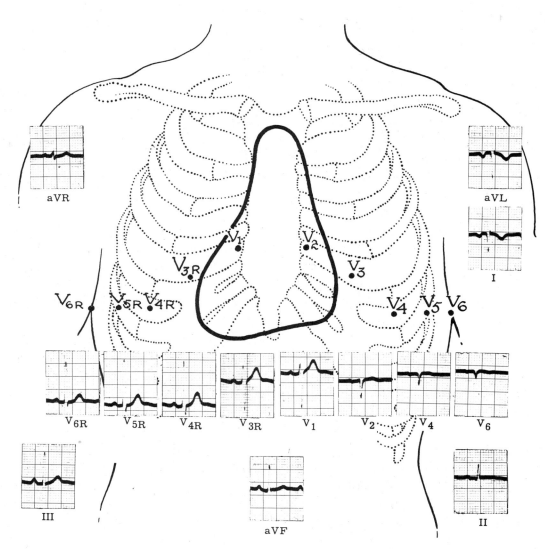

Figure 7–7. Dextrocardia. Lead I complexes are inverted; the patterns in II and III and aVR and aVL are the reverse of normal. Left precordial leads record a right ventricular epicardial complex; right precordial leads record a left ventricular epicardial complex. *Clinical diagnosis:* 30-year-old man with dextrocardia and situs inversus; no evidence of heart disease.

TECHNICAL DEXTROCARDIA

Occasionally a technician will inadvertently interchange the right and left arm electrodes. This will produce a pattern of dextrocardia in the standard and the extremity leads but will not alter the normal pattern in precordial leads.

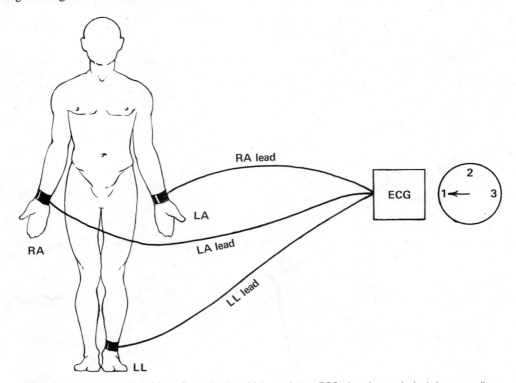

Figure 7–8. Incorrect position of arm leads which produces ECG showing technical dextrocardia.

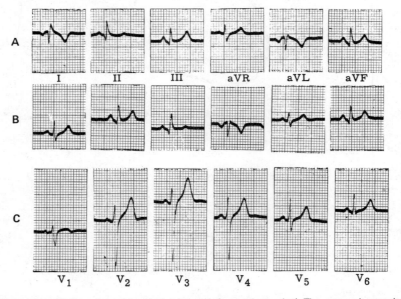

Figure 7–9. Technical dextrocardia (from interchange of right and left arm electrodes). The pattern in standard and extremity leads *(A)* is that of dextrocardia, ie, lead I is completely inverted, and leads II, III, aVR, and aVL are transposed. In *(B)*, standard and extremity leads are taken correctly. However, the precordial leads *(C)* are entirely normal, indicating that this is not a true dextrocardia.

UNUSUAL NORMAL VARIANTS

The "normal" data for electrocardiographic measurements are determined from studies of large groups of clinically normal individuals. If one were to use the 100th percentile range for each measurement, there would be such a large overlap between normal and abnormal conditions as to render electrocardiographic evaluation practically worthless. As a result, arbitrary limits are used that are in the 95–98th percentile range. This corresponds to ±2 standard deviations. Therefore, for any given measurement, 2–5% of normal individuals will be outside the "normal value" and could be considered abnormal. The physician must be aware of this and avoid dogmatic criteria in differentiating between normal and abnormal in electrocardiography.

There are known sources of variability, although in some the cause may not be understood. These include the following: (1) Age. (2) Sex. (3) Body weight and chest configuration. Although statistical significance can be demonstrated when these 3 variables are studied in large groups of a normal population, they are of no major significance in the evaluation of a single record. (4) Race: For unknown reasons, significant differences exist between different races. (5) Food intake: A high-glucose meal can produce electrocardiographic changes that mimic abnormality. These changes are due partly to potassium shift intracellularly. Ideally, all records should be taken under basal conditions. Since this is impractical, the physician must be aware of this possibility. (6) Exercise. (7) Smoking: The patient should be at rest for 15 minutes and abstain from smoking for 30 minutes prior to a routine recording of the ECG. (8) Precordial lead positions: This can be a problem in evaluation of serial records. A change in the location of a precordial electrode can alter the ECG recorded on the given lead. This can be avoided in hospitalized patients in whom serial ECGs are anticipated by correctly marking the precordial positions with India ink at the time of the first recording.

ST SEGMENT ELEVATION

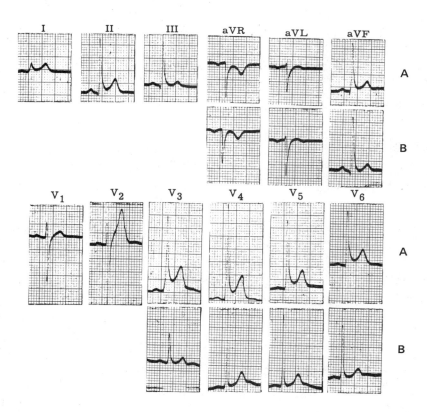

Figure 7–10. Unusual ST segment elevation as a normal variant. Note the marked ST segment elevation in leads V₃–₅. This is 4 mm in V₃–₄ *(A)*. This record was taken on a 24-year-old black man. There was no clinical evidence of organic heart disease. Following exercise *(B)*, the ST segments became isoelectric. (From Goldman MJ: *Am Heart J* 1953;**46**:817.)

ST SEGMENT ELEVATION

On p 25 it was stated that the ST segment may normally be elevated up to 2 mm in the precordial leads. Occasionally, up to 4 mm ST elevation can occur in left precordial leads. The ST segment has an upward concavity, and the T is upright. This has been seen more commonly in young adult blacks. Following exercise, the ST segments return to the isoelectric line.

This phenomenon is considered to represent early repolarization, ie, a major portion of the myocardium is beginning its repolarization before depolarization is completed in other areas of the myocardium. (See Fig 7–10.)

ST SEGMENT ELEVATION & T WAVE INVERSION

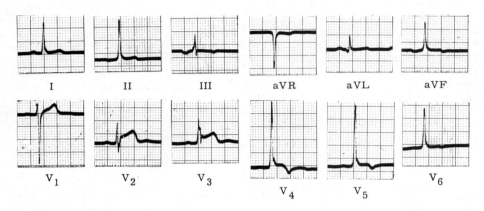

Figure 7–11. Unusual ST segment elevation and T wave inversion as a normal variant. Note the elevated ST segments from V_{2-4}. The T waves are inverted in V_{4-5} and diphasic in V_6 and aVF. This record was taken on a 23-year-old black man. There was no clinical evidence of heart disease, and this electrocardiographic pattern has remained unchanged for 6 years. Because of the electrocardiographic finding alone, this patient had been subjected to exploratory thoracotomy and pericardial biopsy with normal findings. These ST and T variations are not altered by rest, moderate exercise, hyperventilation, and vagal blocking drugs. Although moderate exercise (eg, double Master's test) does not alter the above, maximal exercise (as performed with a treadmill) can temporarily abolish the ST–T changes and normalize the ECG. (From Goldman MJ: *Am Heart J* 1960;**59**:71.)

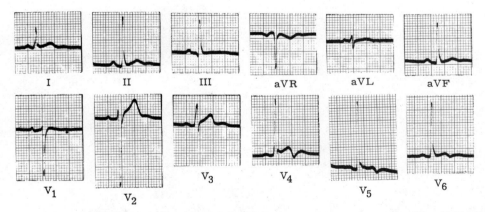

Figure 7–12. Tracing of a 24-year-old black man. The frontal plane leads are within normal limits. Precordial leads reveal ST segment elevation from V_{2-5}. There is late T wave inversion in leads V_{4-6}. The voltage of $SV_1 + RV_5 = 42$ mm. There was no clinical evidence of heart disease. This electrocardiographic pattern remained stationary over a 5-year period of observation and was unchanged by basal conditions, moderate exercise, hyperventilation, or vagal blocking drugs. ¶The recognition of the above normal variants is of utmost clinical importance. The ECG simulates organic heart disease (eg, pericarditis, myocarditis, myocardial infarction). Many healthy young individuals are made cardiac invalids by this electrocardiographic finding alone. Admittedly, a specific diagnosis cannot be made from a single tracing. If the clinical evaluation is entirely normal and serial tracings remain unchanged, a diagnosis of cardiac abnormality should not be made. This illustrates the importance of using total clinical evaluation in electrocardiographic interpretation.

ANXIETY REACTION

In patients with supposedly normal hearts who suffer from anxiety and hyperventilation, the following electrocardiographic abnormalities have been described: (1) prolongation of the P–R interval; (2) sinus tachycardia, less commonly, arrhythmias of various types; and (3) ST segment depression and T wave inversion in left ventricular epicardial leads.

This pattern may simulate coronary insufficiency (see p 144). Such an effect has been documented in individuals with no clinical evidence of heart disease and normal coronary angiograms. The authors who describe these abnormalities ascribe them to imbalance of the autonomic nervous system. Such drugs as ergotamine, atropine, and potassium can revert the ECG to normal. Caution is required, however, since it is dangerous to administer ergotamine to a patient with coronary artery disease. (See Figs 7–13 and 7–14.)

Effect of Oral Potassium on the ECG

The T wave abnormalities discussed above which occur in clinically normal individuals and which are considered as normal variants or "functional" T wave changes may be normalized by oral potassium. This is especially true in those individuals whose electrocardiographic changes are thought to be related to anxiety and hyperventilation. A base-line ECG is obtained in the fasting state. The patient is given 10 g of a potassium preparation (eg, 5 g of potassium citrate and 5 g of potassium bicarbonate), and ECGs are repeated in 60 and 90 minutes. In many such individuals, the T waves will become normal at these times. In patients with organic T wave changes due to coronary artery disease, hypertrophy, and bundle branch block, complete normalization of the T wave does not occur. This test is advised only when the patient has no clinical evidence of any disease or metabolic abnormality which could explain the T wave changes. The serum creatinine and serum potassium must be normal. Although this procedure is of clinical usefulness in evaluating T wave abnormalities of obscure origin, the final decision will depend on sound clinical judgment. (See Fig 7–15.)

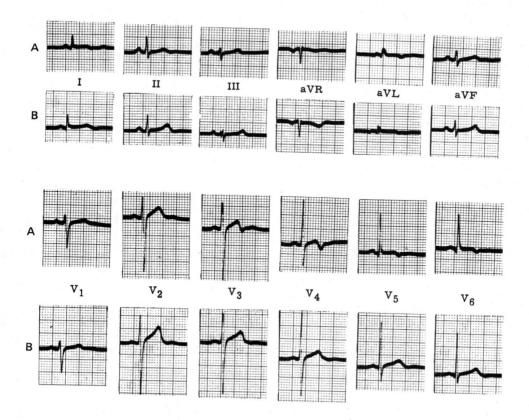

Figure 7–13. Anxiety reaction. The above tracings were taken on a 26-year-old white man with no clinical evidence of heart disease. *A:* Representative of repeatedly "abnormal" ECGs as evidenced by inverted T waves in leads V₄₋₆. *B:* After atropine; the T waves in the above-mentioned leads are now normal.

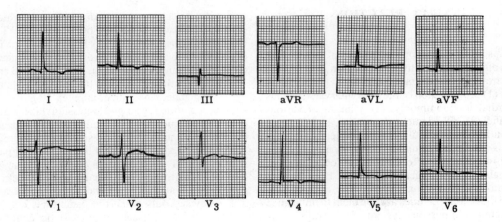

Figure 7–14. Tracing of a 27-year-old man whose clinical diagnosis was anxiety reaction. The T waves are inverted in I, II, aVL, aVF, and V₄₋₆. Serial tracings over several weeks showed no change. There was no evidence of cardiovascular disease or metabolic abnormality.

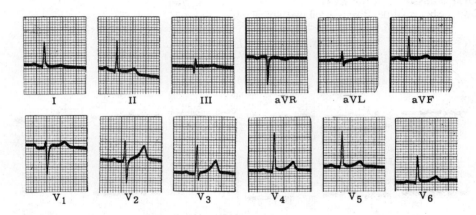

Figure 7–15. Tracing taken 90 minutes after administration of 10 g oral potassium. The T waves are now normal.

EFFECT OF FOOD INTAKE ON THE ELECTROCARDIOGRAM

Following a heavy meal, especially if high in carbohydrate, ST depression or T wave inversion (or both) may occur. This represents a physiologic and not a pathologic phenomenon and is due in part to an intracellular shift of potassium in association with intracellular glucose metabolism. Such electrocardiographic changes may simulate a variety of pathologic states, and the physician should be alert to this possibility. (See Fig 7–16.)

BIPOLAR VERSUS UNIPOLAR CHEST LEADS

The difference between these leads has been discussed above (see p 4). In a vertical heart, because of the relatively high voltage in aVF, the potential of the foot lead (aVF) can appreciably alter the chest potential as recorded in a CF lead. An example of this is seen below. This patient was diagnosed as having organic heart disease on the basis of the CF leads. There was no good clinical evidence of heart disease. Subsequent V leads (taken several years later) were normal. Repeated CF leads still showed the "abnormal" pattern. Unfortunately, the patient had become an incurable cardiac invalid (iatrogenic) in the interval. This illustrates not only the inaccuracy of bipolar chest leads but also the fallacy of diagnosing organic heart disease purely on the basis of "nonspecific" electrocardiographic findings. (See Fig 7–17.)

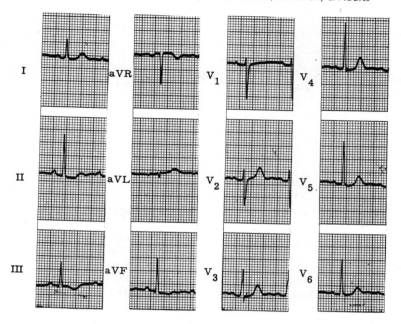

Figure 7–16. Effect of heavy meal. The above ECG was recorded on a clinically normal 30-year-old woman. There is ST depression in leads I, II, III, aVF, and V_{3-6}. The T waves are inverted in leads II and aVF. This tracing was taken 60 minutes after a heavy meal. Repeat ECGs recorded under basal conditions and at least 3 hours postprandially were consistently normal. In this ECG, leads I-II-III, aVR-aVL-aVF, V_{1-3}, and V_{4-6} are recorded simultaneously.

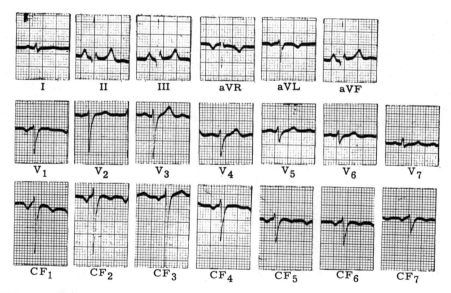

Figure 7–17. Difference between CF and V precordial leads. CF leads reveal inversion of the T waves in precordial leads through CF_7. V leads show normally upright T waves. The "abnormality" in the CF leads is a result of the influence of the potential in aVF, ie, the T in aVF being taller than the T in V_{5-7} results in inverted T waves in CF_{5-7}.

8 | Hypertrophy Patterns

ATRIAL HYPERTROPHY

Etiology & Pathology

Atrial hypertrophy may arise under the following pathologic conditions (in order of incidence): (1) As the result of AV valvular stenosis, eg, left atrial hypertrophy associated with mitral stenosis. (2) Secondary to pulmonary hypertension, eg, right atrial hypertrophy resulting from chronic diffuse pulmonary disease. (3) In association with various congenital heart lesions, eg, right atrial hypertrophy associated with an interatrial septal defect. (4) Secondary to ventricular hypertrophy, eg, left atrial hypertrophy secondary to left ventricular hypertrophy of hypertensive cardiovascular disease.

Incidence

From the standpoint of electrocardiographic diagnosis, atrial hypertrophy can frequently be diagnosed in mitral stenosis, chronic pulmonary disease producing pulmonary hypertension, and certain congenital lesions. It is less commonly diagnosed when associated with left ventricular hypertrophy.

Electrocardiographic Criteria

The normal P wave is not over 0.11 s in width and 2.5 mm in height. Any increase in these values is suggestive of atrial hypertrophy. Although it is not always possible to differentiate electrocardiographically between left and right atrial hypertrophy, the criteria given below and in Figs 8–2 and 8–3 are helpful.

Clinical Significance

This will depend on the etiology and course of the underlying heart disease.

A. Left Atrial Hypertrophy: (As seen in mitral stenosis.) This is manifested by broad, notched P waves ("P mitrale"), usually best seen in leads I and II. Lead V_1 characteristically has a wide, slurred, diphasic P wave in which the downward component of the wave is most prominent. The second notch of the P (upright in I and inverted in V_1) is the result of delayed activation of the hypertrophied left atrium, which is oriented in a leftward and posterior direction. Electrophysiologically, this represents a left atrial conduction delay (also referred to as left atrial abnormality), and, although commonly associated with left atrial hypertrophy, it is not pathognomonic of that condition.

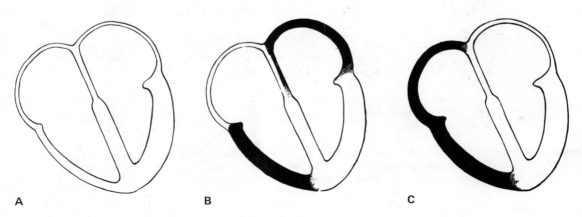

Figure 8–1. Diagrammatic illustration of the normal heart and the heart in hypertrophy. *A:* The normal heart. Diagrammatic illustration of the 4 cardiac chambers. Both atria are thin-walled; the normal left ventricle is considerably thicker than the right. *B:* Hypertrophy of the left atrium and right ventricle (mitral stenosis). *C:* Hypertrophy of the right atrium and right ventricle (chronic pulmonary disease).

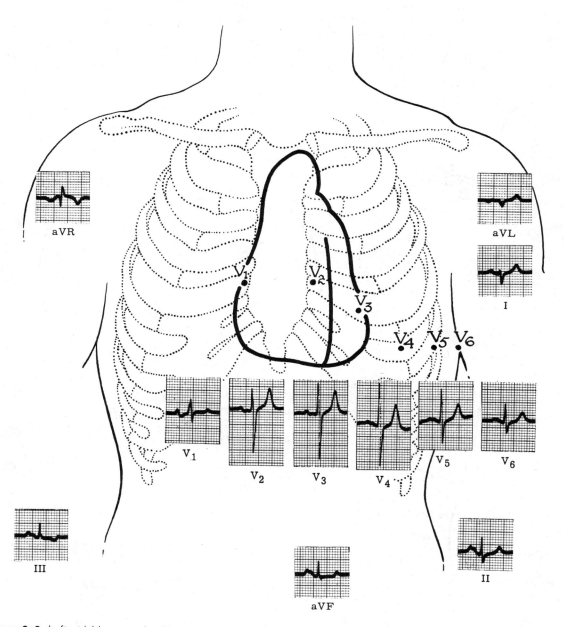

Figure 8–2. Left atrial hypertrophy. Note the broad, notched P waves in standard and extremity leads and V$_{4-6}$. The characteristic diphasic P wave with a wide negative component is seen in V$_1$. Right axis deviation (+110 degrees) and tall R in V$_1$ are indicative of right ventricular hypertrophy (see p 100). *Clinical diagnosis:* Mitral stenosis.

B. Right Atrial Hypertrophy: (As seen in chronic pulmonary disease.) This is manifested by tall, slender, peaked P waves in leads II, III, and aVF (greater than 2.5 mm) and prominent peaked, diphasic, or inverted P waves in V₁.

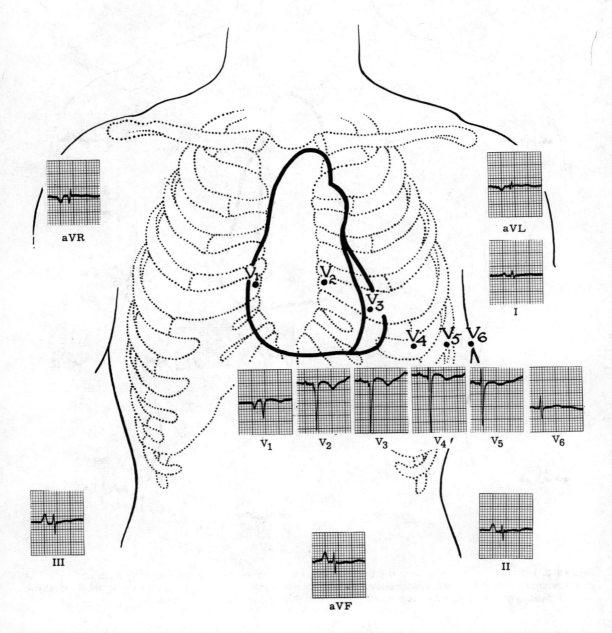

Figure 8–3. Right atrial hypertrophy. There are tall, peaked P waves in II, III, and aVF. A deeply inverted and slender P wave is seen in V₁. The QRS and T abnormalities are indicative of right ventricular hypertrophy (see p 100). *Clinical and autopsy diagnosis:* Severe chronic obstructive lung disease; right atrial and ventricular hypertrophy.

T_a Waves

A prominent T_a wave may be seen in atrial hypertrophy. This produces a depression of the PR segment. This finding alone is not diagnostic of atrial hypertrophy. It is commonly seen in association with sinus tachycardia in normal individuals.

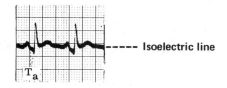

Figure 8–4. T_a wave in atrial hypertrophy.

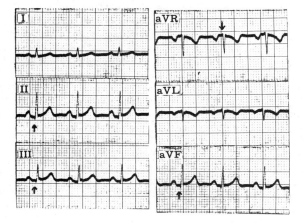

Figure 8–5. T_a waves (simulating ST segment elevation). There appears to be ST segment elevation in II, III, and aVF and ST depression in aVR. However, one should compare an ST segment in its relation to the interval between the T and the P. In doing so, it is seen that the ST segments are isoelectric. The pattern results from the presence of a prominent T_a wave. Although a visible T_a wave may result from atrial hypertrophy, this finding alone is not sufficient to warrant such an electrocardiographic diagnosis.

VENTRICULAR HYPERTROPHY

Pathology

Ventricular hypertrophy results from any pathologic process that produces a sufficient load on either ventricle. Myocardial fibrosis of varying degrees may develop later, especially in the subendocardial layer.

Anatomic & Physiologic Abnormalities That Produce the Electrocardiographic Pattern

The electrocardiographic pattern of ventricular hypertrophy is dependent upon the following:

A. Thickness of Muscle Mass: There is a definite correlation between the thickness of the ventricular muscle mass and the height of the R wave. The reason for the increased voltage is not clearly understood. The action potential of a hypertrophied muscle cell is normal, and there is no increase in the number of cells per unit of muscle mass in the hypertrophied heart. The increased voltage recorded on the body surface is probably related to the altered geometric projection of electrical forces.

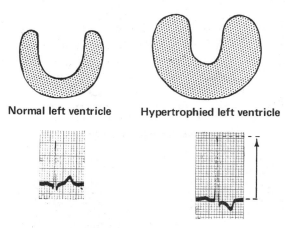

Figure 8–6. Height of R wave increased by thickness of muscle mass.

B. Delay in Conduction: Owing to the increased muscle mass, there is a delay and alteration of conduction, resulting in an increased width of the QRS complex. Usually this does not exceed 0.12 s but may occasionally do so. This also will increase the VAT.

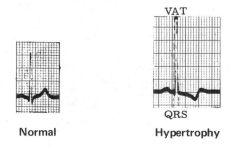

Figure 8–7. VAT and QRS interval increased.

C. Endocardial Changes: ST segment depression may be seen in a lead reflecting epicardial potential. This is probably due to endocardial changes, which are initially ischemic and later fibrotic. (See Fig 8–8.)

D. Changes in Repolarization: Owing to changes in repolarization (the reasons for which are not clearly understood), the T wave is inverted in those leads which record the tall R waves. The inversion characteristically begins after a definite ST interval and is asymmetric. The inversion may be shallow or deep. (See Fig 8–9.)

Electrocardiographic Criteria

The typical pattern which reflects the epicardial surface of a hypertrophied ventricle will be (1) a tall R wave, (2) slight prolongation of the QRS interval, (3) prolongation of the VAT, (4) ST segment depression, and (5) an inverted T wave.

A lead reflecting cavity potential or the potential recorded from a lead overlying the opposite nonhypertrophied ventricle will show (1) a deep S wave (or QS complex), (2) an elevated ST segment, and (3) an upright T wave.

Not all of the foregoing criteria are necessary for making a diagnosis of ventricular hypertrophy.

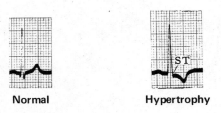

Figure 8–8. ST segment depressed.

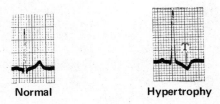

Figure 8–9. T wave inverted.

VENTRICULAR STRAIN

The term ventricular strain is used to describe an electrocardiographic pattern in which the only abnormalities are the ST and T wave changes described above. It is a poor term, though it is traditional. Its electrocardiographic definition is not the same as that given to "strain" by the physicist and the cardiac physiologist. Clinically, the term is used to describe more acute and possibly reversible changes which affect the ventricular musculature.

The correlation between electrocardiographic and anatomic findings is not close. Only nonspecific ST and T wave changes may be evident in the ECG of a patient with definite ventricular hypertrophy. Furthermore, patients who show clinical and anatomic evidence of acute ventricular strain may have abnormally tall R waves. An incomplete (or complete) bundle branch block (Fig 8–30) may be the electrocardiographic pattern of clinical acute heart strain.

A more acceptable term to describe either hypertrophy or strain is ventricular overload.

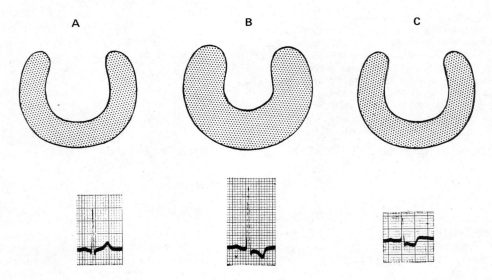

Figure 8–10. ECG in left ventricular hypertrophy and left ventricular strain. *A:* Normal: The QRS voltage and ST–T complex are normal. *B:* Left ventricular hypertrophy: The QRS voltage is increased, the ST segment is depressed, and the T wave is inverted. *C:* Left ventricular strain: The QRS voltage is not increased. The ST segment is depressed and the T wave inverted. The latter are very nonspecific but could result from strain of the left ventricle.

LEFT VENTRICULAR HYPERTROPHY

Etiology

Left ventricular hypertrophy commonly results from the following clinical states: (1) hypertension (essential, renal, or hormonal), (2) aortic valvular disease (aortic stenosis or aortic insufficiency [or both]), (3) mitral insufficiency due to various causes, (4) long-standing coronary artery disease, (5) nutritional and idiopathic hypertrophies (beriberi heart disease and the chronic myocarditides and myocardiopathies), and (6) congenital heart disease (patent ductus arteriosus, coarctation of the aorta, tricuspid atresia). It can also occur in normal individuals as a physiologic response to prolonged periods of strenuous exercise, as in athletes and marathon runners.

Electrocardiographic Criteria

The criteria discussed under ventricular hypertrophy (see p 99), when applied to those leads which reflect a left ventricular epicardial complex, will allow for the diagnosis of left ventricular hypertrophy. The specific leads in which the pattern is seen will depend upon the heart position.

Clinical Significance & Prognosis

This will depend upon the underlying disease. The electrocardiographic pattern will persist unless the course can be corrected. In left ventricular hypertrophy secondary to hypertension, the ECG may improve or revert to normal following successful medical or surgical treatment of the hypertension.

Electrocardiographic evidence of left ventricular hypertrophy in a patient being considered for mitral commissurotomy is an exceedingly important finding. It indicates either functionally significant mitral insufficiency, associated aortic valvular disease, or another disease (eg, hypertension).

(see p 131). There is a tall R in lead I and a deep S in lead III; the voltage of $R_1 + S_3$ is over 26 mm; and ST depression and T wave inversion in leads I and II.

2. Extremity leads–Since a left ventricular epicardial complex is recorded in aVL, a tall R with depressed ST and inverted T will be seen in this lead. In general, an R wave of over 11 mm is consistent with left ventricular hypertrophy. This is the most specific of all voltage criteria. The one exception is in association with left anterior fascicular block (see p 131). In the latter situation, a value of 16 mm or more is necessary for the recognition of left ventricular hypertrophy.

3. Precordial leads–In the absence of unusual rotation on the long axis, abnormally tall R waves with depressed ST segments and inverted T waves will be seen in leads V_{4-6}. The QRS interval may be over 0.1 s and the VAT greater than 0.05 s. Since the S wave in right precordial leads (eg, V_1) is a reflection of the greater left ventricular potential, these waves will be abnormally deep. As a general rule, the total voltage of $[SV_1 + RV_5]$ or $[SV_1 + RV_6]$ is greater than 35 mm, or an R of over 27 mm in V_5 or V_6 is indicative of left ventricular hypertrophy. This is only applicable to adults over age 35. Furthermore, fever, anemia, thyrotoxicosis, or other high-output states can increase this voltage without representing left ventricular hypertrophy. Therefore, an electrocardiographic diagnosis of left ventricular hypertrophy on the basis of voltage alone should be made only if these variables do not exist.

4. Vector analysis–The magnitude of the mean QRS vector is increased. There is only a slight change in direction, being slightly more superior and posterior. The ST and T vectors are oriented approximately 180 degrees from the mean QRS axis.

[Text cont'd on p 95.]

ELECTROCARDIOGRAPHIC PATTERNS OF LEFT VENTRICULAR HYPERTROPHY

An electrocardiographic diagnosis of left ventricular hypertrophy can very often be made when left ventricular hypertrophy is anatomically present. In fact, the ECG may be diagnostic before any roentgenographic evidence is present.

Rotation on the Anteroposterior Axis

A. Horizontal Heart: This is the most common position in left ventricular hypertrophy.

1. Standard leads–The frontal plane QRS axis is usually between 0 degrees and −30 degrees. If greater than −30 degrees (superior axis or left axis deviation), it indicates an associated left anterior fascicular block

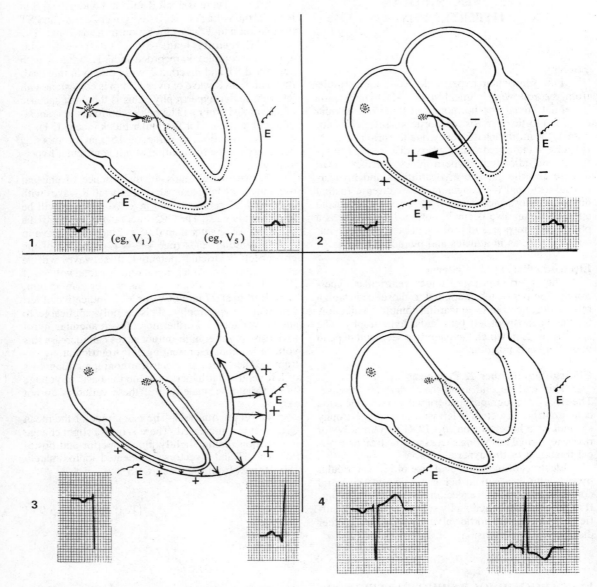

Figure 8–11. Left ventricular hypertrophy. *(1)* Spread of impulse from SA node to AV node. *(2)* Activation of interventricular septum. *(3)* Activation of both ventricles. *(4)* Repolarization.

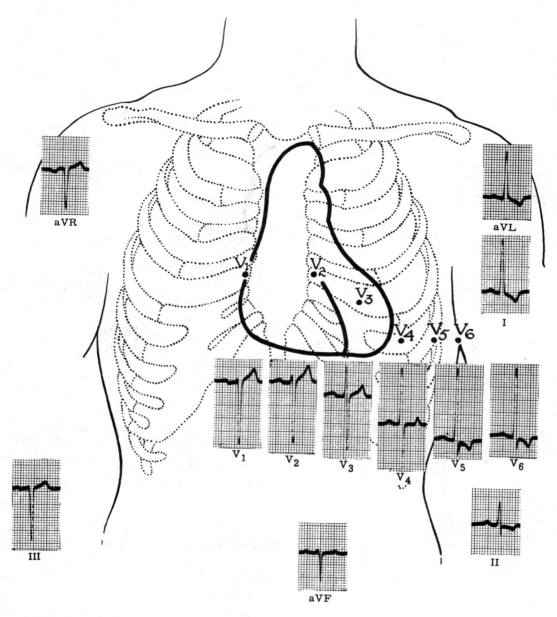

Figure 8–12. Left ventricular hypertrophy, horizontal heart. *Standard leads:* Frontal plane axis = −20 degrees, $R_1 + S_3 = 38$ mm; the T is inverted in I. *Extremity leads:* Horizontal heart position; the R in aVL measures 18 mm; the T is inverted in aVL. *Precordial leads:* $SV_1 + RV_5 = 49$ mm. There is ST depression and T wave inversion in V_5 and V_6. *Clinical diagnosis:* Hypertensive cardiovascular disease.

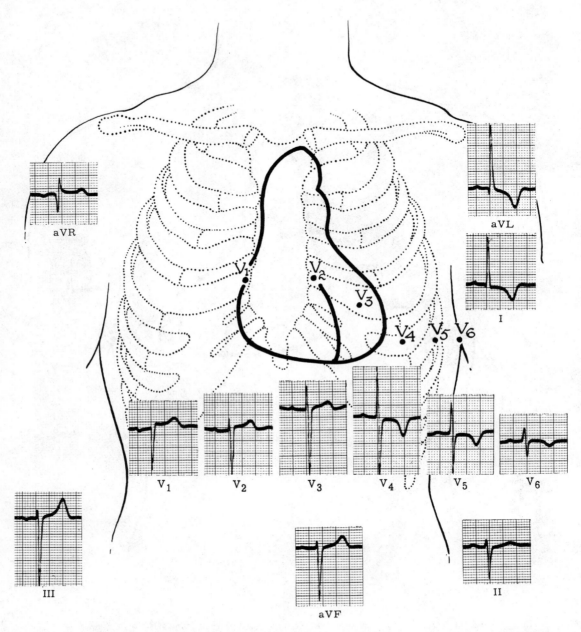

Figure 8–13. Left ventricular hypertrophy. The frontal plane QRS axis = −47 degrees. This is evidence of an associated left anterior fascicular block (see p 131). R = 24 mm in aVL; ST depression and T wave inversion in I and aVL. The above are indicative of left ventricular hypertrophy. Precordial leads do not have voltage criteria ($SV_1 + RV_5$ or RV_6) for left ventricular hypertrophy. This is in part due to the marked superior (left) axis, as a result of which the lead axes of V_{5-6} are far removed from the mean QRS. The T waves are inverted in leads V_{4-6}, but this itself is not diagnostic of left ventricular hypertrophy. *Autopsy diagnosis:* Left ventricular hypertrophy due to hypertension; no evidence of myocardial infarction.

B. Vertical Heart:

1. Standard leads–Frontal plane axis between +45 degrees and +90 degrees; tall R waves with depressed ST segments and inverted T waves in leads II and III.

2. Extremity leads–Since a left ventricular complex is recorded in aVF, this lead will show a tall R wave with depressed ST and inverted T. Although some authors state that an R wave of over 20 mm in aVF is diagnostic of left ventricular hypertrophy, most authorities believe that this in itself is insufficient evidence for such a diagnosis.

3. Precordial leads–In the absence of any unusual rotation on the long axis, the pattern in the precordial leads will be the same as described for a horizontal heart.

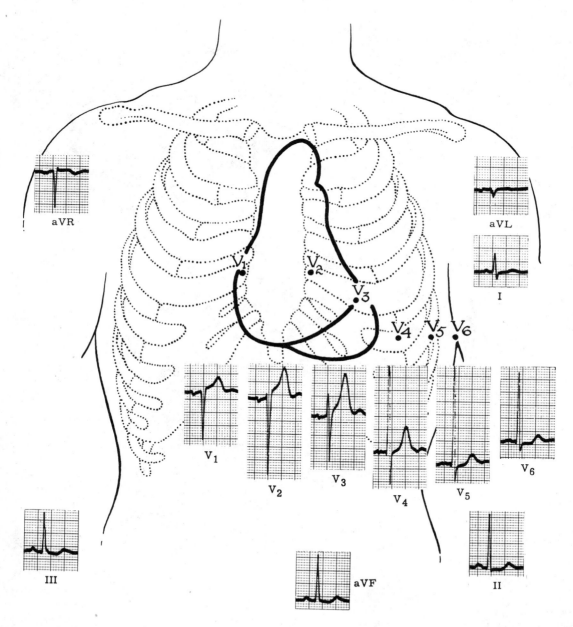

Figure 8–14. Left ventricular hypertrophy, vertical heart. The frontal plane axis is +75 degrees; there are tall R waves with depressed ST segments in leads II, III, and aVF. $SV_1 + RV_5 = 55$ mm; there is ST depression in V_{5-6}. The P waves are notched in all leads. *Clinical and autopsy diagnosis:* Left ventricular and left atrial hypertrophy. The patient was not receiving digitalis at the time this tracing was taken.

Clockwise Rotation on the Long Axis

This may be associated with a vertical or a horizontal heart position.

A. Standard and Extremity Leads: The pattern in these leads will mainly be dependent upon the degree of rotation in the frontal plane.

B. Precordial Leads: The transitional zone is shifted to the left, so that a typical left ventricular hypertrophy pattern may not be seen until leads V_{7-9} are taken.

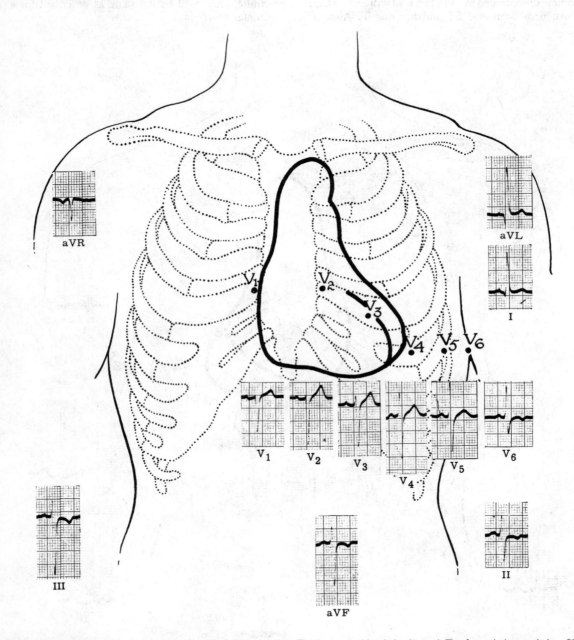

Figure 8–15. Left ventricular hypertrophy, clockwise rotation. The heart position is horizontal. The frontal plane axis is −37 degrees. The tall R in aVL (17 mm) is indicative of left ventricular hypertrophy. Precordial leads show clockwise rotation (persistent S in V_6), which in this case is a result of the superior frontal plane axis. The T is inverted in V_6. *Clinical diagnosis:* Hypertensive cardiovascular disease.

Counterclockwise Rotation on the Long Axis

This is more commonly associated with a horizontal heart position.

A. Standard and Extremity Leads: The pattern will be dependent upon the degree of rotation on the anteroposterior axis.

B. Precordial Leads: Since the transitional zone is shifted to the right, a left ventricular hypertrophy pattern may be seen in leads as far to the right as V_2 or V_3.

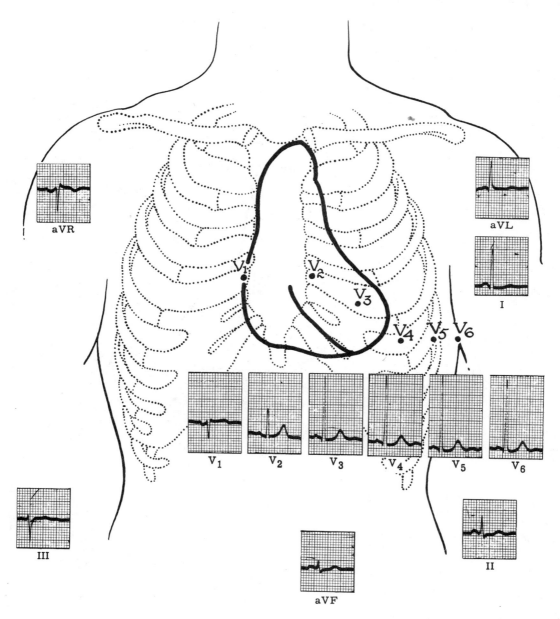

Figure 8–16. Left ventricular hypertrophy, counterclockwise rotation. The heart position is semihorizontal; the frontal plane axis is 0 degrees; the T is flat in aVL. Precordial leads reveal a left ventricular epicardial complex in V_2. Tall R waves are seen in V_{3-6}. R = 28 mm in V_5. *Clinical diagnosis:* Hypertensive cardiovascular disease.

LEFT VENTRICULAR STRAIN

The electrocardiographic pattern of left ventricular strain is that of ST segment depression and T wave inversion in those leads which record a left ventricular epicardial complex. There are no abnormally tall R waves and no prolongation of the QRS interval or VAT. Since these ST–T changes are "nonspecific" and can be produced by many other conditions (see Chapter 18), a positive electrocardiographic diagnosis cannot be made. Proper electrocardiographic interpretation will depend upon correlation with the clinical findings.

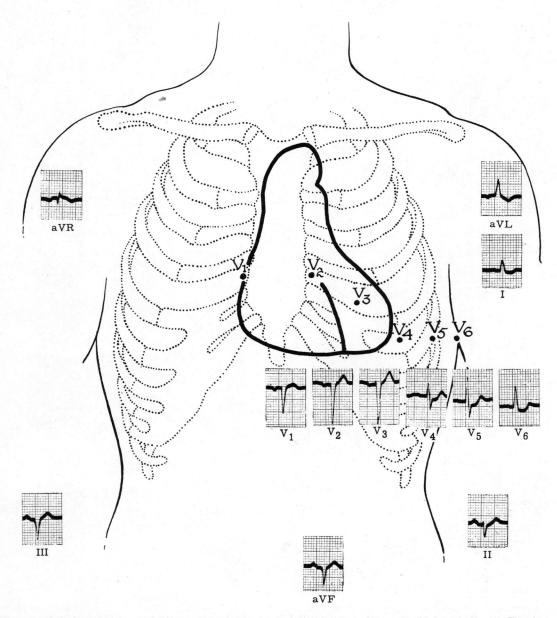

Figure 8–17. Left ventricular strain. ST segment depression is seen in I, aVL, and V_{4-6}; the T is inverted in aVL. The changes are not diagnostic of left ventricular strain. *Clinical diagnosis:* Hypertensive cardiovascular disease. The patient was not receiving digitalis, and there was no clinical evidence of angina, infarction, or electrolyte disturbance. *Autopsy diagnosis:* Left ventricular hypertrophy.

SUMMARY OF ELECTROCARDIOGRAPHIC CRITERIA OF LEFT VENTRICULAR HYPERTROPHY

A. Precordial Leads:

1. Voltage–R waves in V_5 or V_6 over 27 mm. S in V_1 + R in V_5 or V_6 over 35 mm (over age 35).

2. VAT over 0.05 s in V_{5-6}.

3. QRS interval–May be prolonged over 0.1 s in V_{5-6}.

4. ST segment depression and T wave inversion in V_{5-6}.

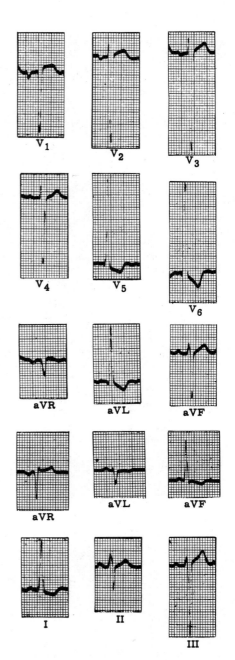

B. Extremity Leads:

1. **Horizontal heart**–R wave of 13 mm or more in aVL (except when frontal plane axis is superior to −30 degrees); VAT, QRS interval, ST–T changes as described for precordial leads.

2. **Vertical heart**–R wave of over 20 mm in aVF; VAT, QRS interval, ST–T changes as described for precordial leads. Unless confirmed by precordial leads, this pattern in aVF is not diagnostic of left ventricular hypertrophy (since right ventricular hypertrophy can give a similar pattern in aVF).

C. Standard Leads: These reflect the same pattern of the extremity leads.

Horizontal heart–Frontal plane QRS axis is usually less than −30 degrees. R_1 + S_3 over 26 mm; pattern in I similar to aVL.

Minimal Criteria

R in aVL > 11 mm; or R in V_{5-6} > 27 mm; or S in V_1 + R in V_{5-6} > 35 mm (if other variables mentioned on p 91 do not exist).

Equivocal Criteria

ST depression and T wave inversion in left precordial leads in the absence of definite voltage criteria.

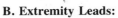

RIGHT VENTRICULAR HYPERTROPHY
(See Figs 8–18 to 8–22.)

Etiology

Right ventricular hypertrophy may occur in association with mitral stenosis or chronic diffuse pulmonary disease (eg, emphysema, bronchiectasis, tuberculosis), and congenital heart disease (eg, tetralogy of Fallot, pulmonary stenosis, Eisenmenger's syndrome, reverse patent ductus arteriosus), or it may be due to nutritional deficiencies or an idiopathic finding, usually in association with left ventricular hypertrophy.

Incidence

An electrocardiographic diagnosis of right ventricular hypertrophy can be made less frequently in the above-mentioned diseases than can the electrocardiographic diagnosis of left ventricular hypertrophy in the presence of a pathologically hypertrophied left ventricle. The incidence of correct electrocardiographic diagnosis is highest in the congenital heart group; diagnosis is less accurate in older patients with mitral stenosis and chronic pulmonary disease.

Electrocardiographic Criteria

The criteria mentioned for the diagnosis of ventricular hypertrophy (see p 89) are applicable to the leads recording a right ventricular complex (most commonly aVR, V_{3R}, and V_1).

Clinical Significance & Prognosis

A definite electrocardiographic diagnosis of right ventricular hypertrophy is as a general rule a more ominous sign than is left ventricular hypertrophy. The prognosis will of course depend upon the underlying disease. The electrocardiographic pattern can improve or revert to normal following successful surgical correction of the congenital lesions and mitral stenosis.

Electrocardiographic Patterns

A. Standard Leads: There may be no unusual axis deviation or there may be right axis deviation. Axis deviation of greater than +110 degrees in an adult, in the absence of an intraventricular conduction defect, is good presumptive evidence of right ventricular hypertrophy. Tall R waves with depressed ST segments and inverted T waves are seen in leads II and III. This is the identical pattern that may be seen in standard leads in left ventricular hypertrophy with a vertical heart. Therefore, one cannot always differentiate electrocardiographically left and right ventricular hypertrophy by the standard leads, in the absence of an abnormal frontal plane axis.

B. Extremity Leads: The pattern will vary with the degree of rotation in the frontal plane. The most common heart position is vertical.

Lead aVR will frequently show a tall R wave, either as a QR, qR, or R complex. This is the result of the abnormal right axis deviation. Although aVR may suggest right ventricular hypertrophy, confirmatory evidence should be present in right precordial leads to make such a diagnosis.

Occasionally, the hypertrophied right ventricle will overlie the left diaphragm and thereby reflect its pattern in aVF. Thus, one will see a small q, tall R, depressed ST, and inverted T in aVF. Such a pattern, as mentioned above under standard leads, is identical with that seen in left ventricular hypertrophy in a vertical heart. Here again, the proper diagnosis of right ventricular hypertrophy will depend upon the findings in right precordial leads.

C. Precordial Leads: Right precordial leads will typically show tall R waves; the VAT is increased to over 0.03 s; the QRS interval may be widened, but rarely up to 0.12 s; the ST segments are depressed and the T waves inverted.

Instead of an initial tall R wave in V_1 (or V_{3R}), one may see a small q preceding the R. This is probably the result of a slight delay in activation of the right ventricle, resulting from hypertrophy.

Although voltage criteria have been assigned to the height of the R waves in right precordial leads as an index of right ventricular hypertrophy, a better criterion is the progressive changes from right to left precordial leads. In right precordial leads one sees R waves of greater voltage than the S. The R:S ratio is usually greater than 1:1 in V_1 or V_{3R}. As leads are taken progressively to the left, the R decreases and the S increases in amplitude. This latter finding of prominent S waves in V_6 is a result of the late rightward forces.

D. Vector Analysis: The mean QRS vector is oriented to the right (110 degrees or more), anteriorly, and either inferiorly or superiorly.

RIGHT VENTRICULAR STRAIN
(Acute Cor Pulmonale)
(See Figs 8–23 to 8–25.)

Right ventricular strain is the electrocardiographic term which is used to describe a pattern in which only the ST segment and T wave changes described on p 90 are seen in right ventricular leads. Such a pattern often occurs in acute pulmonary infarction and during acute exacerbations of chronic pulmonary disease.

ST segment depression with inverted T waves is seen in right precordial leads. The R waves are not abnormal. There frequently is right axis deviation. Electrocardiographically, such a pattern is consistent with but not absolutely diagnostic of right ventricular strain since other conditions can give a similar pattern (eg, coronary artery disease; normal pattern in children and some adult blacks). (See Fig 8–24.)

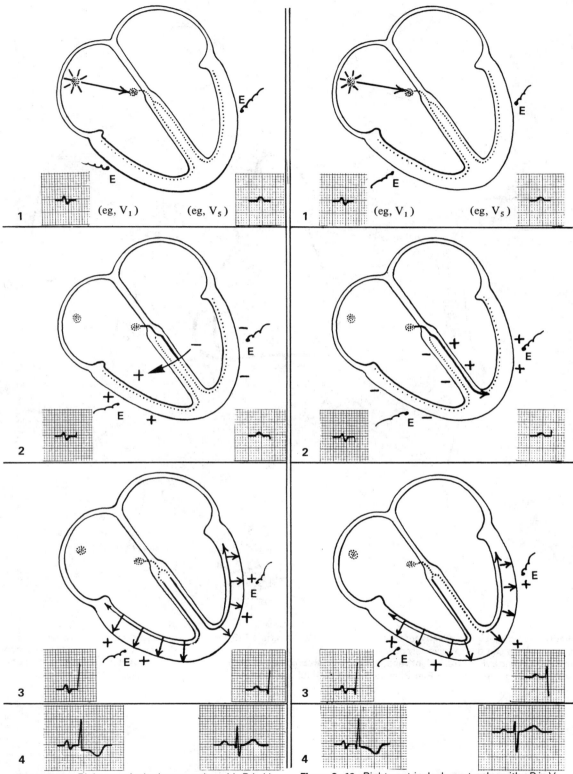

Figure 8–18. Right ventricular hypertrophy with R in V₁. *(1)* Atrial activation. *(2)* Normal interventricular septal activation. *(3)* Activation of both ventricles. *(4)* Repolarization.

Figure 8–19. Right ventricular hypertrophy with qR in V₁. *(1)* Atrial activation. *(2)* Delay in activation of hypertrophied right ventricle. *(3)* Activation of both ventricles. *(4)* Repolarization.

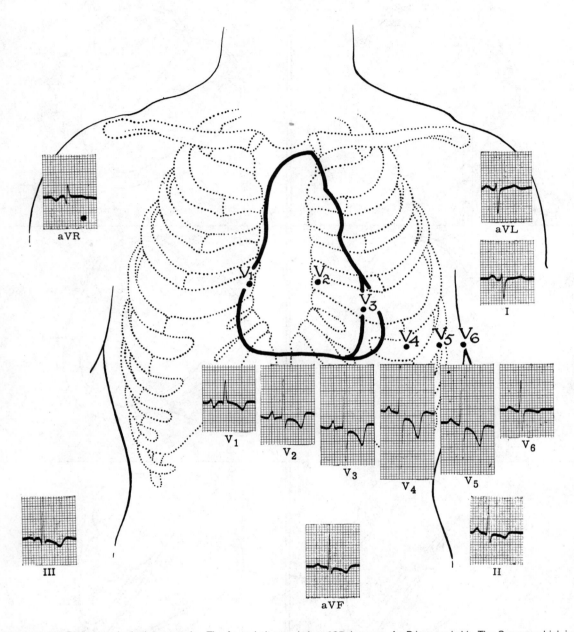

Figure 8–20. Right ventricular hypertrophy. The frontal plane axis is +125 degrees. A qR is seen in V_1. The S wave which is absent in V_1 becomes progressively deeper from V_{2-6}. The T waves are inverted from V_{1-6} and the ST segments depressed from V_{2-5}. Lead aVF records a right ventricular epicardial complex similar to V_1. The mean QRS vector is directed to the right, anteriorly, and inferiorly. The P in V_1 is consistent with left atrial hypertrophy. *Clinical diagnosis:* Mitral stenosis.

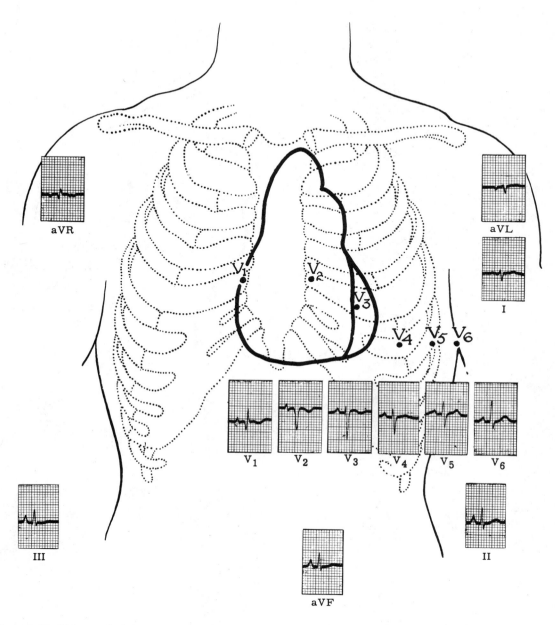

Figure 8–21. Right ventricular hypertrophy. A QR is present in V_1; VAT = 0.05 s. In addition, the T waves are inverted in V_{1-3}. The frontal plane axis is +105 degrees. *Clinical diagnosis:* Pulmonary emphysema with right heart failure. *Autopsy diagnosis:* Right ventricular hypertrophy.

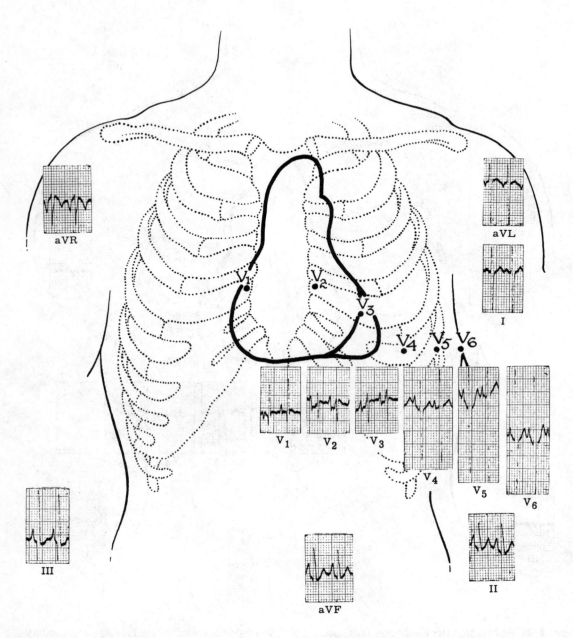

Figure 8–22. Right ventricular hypertrophy, congenital heart disease (4-month-old infant). The heart rate is 177. The slight variation in rate in the various leads is due to sinus arrhythmia. This rapid rate in an infant is an indication of sinus tachycardia and does not indicate a paroxysmal atrial tachycardia. Prominent P waves are seen in II, III, and aVF, suggesting right atrial hypertrophy. A qR pattern is seen in V_1. The VAT is 0.03 s. The tall R wave could be a normal finding in an infant. However, an initial q wave is never normally present in infancy. This pattern is therefore indicative of right ventricular hypertrophy. *Clinical findings:* Cyanotic infant with cardiac enlargement. *Clinical diagnosis:* Tetralogy of Fallot.

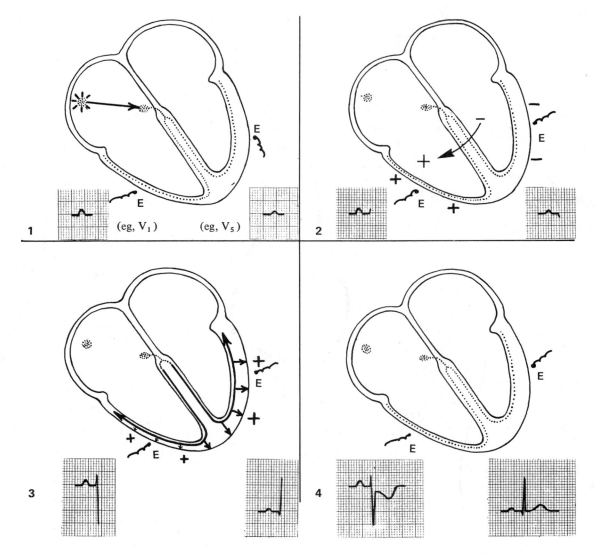

Figure 8–23. Right ventricular strain. *(1)* Atrial activation. *(2)* Interventricular septal activation. *(3)* Activation of both ventricles. *(4)* Repolarization.

VARIANTS OF RIGHT VENTRICULAR HYPERTROPHY PATTERNS

A. Questionable Right Ventricular Hypertrophy: Prominent P waves suggestive of right atrial hypertrophy may be indirect evidence of associated right ventricular strain or hypertrophy. (See Fig 8–24.)

B. Right Ventricular Hypertrophy in Older Adults: As stated above, the typical electrocardiographic expression of right ventricular hypertrophy is a mean QRS vector oriented to the right (right axis deviation) and anteriorly (tall R waves in right precordial leads). However, it is common in elderly patients with chronic lung disease and cor pulmonale to see the mean QRS vector oriented to the right and posteriorly.

As such, right axis deviation is evident, but right precordial leads will not show tall R waves. Instead, the R waves in V_{1-3} may be normal, small, or absent. In the latter instance, these leads will simulate anterior myocardial infarction (see pp 191 and 192). A similar pattern may be seen in older adults with mitral stenosis. The presence of P waves consistent with right or left atrial hypertrophy or inverted T waves in V_{1-3} will aid in the diagnosis of right ventricular hypertrophy. (See Fig 8–27.)

C. The ECG in Pulmonary Emphysema: Pulmonary emphysema commonly produces changes in the ECG which are secondary to the hyperinflation of the lungs and which need not indicate associated right ventricular hypertrophy or strain. These are as follows: (See also Figs 8–28 to 8–30.)

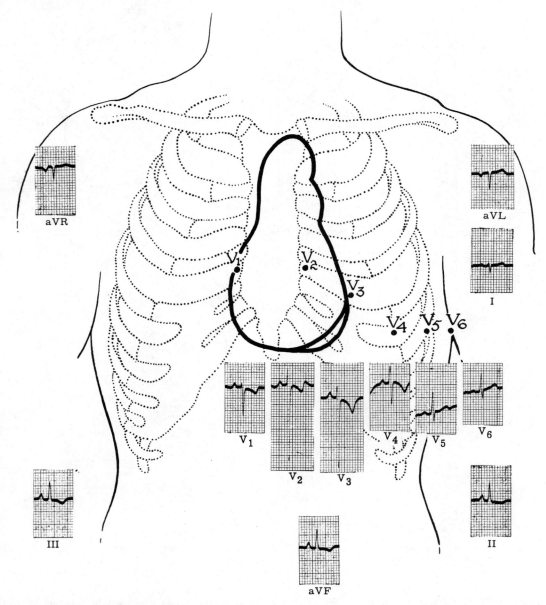

Figure 8–24. Right ventricular strain. Right axis deviation (+100 degrees); vertical heart position; inverted T waves in II, III, and aVF; normal R waves in precordial leads; inverted T waves and depressed ST segments in V_{1-4}. *Clinical diagnosis:* Pulmonary sarcoidosis, before therapy. See Fig 8–25 for change after therapy.

1. Low voltage in frontal plane (standard bipolar and extremity) leads—Low voltage is defined as a total QRS magnitude that does not exceed 5 mm in any of the above leads. Since air is a relatively poor conductor of electricity, it is understandable that the hyperinflated lungs will reduce the electrical potential of the heart as recorded on the body surface.

2. Abnormalities in frontal plane QRS axis—

a. The frontal plane QRS axis may be between +90 degrees and +110 degrees. This degree of rightward axis is not in itself diagnostic of right ventricular hypertrophy in a patient with emphysema.

b. The terminal QRS forces in the frontal plane may be directed rightward (producing an S wave in I) and superiorly (producing S waves in II, III, and aVF). This has been known as the S_1, S_2, S_3 syndrome. The cause for this is not known. Although it is seen in patients with emphysema, it is also seen as a normal variant in children and young adults.

c. The terminal QRS forces in the frontal plane

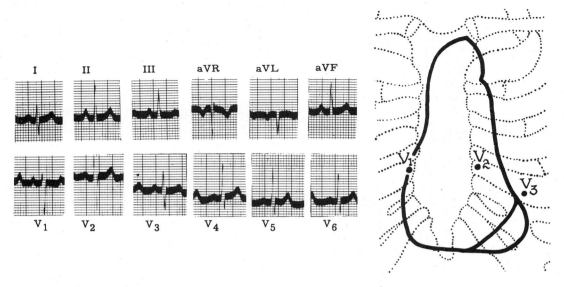

Figure 8–25. Right ventricular strain or hypertrophy. Reversion to normal. *Clinical diagnosis:* Pulmonary sarcoidosis after therapy with cortisone, which resulted in clearing of the lung lesions and disappearance of right heart failure. For ECG before therapy, see Fig 8–24.

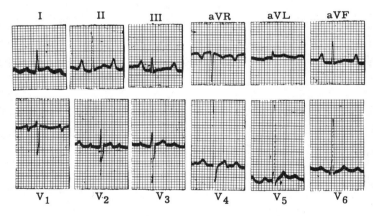

Figure 8–26. Questionable right ventricular hypertrophy. There are no criteria in the QRS–T complexes to suggest right ventricular hypertrophy. Tall P waves in II, III, and aVF are consistent with right atrial hypertrophy. Clinically, the patient had diffuse pulmonary fibrosis and early signs of right heart failure. Only in combination with the clinical findings is one justified in making a diagnosis of right ventricular hypertrophy.

may be directed leftward (R in I) and superiorly (S waves in II, III, and aVF), resulting in a mean frontal plane QRS axis superior to −30 degrees and simulating a left anterior fascicular block (see p 131).

3. Abnormalities in precordial leads–See B, above.

D. Right Bundle Branch Block: An incomplete (or complete) right bundle branch block may be a manifestation of right ventricular strain (see Fig 8–30 and pp 114–122).

Clinical Significance & Prognosis of the Foregoing Patterns

All of the above patterns can be seen in association with true pathologic right ventricular hypertrophy. Therefore, one cannot differentiate, in a single electrocardiographic record, between strain and hypertrophy. For this reason, many physicians prefer the term right ventricular overload. The clinical findings and serial electrocardiographic changes (such as reversion to normal) are necessary for proper interpretation.

The prognosis will depend upon the nature of the underlying disease.

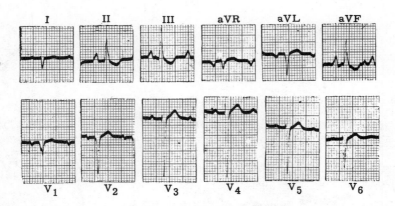

Figure 8–27. Right ventricular hypertrophy in older adults. Tall P waves in II, III, and aVF are consistent with right atrial hypertrophy. The frontal plane axis is +115 degrees. There is marked clockwise rotation with QS complexes in V$_{1-2}$ and very small r waves in V$_{3-6}$. The combination of these 3 findings is strongly suggestive of right ventricular hypertrophy. *Clinical diagnosis:* Pulmonary emphysema and bronchiectasis with right heart failure in a 70-year-old man.

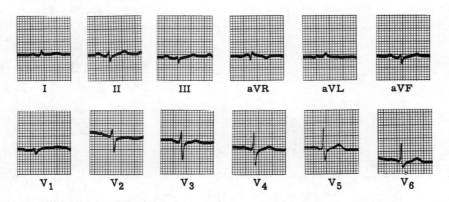

Figure 8–28. Pulmonary emphysema. The QRS complexes are of low voltage. The mean frontal plane QRS axis is −35 degrees. The persistent S waves in V$_{5-6}$ meet the criteria for clockwise rotation and are a result of the superior axis. The above features are typical of pulmonary emphysema but are not indicative of right ventricular hypertrophy.

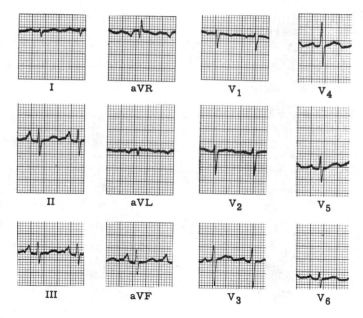

Figure 8–29. Pulmonary emphysema and cor pulmonale. The tall peaked P waves in II, III, and aVF are consistent with right atrial hypertrophy. There are small initial QRS forces to the left (r in I) with greater terminal forces to the right (S in I). These terminal forces are directed superiorly (S in II, III, and aVF). This is an example of the S_1, S_2, S_3 syndrome. The tracing is consistent with pulmonary emphysema. The prominent P waves are the only positive evidence of right heart overload.

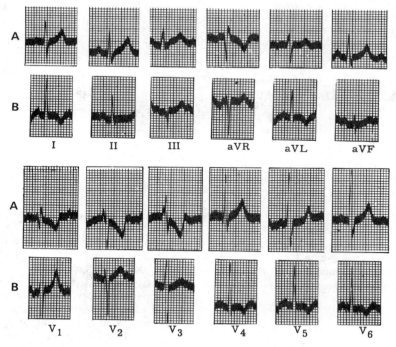

Figure 8–30. Incomplete right bundle branch block as a manifestation of acute right ventricular strain. *A:* The pattern is that of an incomplete bundle branch block (rsr′ complexes with depressed ST segments and inverted T waves in V_{1-3}). *B:* Five days after (A): There has been a marked change. The incomplete right bundle branch block is no longer present. In the interval the T waves have become inverted in leads I, aVL, and V_{4-6}. *Clinical status:* At (A) the patient had an episode of acute pulmonary infarction. Five days later he had markedly improved. The ECG in (A) was a reflection of acute right ventricular strain. The pulmonary hypertension had clinically subsided by (B), and the second ECG demonstrated the abnormalities associated with the basic heart disease, beriberi.

SUMMARY OF ELECTROCARDIOGRAPHIC CRITERIA OF RIGHT VENTRICULAR HYPERTROPHY

A. Precordial Leads: These are the best leads for diagnosis.
1. R wave of greater voltage than S in V_1 or V_{3R}.
2. qR pattern in V_1 or V_{3R}.
3. VAT over 0.03 s in V_1 or V_{3R}.
4. Persistent S waves in V_{5-6}.
5. ST segment depression and T wave inversion in V_{1-3}.

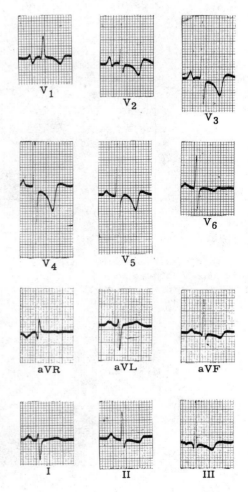

B. Extremity Leads:
1. Tall R in aVR; unless accompanied by the criteria in A, this alone is not indicative of right ventricular hypertrophy.
2. Tall R with depressed ST and inverted T in aVF; unless confirmed by precordial leads, this pattern in itself is in no way diagnostic of right ventricular hypertrophy.

C. Standard Leads: Right axis deviation (+110 degrees or more); depressed ST and inverted T in II and III.

Minimal Criteria
Rs or qR complex in V_1 or V_{3R} with VAT > 0.03 s. Right axis deviation.

Helpful Criteria
Abnormally tall or notched P waves and clockwise rotation; or ST depression with T wave inversion in V_{3R}, and V_{1-3} in the absence of a tall R in these leads; or incomplete or complete right bundle branch block.

COMBINED RIGHT & LEFT VENTRICULAR HYPERTROPHY

The electrocardiographic diagnosis of ventricular hypertrophy is far from perfect. Correlation of the ECG with autopsy findings has furnished the following results: A correct electrocardiographic diagnosis of left ventricular hypertrophy (proved at autopsy) can be made in 85% of cases using the criteria discussed above. However, using the same criteria, a false-positive diagnosis has been made in 10–15% of cases. The electrocardiographic diagnosis of autopsy-proved right ventricular hypertrophy is less reliable. The correlation has ranged from 23–100%, the latter figure occurring only in analysis of patients with congenital heart disease. Combined right and left ventricular hypertrophy commonly is not diagnosed electrocardiographically. The autopsy correlation is only 8–26%.

This is understandable on the basis of opposing right and left electrical forces. In most patients with left ventricular hypertrophy and right heart failure with autopsy documentation of associated right ventricular hypertrophy, the predominance of the left ventricular forces counterbalances the increased rightward forces of the right ventricular hypertrophy, so that the mean forces are those of left ventricular hypertrophy. It is possible that "balanced" left and right ventricular hypertrophy can result in cancellation of forces to result in a normal QRS vector. Increasing right ventricular forces can cancel some of the leftward forces of the associated left ventricular hypertrophy and thereby result in a loss of QRS criteria for left ventricular hypertrophy.

In the author's opinion, the most reliable criteria are the presence of signs of left ventricular hypertrophy in precordial leads plus a frontal plane axis of more than +90 degrees. This is especially valid if serial ECGs demonstrate a progressive change of frontal plane axis to the right of +90 degrees in the presence of precordial lead criteria of left ventricular hypertrophy.

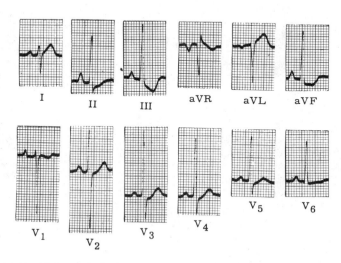

Figure 8–31. Combined right and left ventricular hypertrophy. The mean frontal plane axis is +105 degrees; there is ST depression in leads II, III, aVF, and V_{5-6}; the T is flat in II and V_6, inverted in III and aVF. $SV_1 + RV_5 = 39$ mm. *Clinical and autopsy diagnosis:* Right and left ventricular hypertrophy, idiopathic.

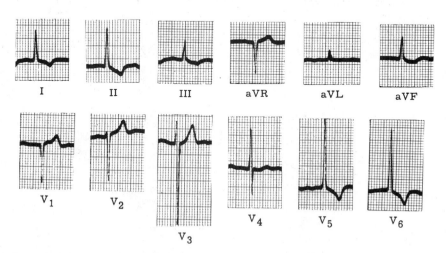

Figure 8–32. Left ventricular hypertrophy. The rhythm is atrial fibrillation. The frontal plane axis is +50 degrees. $SV_1 + RV_5 = 42$ mm; there is ST depression and T wave inversion in I, II, III, aVF, and V_{5-6}. Some of the ST–T changes are the result of digitalis therapy. *Clinical diagnosis:* Hypertensive cardiovascular disease.

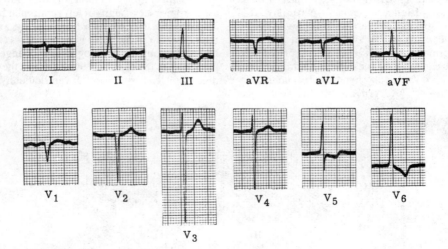

Figure 8–33. Combined right and left ventricular hypertrophy. This ECG was taken on the same patient 6 years after the above tracing (Fig 8–32). In the interval the patient had developed progressive right heart failure. The frontal plane axis has changed to +100 degrees. Voltage criteria (SV_1 + RV_5 or RV_6) are no longer present for the diagnosis of left ventricular hypertrophy. The ST–T abnormalities in II, III, aVF, and V_{5-6} are the result of digitalis therapy plus left ventricular hypertrophy.

Intraventricular Conduction Defects | 9

An intraventricular conduction defect is the result of an abnormality of conduction through one or more of the divisions of the intraventricular conduction system distal to the bundle of His or involvement of specific longitudinal tracts in the bundle of His (see p 37). The anatomic structures are (1) the right bundle branch, (2) the left bundle branch, (3) the left anterior fascicle, (4) the left posterior fascicle, (5) the septal fibers from the left bundle branch and its fascicles that enter the left septal myocardium, and (6) the peripheral Purkinje fibers.

Classification of Intraventricular Conduction Defects

A. Bundle Branch Block:
1. Right bundle branch block–
   a. Complete.
   b. Incomplete.
2. Left bundle branch block–
   a. Complete.
   b. Incomplete.

B. Peripheral Left Ventricular Conduction Defects:
1. Left anterior fascicular block.
2. Left posterior fascicular block.
3. Left septal block.
4. Left anterior conduction delay.
5. Peri-infarction blocks.

C. Bilateral Bundle Branch Block:
1. Right bundle branch block with left anterior fascicular block.
2. Right bundle branch block with left posterior fascicular block.
3. Right or left bundle branch block with prolonged AV conduction (P–R interval > 0.21 s).
4. Alternating right and left bundle branch block.

D. Trifascicular Block.

E. Indeterminate Intraventricular Conduction Defects.

BUNDLE BRANCH BLOCK

The term bundle branch block denotes a specific type of electrocardiographic pattern resulting either from complete failure of conduction or from delayed conduction through either the right bundle or the main division of the left bundle. Since the ECG does not distinguish between total block or delayed conduction, many prefer the more general term intraventricular conduction defect (right or left). It is not a clinical diagnosis, although it can be suspected on physical examination—on the basis of wide splitting of the second sound (right bundle branch block) or paradoxic splitting of the second sound (left bundle branch block).

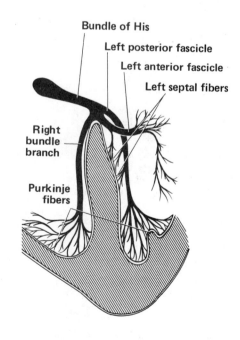

Figure 9–1. Diagrammatic illustration of the intraventricular conduction system.

Electrocardiographic Criteria

A. Complete:

1. Delay of excitation and abnormal spread of excitation through the ventricle whose bundle is "blocked," resulting in an abnormal QRS configuration. (The term "QRS" is used because it is the traditional electrocardiographic identification of ventricular depolarization. The actual pattern discussed here is not QRS but rSR'.)

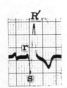

2. Prolongation of the QRS interval to 0.12 s or longer.

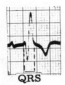

3. VAT (measured to the peak of the R') is prolonged.

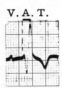

4. The ST segments are depressed and the T waves inverted in leads that record the abnormal R' waves.

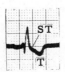

B. Incomplete: An incomplete bundle branch block is an arbitrary subclassification of the above in which the same abnormalities are present except that the QRS interval is less than 0.12 s, and the VAT is less than that seen in a complete bundle branch block. The term incomplete does not imply that conduction is incomplete.

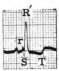

RIGHT BUNDLE BRANCH BLOCK

Etiology

A right bundle branch block may be present in almost any type of heart disease, including coronary artery disease, hypertensive cardiovascular disease, any of the diseases that produce right ventricular hypertrophy, and congenital lesions involving the septum. It may also be found in normal individuals with no clinical evidence of heart disease.

Incidence

Right bundle branch block is a fairly common electrocardiographic finding. It is not diagnostic of heart disease as such or of any type of heart disease.

Mechanism

The spread of excitation from the SA node to the AV node and through the main bundle of His occurs in a normal fashion. Septal activation occurs normally from left to right.

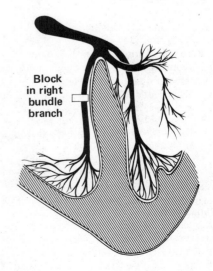

Block in right bundle branch

Figure 9–2. Right bundle branch block.

RIGHT BUNDLE BRANCH BLOCK
ELECTROCARDIOGRAPHIC CRITERIA

A. Right Ventricular Epicardial Complex (eg, V₁):

1. As a result of the normal septal activation, which is oriented to the right and anteriorly, a small initial r will be recorded.

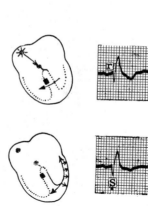

2. Since the right bundle is "blocked," the excitation wave will next spread down the left bundle and through the left ventricular myocardium, resulting in an S wave.

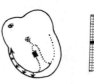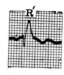

3. The impulse will then pass around the "blocked" right bundle into the right ventricular myocardium, producing a wide R' wave. Thus, a typical pattern will be an rsR' complex.

4. Occasionally, the s wave is small or absent, resulting in an rsR' or rR' complex.

5. The ST segment is depressed and the T wave is inverted.

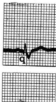

B. Left Ventricular Epicardial Complex (eg, V₅):

1. An initial small q will be seen as a result of septal activation.

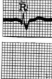

2. This will be followed by an R resulting from left ventricular activation.

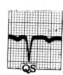

3. There will follow a wide S wave resulting from delayed activation of the right ventricle. The ST segment is usually isoelectric and the T upright.

C. Left Ventricular Cavity Complex (eg, aVL in a Vertical Heart): A QS complex will be present as under normal conditions but will be wide. The ST segment is isoelectric, and the T wave is inverted.

D. Right Ventricular Cavity Complex (eg, aVR): An initial r may be recorded as occurs normally. This will be followed by an S resulting from the spread of the excitation through the left ventricle (as in a normal heart). A late, wide R' wave may follow as a result of the late activation of the right side of the interventricular septum. The ST segment is isoelectric or elevated; the T is inverted.

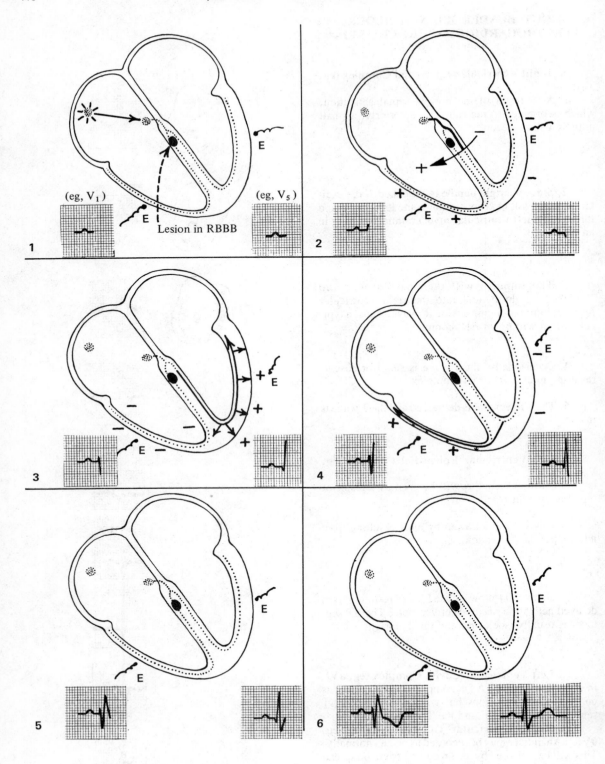

Figure 9–3. Development of right and left ventricular epicardial complexes in right bundle branch block. *(1)* Atrial activation. *(2)* Normal interventricular septal activation. *(3)* Right bundle branch blocked; therefore, the left ventricle is activated first. *(4)* Delayed activation of the right ventricle "around" the block. *(5)* Depolarization complete. *(6)* Repolarization complete.

Electrocardiographic Pattern

The characteristic feature of a right bundle branch block is the late and delayed electrical force of right ventricular depolarization oriented to the right and anteriorly. This late right vector force produces the wide S wave in leads I, V_{4-6} (left ventricular epicardial complex) and the wide R or R′ in aVR. The anterior component of this late force will produce the wide R′ waves in right precordial leads, V_{3R}, V_1, and V_2 (right ventricular epicardial complex). This same late force may be directed superiorly or inferiorly. If superior, it will produce a wide S in aVF; if inferior, a

wide R′ in aVF. The ST segment and the T wave are opposite in direction to this late force of ventricular depolarization, resulting in ST depression and T wave inversion in right precordial leads. The QRS interval is 0.12 s or greater.

The pattern of septal and left ventricular depolarization in an uncomplicated right bundle branch block will be normal. Therefore, these will vary with heart position within the range of normal. In a right bundle branch block it will be of little significance to determine the mean frontal plane axis of the entire QRS. Instead, one should evaluate the initial 0.04–0.06 s of

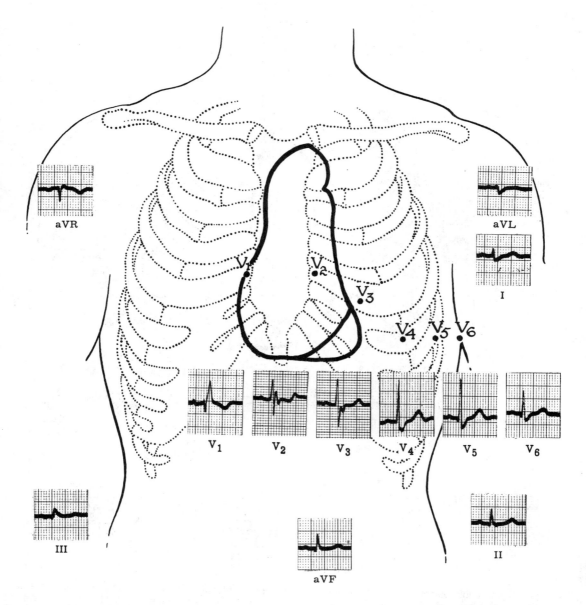

Figure 9–4. Complete right bundle branch block, vertical heart. The mean frontal plane axis of the initial 0.04 s of the QRS (determined by measuring r in I and qr in III, disregarding the wide s in I and wide r in III) = +60 degrees. The QRS interval = 0.14 s. The wide s waves in I and V_{4-6} and the R′ waves in V_{1-2} are typical of right bundle branch block.

the QRS (representing normal septal and left ventricular depolarization) in frontal plane leads and determine the frontal plane axis therefrom (Fig 4–5).

A. Vertical Heart: The mean of the forces resulting from septal and left ventricular depolarization will be oriented between +45 degrees and +110 degrees in the frontal plane (including semivertical heart position). Thus, this portion of the QRS complex in an uncomplicated right bundle branch block will be the same as in any normal vertical (or semivertical) heart. The factors that produce the right

bundle branch block are as given above.

B. Horizontal Heart: The mean of the forces resulting from septal and left ventricular depolarization will be oriented between +15 degrees and −30 degrees in the frontal plane (including semihorizontal heart position). Thus, this portion (the initial 0.04–0.06 s) of the QRS complex in an uncomplicated right bundle branch block will be the same as in any normal horizontal (or semihorizontal) heart. The factors producing right bundle branch block are as stated on p 117.

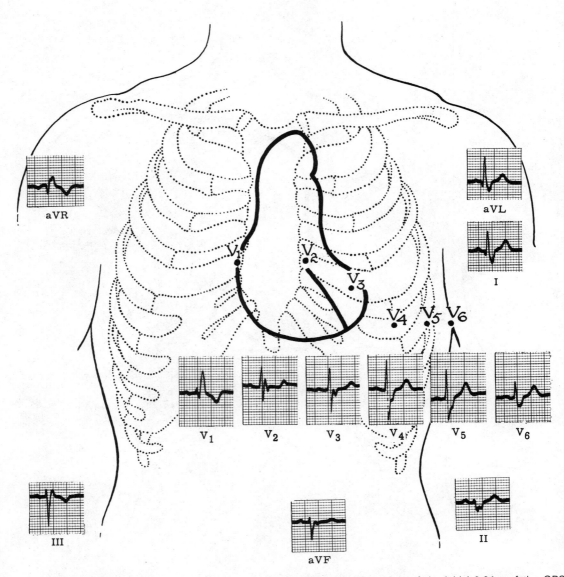

Figure 9–5. Right bundle branch block, horizontal heart. The mean frontal plane axis of the initial 0.04 s of the QRS (determined by measuring q and R in I and r and S in III, disregarding the wide S in I and wide r in III) = −40 degrees and therefore, by definition (see p 33), is left axis deviation and is abnormal. The QRS interval = 0.14 s. The wide S waves in I, II, aVL, and V$_{4-6}$, the wide r in III and aVR, and the wide R′ in V$_{1-2}$ are typical of right bundle branch block. The combination of left axis deviation and right bundle branch block is indicative of bilateral bundle disease (see p 134).

Right Bundle Branch Block With Left Ventricular Hypertrophy

In this situation, the tracing may show—in addition to the right bundle branch block pattern—the typical characteristics of left ventricular hypertrophy in leads I, aVL, and V4–6. Thus, these leads will show abnormally tall R waves and ST–T changes. The heart position is usually horizontal, resulting in an abnormally tall R wave in aVL.

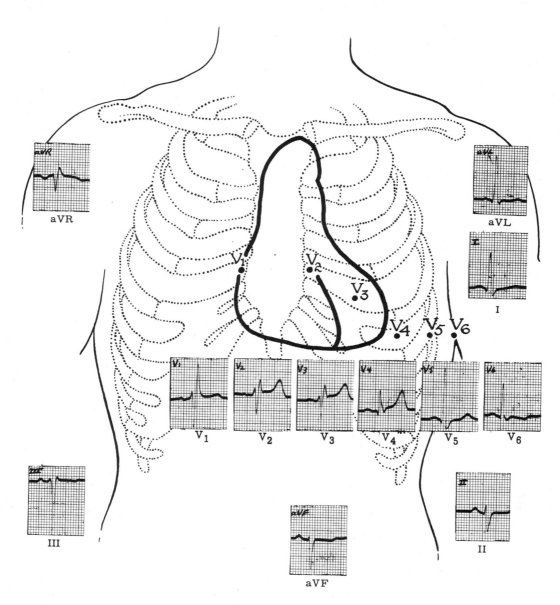

Figure 9–6. Right bundle branch block and left ventricular hypertrophy. Precordial leads show the typical pattern of a right bundle branch block. The R in aVL = 17 mm. This is indicative of left ventricular hypertrophy. The inverted T in V6 is probably also a manifestation of this latter diagnosis. The frontal plane QRS axis is oriented superiorly (−50 degrees). This indicates a lesion in the anterior fascicle of the left bundle, and in combination with the right bundle branch block is indicative of bilateral bundle disease (see p 134). *Clinical diagnosis:* Hypertensive cardiovascular disease.

Incomplete Right Bundle Branch Block

The pattern is similar to that of a complete right bundle branch block with the following exceptions: The QRS interval is under 0.12 s, and the VAT in V_1 is under 0.06 s. An incomplete right bundle branch block may occur as a result of right ventricular hypertrophy or strain (see pp 107 and 122 and Fig 8–30).

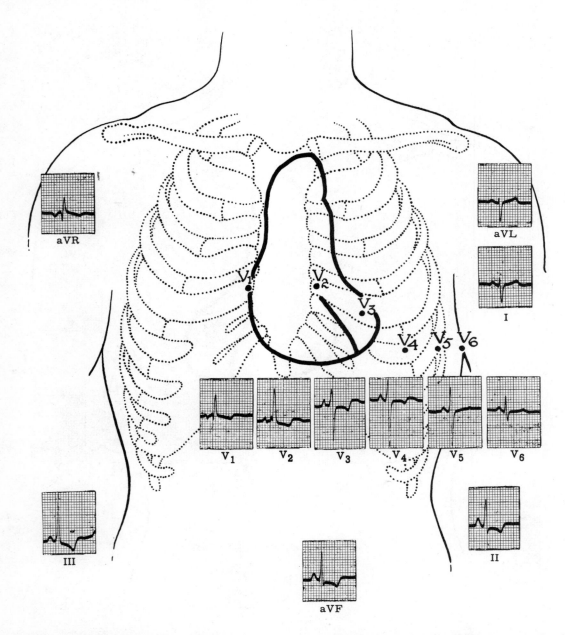

Figure 9–7. Incomplete right bundle branch block. The pattern is similar to that of a right bundle branch block except that the QRS interval = 0.08–0.1 s. The right axis deviation (+110 degrees) and the rR' complex in V_2 indicate associated right ventricular hypertrophy. *Clinical diagnosis:* Pulmonary sarcoidosis with right heart failure.

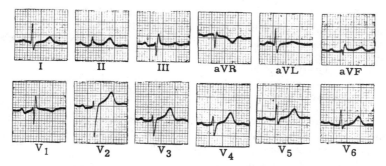

Figure 9–8. Incomplete right bundle branch block or a normal tracing. An rSR' complex is seen in V₁ and aVF. The R' is narrow in V₁ but wide in aVF. This tracing could be interpreted as normal or as an incomplete right bundle branch block. The latter electrocardiographic diagnosis does not necessarily indicate organic heart disease.

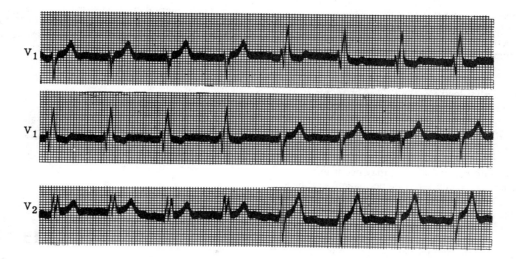

Figure 9–9. Intermittent right bundle branch block. Leads V₁ and V₂ are illustrated. The pattern is changing from a normal complex to that of a right bundle branch block. *Clinical diagnosis:* Arteriosclerotic heart disease. Two months later, the pattern became that of a permanent right bundle branch block.

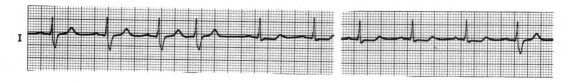

Figure 9–10. Intermittent rate-related right bundle branch block. The first 3 beats are sinus-conducted. There is a wide S wave in lead I, indicative of right bundle branch block. The fourth beat is an atrial ectopic beat with similar right bundle branch block. The pause that follows permits recovery of conduction through the right bundle for the following 5 beats. A slight increase in the heart rate then results in return of the conduction defect.

Normal rSr′ Pattern in V₁

The pattern of an incomplete right bundle branch block can resemble the normal pattern in which an rSr′ is seen in V_1. However, in the latter the r′ in V_1 is narrow, whereas in an incomplete right bundle branch block the r′ in V_1 appears widened. At times, it is impossible to differentiate between these 2 patterns. (See Figs 9–8 and 9–9.)

Differential Diagnosis of Right Bundle Branch Block & Right Ventricular Hypertrophy

A complete or incomplete right bundle branch block may be a manifestation of right ventricular hypertrophy. However, it may be impossible to diagnose right ventricular hypertrophy in the presence of a right bundle branch block from the ECG alone.

Typically, the following points are of differential value:

(1) In right bundle branch block the QRS interval is 0.12 s or longer; in right ventricular hypertrophy the QRS interval is under 0.12 s.

(2) In right bundle branch block a right precordial lead (such as V_1) shows an rSR′ complex. In right ventricular hypertrophy only an R wave, qR complex, or rR′ complex is seen.

(3) In right bundle branch block the VAT in a right precordial lead (V_1) is 0.06 s or more. In right ventricular hypertrophy the VAT is between 0.03 and 0.05 s.

Clinical Significance

Right bundle branch block does not necessarily imply organic heart disease; it may occur in a normal individual. The pattern may be permanent or transient (in serial tracings or in the same tracing), depending upon the cause. Pulmonary embolism or an acute exacerbation of some chronic pulmonary disease can produce a transient right bundle branch block.

A complete or incomplete right bundle branch block is a typical finding in the patient with an interatrial septal defect. It does not indicate a lesion in the main right bundle but is the result of delayed depolarization of the outflow tract of the right ventricle secondary to hypertrophy. In the presence of this congenital anomaly, left axis deviation of the initial 0.04–0.06 s of the QRS is strongly suggestive of an ostium primum defect. A normal frontal plane axis of the initial 0.04–0.06 s QRS favors the presence of an ostium secundum.

Right bundle branch block may occur as a rate-related phenomenon. As the heart rate increases, the refractory period of the bundle will be encountered and result in block. (See Fig 9–10.)

SUMMARY OF ELECTROCARDIOGRAPHIC CRITERIA OF RIGHT BUNDLE BRANCH BLOCK

A. Precordial Leads:

1. RSR′ or rsR′ complexes in V_{3R} and V_{1-2}. An initial q wave is never present in these leads unless there is associated infarction, right ventricular hypertrophy or dilatation, or additional left anterior fascicular block.

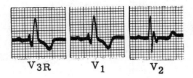

V_{3R} V_1 V_2

2. Wide S waves in V_{5-6}.
3. QRS interval = 0.12 s or more.
4. VAT = 0.06 s or more in V_{3R} and V_{1-2}.
5. ST depression and T wave inversion in V_{1-3}; these findings are common but are not essential for the diagnosis.

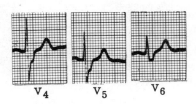

V_4 V_5 V_6

B. Extremity Leads:

1. Wide rSr′ complex in aVR.
2. Patterns in aVL and aVF will depend on heart position.

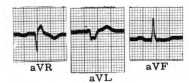

aVR   aVL   aVF

C. Standard Leads: A wide S wave is invariably present in lead I.

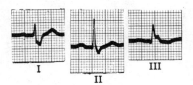

I   II   III

Minimal Criteria

rsR′ complex in a right precordial lead (V_{3R}, V_1, V_2) with QRS interval > 0.12 s and a wide S wave in lead I.

LEFT BUNDLE BRANCH BLOCK

Etiology & Incidence

Left bundle branch block may occur in almost any form of heart disease, including coronary artery disease, any of the diseases that produce left ventricular hypertrophy, and congenital lesions involving the septum.

Left bundle branch block is a common finding in coronary artery disease. It may be seen as an electrocardiographic finding in those diseases that produce left ventricular hypertrophy, eg, hypertension and aortic valvular disease. It is a rare finding in rheumatic heart disease with isolated mitral valvulitis. It is a much less common finding in congenital heart disease than is right bundle branch block. It is rarely seen in an individual with no clinical evidence of organic heart disease.

Mechanism

The spread of excitation from the SA node to the AV node and the bundle of His occurs in a normal fashion. The impulse cannot enter the left bundle system and activate the left septal fibers. Therefore, the septum is initially depolarized from fibers arising from the distal portion of the right bundle branch, resulting in an initial vector oriented to the left.

A. Left Ventricular Epicardial Complex (eg, V₅):

1. As a result of septal activation from right to left, a small initial r wave will be recorded. No q wave will be present.

2. Since the left bundle is "blocked," the excitation wave will next spread down the right bundle and through the right ventricular myocardium, resulting in an s wave.

3. Because of the relative thinness of the right ventricle, this s wave may not go below the isoelectric line but may merely produce a notch in the R wave.

4. The impulse then passes around the "blocked" left bundle into the left ventricular myocardium, producing a wide R' wave.

5. Thus, a typical pattern will be an rsR' or notched or slurred widened R.

The VAT is prolonged to 0.09 s or longer; the QRS interval is 0.12+ s; the ST segments are usually depressed and the T waves inverted.

B. Right Ventricular Epicardial Complex (eg, V₁):

1. An initial small q wave resulting fom septal activation (right to left).

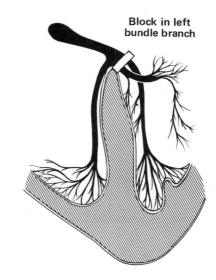

Block in left bundle branch

Figure 9–11. Left bundle branch block.

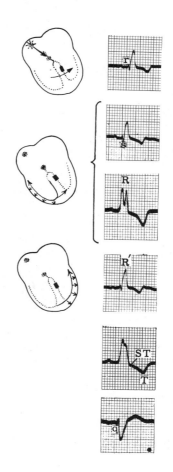

2. This is followed by a small r wave resulting from the normal activation of the right ventricle.

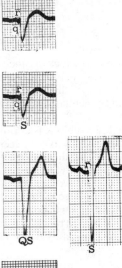

3. The impulse then passes around the "blocked" left bundle and into the left ventricular myocardium, producing a deep, wide S wave.

4. Occasionally, either the small initial q or r may not be recorded.

The patterns are therefore either qrS (¶B 1, 2, and 3, above), rS, or QS complexes. The ST segment may be elevated, and the T is upright.

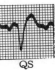

C. Right Ventricular Cavity Complex: Since septal activation is from right to left, the cavity will be negative throughout ventricular depolarization, producing a wide QS complex. The ST segment may be elevated, and the T is upright.

D. Left Ventricular Cavity Complex: Initial septal depolarization from right to left produces an initial small r wave. Ventricular depolarization, proceeding from the endocardial to the epicardial surfaces, results in a larger negative deflection, an S wave. The left ventricular cavity complex is therefore rS.

Clinical Significance & Prognosis

A left bundle branch block may be permanent or transient in the same tracing or in serial tracings. Transient left bundle branch block may occur in the course of myocardial infarction, heart failure, acute myocarditis, and as the result of quinidine therapy. Permanent left bundle branch block is practically always the result of organic heart disease. The prognosis will depend on the nature of the underlying heart disease. In the rare instance in which a left bundle branch block is found in a "normal" person, it has been assumed that a congenital lesion of the left bundle branch exists.

Left bundle branch block may be rate-related. With increasing heart rates, the refractory period of the left bundle branch is exceeded, resulting in block. (See Fig 9–15.)

Electrocardiographic Pattern

The patterns in standard leads and unipolar extremity leads will vary with heart positions. The pattern in the precordial leads will vary much less with change in heart position.

A. Horizontal Heart: This is the most common heart position.

1. Standard leads–Frontal plane QRS axis = 0 to −30 degrees; QRS interval = 0.12+ s; wide and slurred R waves in I and II; depressed ST segments and inverted T waves in I and II.

On occasion, the mean frontal plane QRS axis is superior to −30 degrees.

Although there is significant conduction delay in the entire left bundle system, there is more delay in conduction through the left anterior than the left posterior fascicle. This causes the terminal forces of the left bundle branch block to be oriented superiorly, as in uncomplicated left anterior fascicular block.

On rare occasions, an abnormal right axis deviation is seen in association with left bundle branch block. This could be the result of more delay in conduction through the left posterior fascicle (as in uncomplicated left posterior fascicular block) or additional right ventricular hypertrophy (Fig 9–33).

2. Extremity leads–Lead aVL records a left ventricular epicardial complex, producing an rsR' or wide slurred R; the ST is depressed and the T inverted. Lead aVF records a right ventricular epicardial complex, producing a qrS, QS, or rS complex with an elevated or isoelectric ST segment and upright T wave.

3. Precordial leads–Left precordial leads (V_{4-6}) will show the typical left ventricular epicardial pattern of a wide, notched R wave or rsR' complex. The VAT is prolonged to more than 0.09 s. The ST segments are depressed and the T waves inverted. Right precordial leads reflect a right ventricular epicardial complex.

4. Vector analysis–The normal initial QRS vector (directed to the right and anteriorly) is absent. Instead, the initial QRS vector is directed to the left and posteriorly, which explains the absence of a normal septal q wave in lead I and left precordial leads. Conduction delay is present through most of the QRS vector, producing the broad and slurred R waves in left precordial leads. The ST and T vectors are oriented to the right and anteriorly.

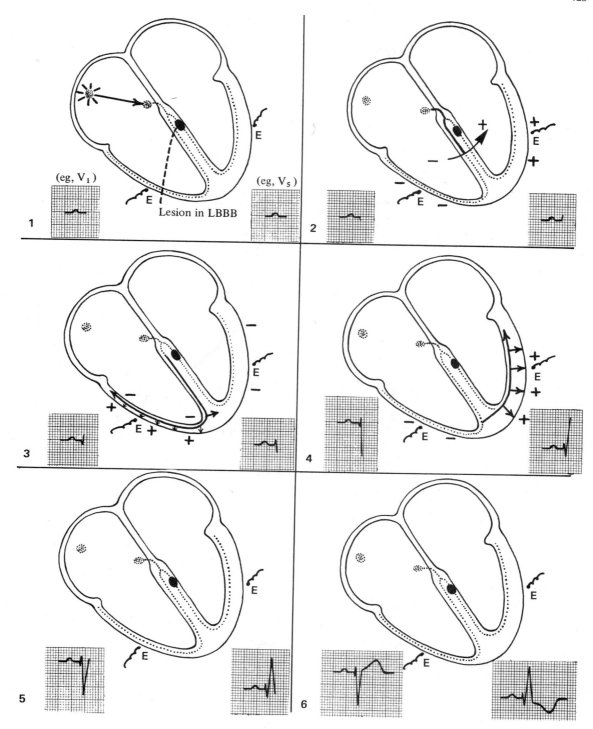

Figure 9–12. Development of left and right ventricular epicardial complexes in left bundle branch block. *(1)* Atrial activation. *(2)* Interventricular septal activation from right to left. *(3)* Left bundle branch blocked; therefore, right ventricle activated first. *(4)* Delayed activation of the left ventricle "around" the blocked bundle. *(5)* Depolarization complete. *(6)* Repolarization complete.

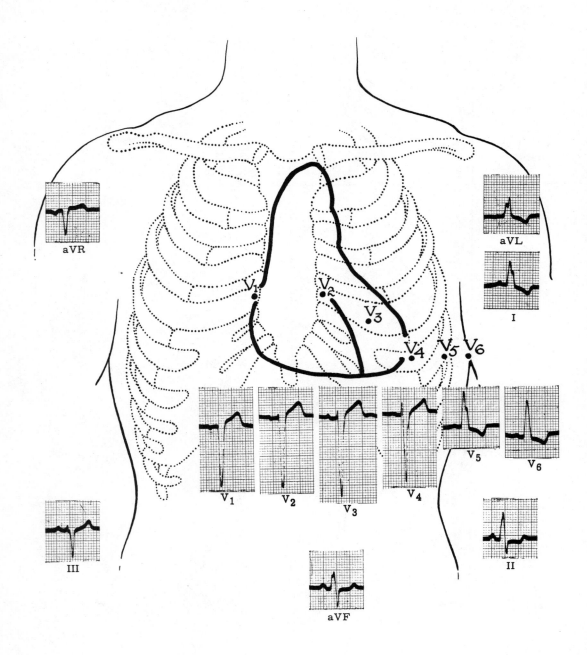

Figure 9–13. Left bundle branch block, horizontal heart position. Frontal plane QRS axis = 0 degrees. Precordial leads show the typical pattern of left bundle branch block. A wide, notched R wave with depressed ST and inverted T is seen in V_{5-6}; QRS interval = 0.12 s; VAT = 0.1 s. Lead aVL records a left ventricular epicardial complex and resembles V_{5-6}. *Clinical diagnosis:* Hypertensive and arteriosclerotic heart disease.

Vertical Heart

A. Standard Leads: Normal vertical frontal plane axis; wide, slurred R waves with depressed ST and inverted T in I, II, and III.

B. Extremity Leads: The typical left ventricular epicardial complex is recorded in aVF.

C. Precordial Leads: The same as stated for a horizontal heart. As in right bundle branch block, the diagnosis of a left bundle branch block is best made from a study of the precordial leads.

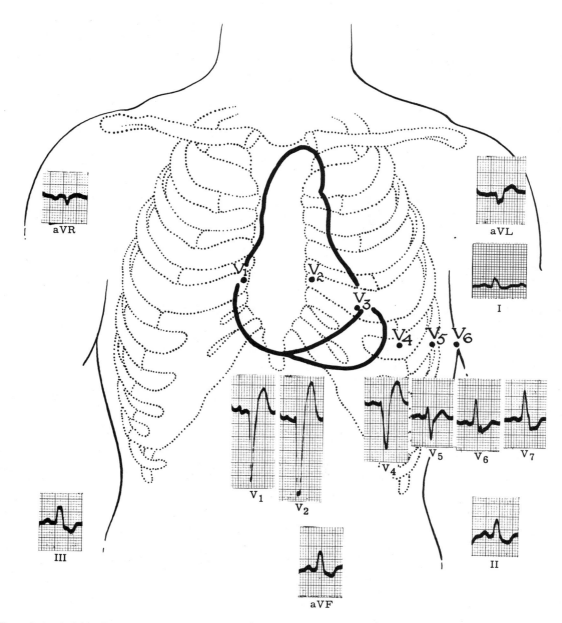

Figure 9–14. Left bundle branch block, vertical heart. Frontal plane QRS axis = +70 degrees. The pattern in precordial leads is that of a left bundle branch block. Lead aVF records a left ventricular epicardial complex and resembles V₇. *Clinical and autopsy diagnosis:* Hypertensive and arteriosclerotic heart disease; no evidence of myocardial infarction.

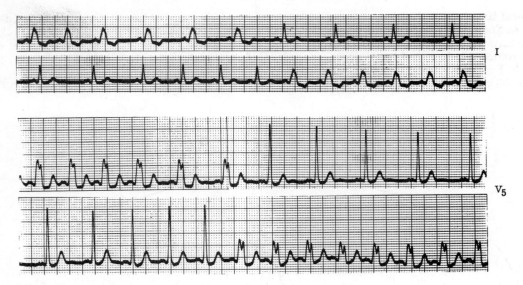

Figure 9–15. Intermittent left bundle branch block, leads I and V₅. The pattern of left bundle branch block periodically changes to normal intraventricular conduction. This is often a rate-related phenomenon, the bundle branch block appearing with a more rapid rate, as illustrated in this tracing.

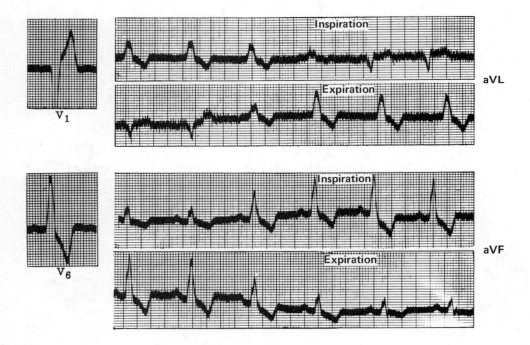

Figure 9–16. Left bundle branch block; change in frontal plane axis with respiration. *aVL:* As a result of deep inspiration, the typical left ventricular epicardial complex is converted into a right ventricular epicardial complex. This results from a change from horizontal to vertical position. *aVF:* As a result of the same change, lead aVF records a more typical left ventricular epicardial complex during deep inspiration. The frontal plane QRS axis shifts from +70 degrees (inspiration) to +20 degrees (expiration). Leads V₁ and V₆ indicate the presence of the left bundle branch block.

Effect of Deep Respiration

Deep inspiration and expiration, by altering the heart position, can greatly modify the electrocardiographic pattern, especially in the extremity leads. (See Fig 9–16.)

Incomplete Left Bundle Branch Block

The pattern is similar to that of a complete left bundle branch block except that the QRS interval is under 0.12 s, and the VAT is under 0.09 s.

T Wave Changes Following Reversion of Left Bundle Branch Block

Following spontaneous reversion of left bundle branch block to normal intraventricular conduction, the ECG may show deep T wave inversions in precordial leads. Such inversions need not be of clinical significance since they occur in the absence of documented heart disease (Fig 9–19).

Differential Diagnosis of Left Bundle Branch Block & Left Ventricular Hypertrophy

A left bundle branch block may be seen in the same clinical conditions that produce left ventricular hypertrophy. The important point in the differential diagnosis of the above 2 conditions is the absence of a q wave in leads that definitely record septal activity in the right-left axis (ie, I, V_{5-6}). The presence of a q wave in leads I and V_{5-6} negates the diagnosis of left bundle branch block or indicates associated infarction. Voltage criteria used for the diagnosis of left ventricular hypertrophy are probably not valid in the presence of left bundle branch block.

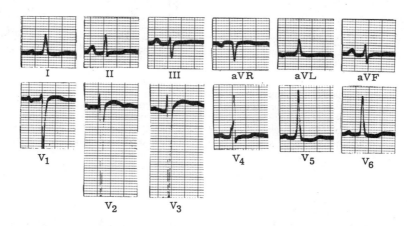

Figure 9–17. Incomplete left bundle branch block. The QRS interval = 0.1 s. There are no q waves in I and V_{5-6}. The R wave is slurred in I, aVL, and V_{5-6} and notched in V_4. There are ST depression and flattened T waves in the above leads. Precordial voltage is high, $SV_1 + RV_5 = 38$ mm. *Clinical diagnosis:* Hypertensive cardiovascular disease.

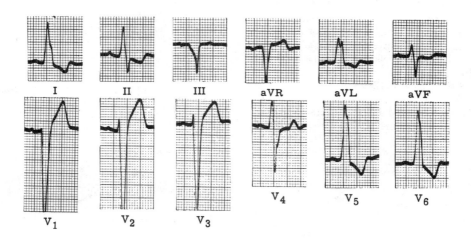

Figure 9–18. Left bundle branch block. The heart position is horizontal; frontal plane QRS axis = −10 degrees; QRS interval = 0.15 s; absent q waves with wide, slurred R waves, depressed ST segments, and inverted T waves in leads I, aVL, and V_{5-6}. $SV_1 + RV_5 = 51$ mm. *Clinical diagnosis:* Syphilitic aortic insufficiency. *Autopsy diagnosis:* Syphilis of the aorta; left ventricular hypertrophy.

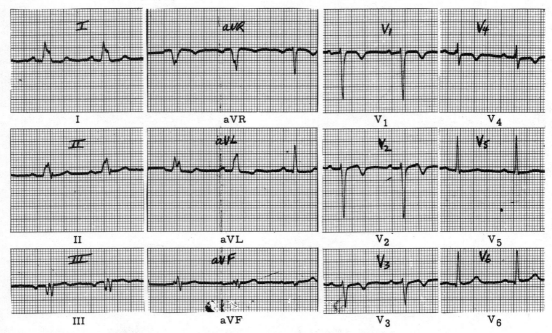

Figure 9–19. Spontaneous reversion of left bundle branch block. The complexes in leads I, II, and III and the first complex in leads aVR, aVL, and aVF are typical of left bundle branch block. The third complex in leads aVR, aVL, and aVF and all complexes in leads V_{1-6} reveal normal intraventricular conduction. The second complex in leads aVR, aVL, and aVF has a lesser degree of intraventricular conduction delay. The heart rate is the same during left bundle branch block and normal intraventricular conduction. Note the inverted T waves in leads V_{1-4}, which could represent ischemia or infarction of the left ventricular anterior wall and septum, explaining the intermittent left bundle branch block. However, it is important to appreciate that such T wave changes can occur in the absence of active heart disease and therefore do not have specific diagnostic significance.

SUMMARY OF ELECTROCARDIOGRAPHIC CRITERIA OF LEFT BUNDLE BRANCH BLOCK

A. Precordial Leads: These are the best leads for diagnosis.

1. Wide, slurred R waves or rsR′ or RsR′ complexes in V_{4-6}; absent q waves in these leads, with the possible exception of one lead (eg, V_4) that borders on the transitional zone.

2. QRS interval = 0.12+ s.

3. VAT = 0.09+ s in V_{4-6}.

4. ST depression and T wave inversion in V_{4-6}; these findings are common but are not essential for the diagnosis.

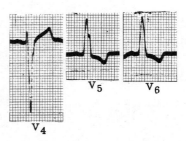

B. Extremity Leads: Pattern similar to that seen in V_{4-6} is present in aVL if heart is horizontal (more common); in aVF if heart is vertical (less common).

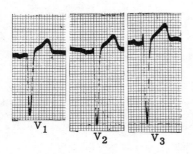

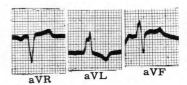

C. Standard Leads: These reflect the same pattern as in extremity leads. Absent q wave; wide and abnormal R wave (or rsR′ complex); ST depression and T wave inversion in lead I.

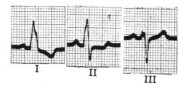

I   II   III

Minimal Criteria

rsR' complex or wide, notched R wave in left precordial leads (V$_{4-7}$) and lead I; absence of q waves in these leads; QRS interval > 0.12 s.

PERIPHERAL LEFT VENTRICULAR CONDUCTION DEFECTS

As stated on p 37, the left bundle branch divides immediately after its origin from the common bundle (His) into 2 major divisions or fascicles: (1) the posterior fascicle, which arises proximally and spreads as a broad band of fibers over the inferior and posterior endocardial areas of the left ventricle; and (2) the anterior fascicle, which arises more distally, is a narrower band of fibers, and spreads over the anterior and superior endocardial areas of the left ventricle. Peripherally, these 2 divisions are connected by intertwining fibers of the Purkinje system. In addition, specialized fibers from the proximal left bundle spread into the left septal region and constitute a third left fascicle.

Normally, conduction spreads simultaneously through both divisions. This results in a normally di-

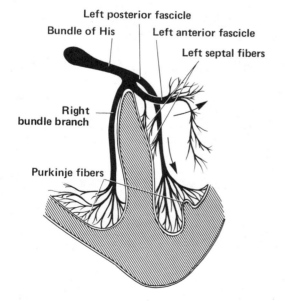

Left posterior fascicle
Bundle of His   Left anterior fascicle
Left septal fibers
Right bundle branch
Purkinje fibers

Figure 9–20. Diagram of the conduction system, illustrating normal left ventricular activation by simultaneous activation of both divisions of the left bundle.

rected QRS vector, between −30 degrees and +110 degrees in the frontal plane (Fig 4–5). However, if one division of the left bundle is damaged by a pathologic process, conduction will first proceed through the undamaged division, thus altering the direction of the mean QRS vector. Since the speed of conduction through the bundle tissues and Purkinje system is rapid, this lesion will not produce a significant prolongation of the QRS interval.

LEFT ANTERIOR FASCICULAR BLOCK

A left anterior fascicular block (left anterior hemiblock, anterolateral parietal block) is the result of a lesion in the anterior fascicle of the left bundle. Therefore, left ventricular conduction initially spreads through the posterior fascicle of the left bundle, resulting in a vector oriented inferiorly (r wave in II, III, and aVF) and rightward (q wave in I). The anterior fascicle will be activated later via interconnecting Purkinje fibers distal to the site of the block resulting in a vector oriented to the left (R in I) and superiorly (S in II, III, and aVF). The mean frontal plane QRS axis is greater than −30 degrees (superior or left axis deviation). There is no appreciable widening of the QRS interval. However, if an ECG is available prior to the appearance of this block, a slight prolongation of the QRS up to 0.02 s may be seen.

The above electrocardiographic pattern is seen in the following clinical conditions:

(1) Coronary artery disease: The abnormal degree of left axis deviation may be the only electrocardiographic finding. On occasion, there may be associated ST segment depression and T wave inversion, thus simulating the pattern of left ventricular strain (Fig 8–17).

(2) Left ventricular hypertrophy: The abnormal degree of left axis deviation is probably not due to the hypertrophied muscle mass as such, but to associated subendocardial fibrosis involving the anterior fascicle of the left bundle. One cannot make an electrocardiographic diagnosis of left ventricular hypertrophy from this finding alone. There must be increased voltage or prolongation of the VAT (or both) (see p 99). The usual criterion of R voltage in aVL of 11 mm is not valid in the presence of left anterior fascicular block. Although not definitely determined, a value of at least 16 mm is required.

(3) Pulmonary emphysema: The mean QRS vector is commonly along the vertical axis and is usually directed inferiorly, ie, close to the +90 degree frontal plane axis. Uncommonly, as a result of abnormal electrical conduction from the surface of the heart to the body surface caused by the diseased lungs and deformed thorax, this same vertical axis may be directed superiorly, ie, close to the −90 degree frontal plane axis, resulting in an abnormal left axis deviation. The voltage of the QRS complexes is low, thus aiding

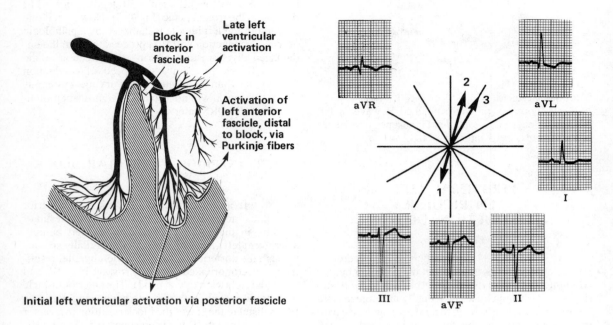

Figure 9–21. Left anterior fascicular block. The initial QRS (1) is oriented to the right (q in I) and inferiorly (r in II, III, and aVF). The terminal QRS (2) is oriented to the left (R in I) and superiorly (S in II, III, and aVF). The mean QRS frontal plane vector = −60 degrees (3).

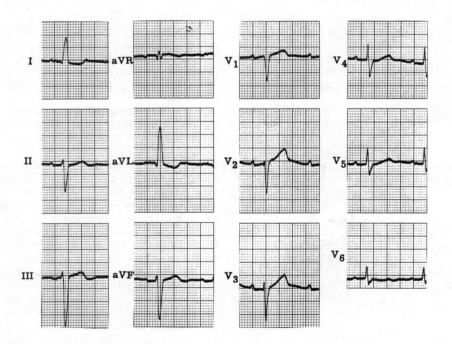

Figure 9–22. Left anterior fascicular block. The mean QRS axis = −50 degrees. The QRS interval = 0.1 s. The R voltage in aVL = 14 mm. In the presence of left anterior fascicular block, this voltage is not diagnostic of left ventricular hypertrophy. There is ST depression in I, aVL, and V₆. Persistent S waves in V₅₋₆ (clockwise rotation) are the result of the superiorly directed late QRS forces. *Clinical diagnosis:* Hypertensive cardiovascular disease.

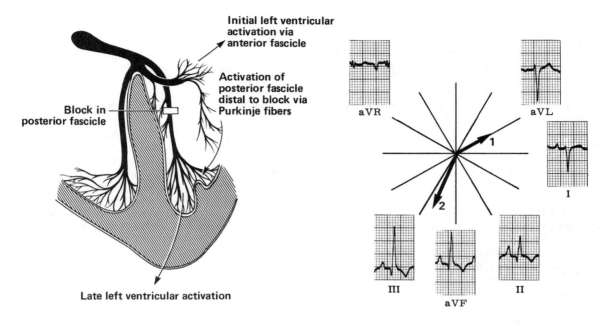

Figure 9–23. Left posterior fascicular block. The initial QRS (1) is oriented to the left (r in I) and superiorly (q in II, III, and aVF). The terminal QRS (2) is oriented rightward (S in I) and inferiorly (R in II, III, and aVF), resulting in a mean frontal plane QRS axis of +110 degrees.

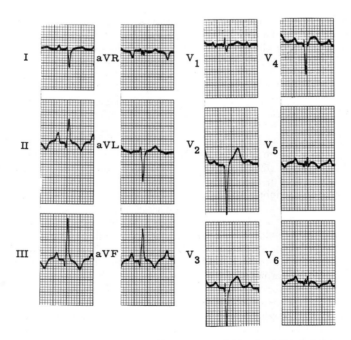

Figure 9–24. Left posterior fascicular block. The mean frontal plane QRS axis = +110 degrees. The QRS interval = 0.1 s. The P waves are tall in II, III, and aVF. The above are consistent with right atrial and right ventricular hypertrophy. However, cardiac catheterization revealed normal right heart pressures. This emphasizes the necessity for excluding right ventricular hypertrophy before an electrocardiographic diagnosis of posterior fascicular block can be made. The precordial leads are indicative of anterior myocardial infarction. *Clinical diagnosis:* Arteriosclerotic heart disease with old myocardial infarction.

in differentiation from an otherwise similar electrocardiographic pattern produced by coronary artery disease. However, the correct differential diagnosis will depend on proper clinical evaluation of the patient. In this situation, there is no pathologic lesion in the left anterior fascicle.

(4) **Peri-infarction block:** See p 207.

(5) **Various myocarditides and myocardiopathies.**

LEFT POSTERIOR FASCICULAR BLOCK

A left posterior fascicular block (left posterior hemiblock) is the result of a lesion in the posterior fascicle of the left bundle. Left ventricular conduction initially spreads through the anterior fascicle, resulting in a vector oriented to the left (R in I) and superiorly (q in II, III, and aVF). The posterior fascicle will be activated later via interconnecting Purkinje fibers distal to the site of the block, resulting in a vector oriented to the right (S in I), inferiorly (R in II, III, and aVF), and posteriorly (S in V_{1-2}). The mean frontal plane QRS axis is +110 degrees or greater. The recognition of this entity as an isolated finding (ie, in the absence of inferior infarction or right bundle branch block) is difficult. A frontal plane QRS axis of +110 degrees can be within the wide range of normal. It can also be a manifestation of right ventricular hypertrophy or lateral wall infarction. Therefore, such an electrocardiographic diagnosis can be made only if there is clinical evidence to exclude the possibility of right ventricular hypertrophy and myocardial infarction. ———

LEFT SEPTAL BLOCK

Normal initial septal depolarization results from impulses transmitted by the septal fibers that arise from the proximal portions of the left bundle branch. The resulting vector is oriented to the right, producing small q waves in leads I, V_5, and V_6. It would be expected that absence of these q waves would indicate interruption of conduction of these septal fibers. As an isolated finding, the ECG would be normal except for the absence of q waves in leads I, V_5, and V_6. Such ECGs have been interpreted as "abnormal septal depolarization" or "indicative of septal fibrosis." Although this cannot be denied, it is known that 20% of clinically normal individuals do not have initial rightward forces, ie, no q wave in I, V_5, and V_6. This does not disprove the concept of septal depolarization from left to right. It indicates that the interventricular septum is parallel to the frontal plane of the body, and, even though the septum is activated from its left to its right, the projection of this force is oriented anteriorly but not rightward.

LEFT ANTERIOR CONDUCTION DELAY

A left anterior conduction delay is believed to result from a delay in conduction through anterior fibers of the left anterior fascicle. Instead of the expected superior (left) frontal plane axis, it is manifested by abnormally prominent anterior QRS forces, resulting in tall R waves in V_1 and V_2 (R greater than S in V_1). In the presence of coronary artery disease, the above is consistent with posterior wall infarction. However, in selected cases, coronary arteriography has revealed left anterior descending coronary artery disease and left ventricular angiography has demonstrated anterior wall motion abnormality with normal posterior wall motion. It is assumed that conduction delay to the anterior wall produces this pattern.

PERI–INFARCTION BLOCKS
(See Chapter 11.)

BILATERAL BUNDLE BRANCH BLOCK

Bilateral bundle branch block indicates disease in both right and left bundle systems. The types of such blocks are listed on p 113. These are of prognostic significance in that they greatly increase the probability of complete heart block in the future. In the elderly patient, bilateral bundle branch block disease is most commonly associated with a degenerative process of unknown cause that involves the upper portion of the interventricular septum (thereby interrupting conduction in the bundle branches) and the anulus structures of the mitral and aortic valves, producing fibrosis and eventual calcification in these areas. Coronary artery disease is the next most common cause. When bilateral block occurs in association with myocardial infarction, the prognosis is very ominous not only because of the high risk of complete heart block but because of severe cardiac insufficiency as a result of extensive infarction.

A. Right Bundle Branch Block With Anterior Fascicular Block: This is one of the most common types of bilateral bundle branch block. It is recognized by the combination of the criteria given above for each type of block, ie, (1) delayed terminal QRS forces oriented to the right and anteriorly, producing wide S waves in I, V_5, and V_6 and wide R or R' waves in V_1 and V_2; plus (2) a mean 0.04–0.06 s QRS vector in the frontal plane greater than −30 degrees.

B. Right Bundle Branch Block With Left Posterior Fascicular Block: The electrocardiographic features that permit recognition of this type of bilateral bundle branch block are (1) typical findings of right bundle branch block and (2) a frontal plane QRS axis of +110 degrees or greater (axis is calculated on magnitude, not area). Right bundle branch block alone does not produce this degree of rightward axis. As in

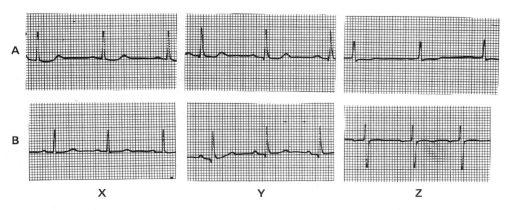

Figure 9–25. Left anterior conduction delay. The above leads are X, Y, and Z of the Frank lead system, comparable to conventional leads I, aVF, and V$_1$, respectively. The patient was a 60-year-old man with intractable angina. Record A reveals an abnormally tall R in Z, indicative of prominent anterior forces. This was initially interpreted as posterior myocardial infarction. Cardiac catheterization and coronary angiography revealed normal pressures (excluding right ventricular hypertrophy) and total occlusion of the proximal left anterior descending artery (LAD) and diagonal branch, with filling of the distal LAD from the right posterior descending and circumflex vessels. Left ventricular angiography revealed hypokinesia of the anterior wall, with good inferior and posterior wall motion. Bypass grafts were inserted into the LAD and diagonal vessels. For the following year, the patient was completely free of angina. Record B is representative of many postoperative ECGs, all of which were normal. The abnormally prominent anterior forces are no longer present (the R:S ratio in lead Z is normal). A repeat study revealed patency of the grafts and normal left ventricular wall motion. The patient died 1 year later from a noncardiac illness. Autopsy revealed no evidence of old or recent myocardial infarction and no right ventricular hypertrophy. In view of all the above data, the only probable explanation for the initially (preoperative) abnormal anterior forces is an anterior conduction delay.

isolated left posterior fascicular block, right ventricular hypertrophy must be excluded by clinical evaluation.

C. Right or Left Bundle Branch Block With Prolonged AV Conduction: A prolonged P–R interval (> 0.21 s) will be present in association with either a right or left bundle branch block. The prolonged P–R interval (ie, first degree AV block; see p 237) could be the result of conduction delay in the AV node. In this instance, it would not indicate bilateral bundle branch disease. However, in most instances, bundle of His recordings have shown that the prolongation of the P–R interval is due to delayed conduction distal to the bundle of His and is therefore evidence of "incomplete" block in the opposite bundle branch.

D. Alternating Right and Left Bundle Branch Block: In this instance, the ECG will demonstrate a typical complete right (or left) bundle branch block at

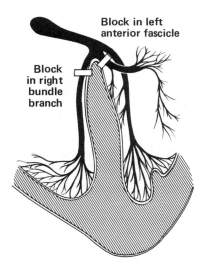

Figure 9–26. Diagram of right bundle branch block plus left anterior fascicular block. It can be seen that a relatively small lesion can produce this type of bilateral bundle branch block.

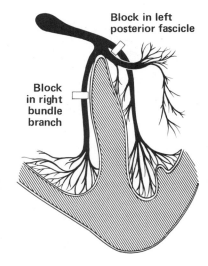

Figure 9–27. Diagram of right bundle branch block plus left posterior fascicular block.

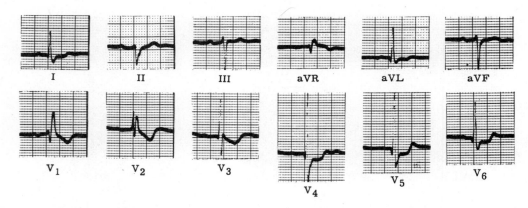

Figure 9–28. Bilateral bundle disease. The initial 0.05 s QRS is directed leftward and superiorly (frontal plane axis = −60 degrees). This indicates a lesion in the anterior fascicle of the left bundle. The terminal portion of the QRS is delayed and oriented to the right and anteriorly (wide S in I and V_{5-6}; wide R' in V_{1-2}), which is typical of right bundle branch block. The combination indicates bilateral bundle disease.

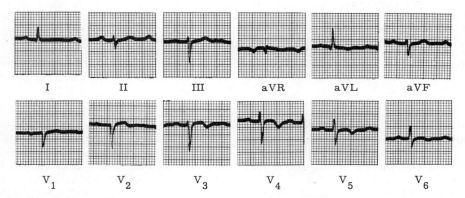

Figure 9–29. Superior axis and anterior infarction. The frontal plane QRS is −45 degrees, indicating a superior axis (left axis) and implying a lesion in the anterior fascicle of the left bundle. The QS complexes in V_{1-2} and the T inversion in aVL and precordial leads are consistent with anterior wall infarction (see p 155). Clinically, the patient had had a myocardial infarction 6 months previously.

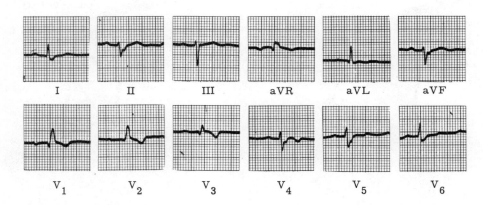

Figure 9–30. Development of bilateral bundle disease. This tracing was taken on the above patient 1 year later. Anginal pain was a frequent complaint. The frontal plane axis of the initial 0.05 s QRS remains superior (−60 degrees). An intraventricular conduction defect is now present, with wide S waves in I, V_{5-6} and late, wide R waves in V_{1-3}, typical of right bundle branch block. The combination indicates bilateral bundle branch disease, ie, block in the anterior fascicle of the left bundle and block in the right bundle. The Q waves in V_{1-3} are indicative of the old anterior infarct.

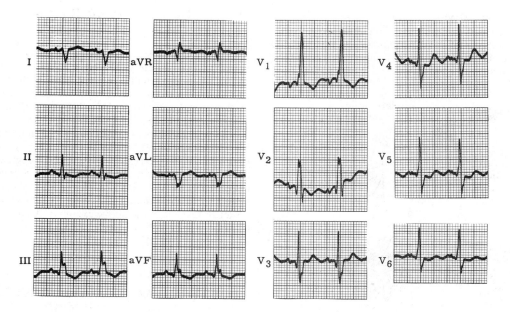

Figure 9–31. Right bundle branch block with left posterior fascicular block. The QRS interval = 0.13 s. The wide S waves in I and the wide R waves in V_{1-2} are indicative of right bundle branch block. The frontal plane QRS axis is +120 degrees, which meets the criterion for an associated left posterior fascicular block. The q waves in V_{1-3} are indicative of associated anterior myocardial infarction. The possibility of right ventricular hypertrophy was excluded by clinical evaluation.

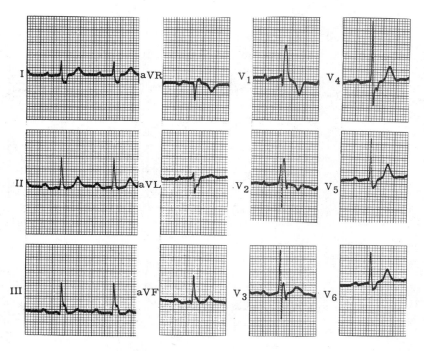

Figure 9–32. Right bundle branch block with first degree heart block. The QRS interval = 0.14 s. The wide S waves in I and V_6 and the wide R′ waves in V_{1-2} are typical of right bundle branch block. The P–R interval = 0.25 s, indicating a first degree AV block. Although the latter could be the result of delay in the AV node, the associated intraventricular conduction defect makes it more likely that the site of block is distal to the bundle of His (see p 235). This would indicate an incomplete block in the left bundle system.

one moment and within minutes or days will show the opposite type of complete bundle branch block. When this does occur, it is very ominous and predictive of complete heart block unless it is due to some reversible factor such as drug toxicity.

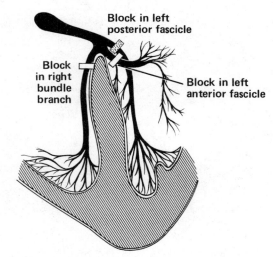

Figure 9–33. Diagram of trifascicular block. Complete blocks in right bundle branch and left anterior fascicle; incomplete block in left posterior fascicle which prolongs the P–R interval.

TRIFASCICULAR BLOCK

If all 3 fascicles of the intraventricular conduction system were completely blocked, it would be impossible for a supraventricular focus to activate the ventricle. Complete heart block with an idioventricular rhythm would occur (see p 241). The term trifascicular block is used to describe an ECG that shows bilateral bundle branch block—most commonly right bundle branch block with left anterior fascicular block—and a prolonged P–R interval indicating first degree AV block. Although the latter could be due to conduction delay in the AV node, it more likely represents incomplete block in the third fascicle, which would be the left posterior fascicle in the above example. A His bundle recording (see p 235) would be necessary to prove the site of the AV block.

INDETERMINATE INTRAVENTRICULAR CONDUCTION DEFECTS

At times, a bizarre intraventricular conduction defect will be seen that cannot be placed in any of the above categories. It is therefore called an indeterminate type of intraventricular conduction defect.

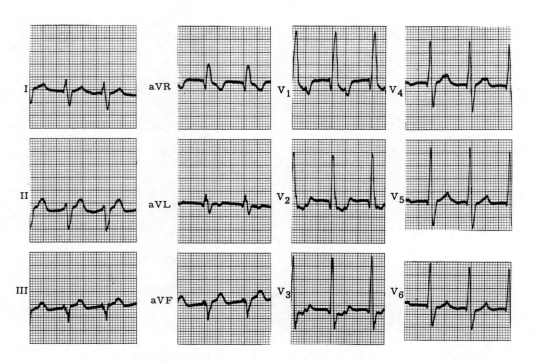

Figure 9–34. Trifascicular block. The QRS interval = 0.13 s. The wide S waves in I and wide R' waves in V_{1-3} are indicative of right bundle branch block. The initial 0.06 s frontal plane QRS vector = −60 degrees, indicating a left anterior fascicular block. The P–R interval = 0.35 s, indicating a first degree heart block which could be due to incomplete block in the left posterior fascicle. The q waves in V_{2-3} do not necessarily indicate anterior wall infarction.

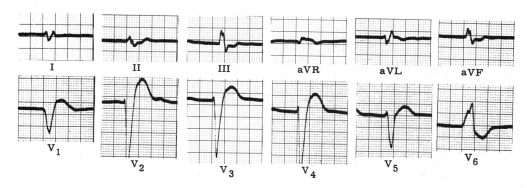

Figure 9–35. Indeterminate intraventricular conduction defect. The QRS interval = 0.18 s. The pattern in precordial leads is typical of left bundle branch block. A significant s wave is seen in lead I, indicating rightward forces. This could be the result of a greater degree of conduction delay in the left posterior fascicle than in the left anterior fascicle, or it could indicate associated right ventricular hypertrophy or myocardial infarction. The rhythm is atrial fibrillation. The only medication was digitalis. *Clinical and autopsy diagnosis:* Idiopathic myocardiopathy; marked left and right ventricular hypertrophy; no myocardial infarction.

10 | Coronary Artery Disease: Myocardial Ischemia

The common clinical and electrocardiographic manifestations of coronary artery disease are myocardial ischemia and myocardial infarction.

Myocardial ischemia (angina, coronary insufficiency) refers to changes in the myocardium resulting from a temporarily insufficient blood supply. These changes are commonly seen during spontaneous angina and induced myocardial ischemia (exercise test).

Etiology & Incidence

Arteriosclerosis of the coronary arteries is the most frequent cause of myocardial ischemia. Patients with marked left ventricular hypertrophy may develop angina with exertion since the coronary vessels, even though not seriously diseased, cannot supply enough oxygen to the hypertrophied myocardium during periods of stress. Aortic stenosis with its low cardiac output reduces the coronary blood flow and therefore can produce myocardial ischemia. Syphilitic aortitis, by encroaching upon the orifices of the coronary arteries, can result in angina. Pulmonary hypertension, such as results from mitral stenosis and chronic diffuse pulmonary disease, reduces the left ventricular cardiac output and can produce angina. Polycythemia, by increasing the viscosity of the blood and slowing its circulation, can produce myocardial ischemia. Rarely, other arteritides such as Buerger's disease, rheumatic fever, and other collagen diseases involve the coronary arteries and result in coronary insufficiency. Diabetes mellitus and myxedema, by increasing the degree of arteriosclerosis, are often associated with coronary artery disease. Other conditions that can cause myocardial ischemia are anemia, hyperthyroidism, and rapid paroxysmal arrhythmias.

Differential Diagnosis of the ECG

Since the electrocardiographic findings of myocardial ischemia are ST segment and T wave changes, a single ECG is not pathognomonic of myocardial ischemia. Similar changes can be produced by a variety of conditions, eg, left ventricular hypertrophy, drug effect, hypokalemia, pericarditis, and myocarditis. The diagnosis is dependent upon the clinical evaluation of the patient and electrocardiographic changes during spontaneous angina or myocardial ischemia induced by exercise tests.

Clinical Significance

The diagnosis of myocardial ischemia must never depend entirely upon the ECG. A normal resting record and even a normal exercise tracing does not exclude the diagnosis. A careful history is frequently of more value in diagnosis than the ECG.

Prognosis

Although a patient with angina is subject to sudden death, he must not be made a permanent invalid since most patients can lead useful and productive lives for many years under sensible management.

A sudden appearance of angina in a previously asymptomatic individual or a sudden increase in the severity of symptoms is an indication of impending myocardial infarction. It is wise to treat such patients as one would a definite case of myocardial infarction.

Mechanism of the Electrocardiographic Pattern

The electrocardiographic changes resulting from myocardial ischemia are transitory ST segment deviations and T wave changes.

A. ST Segment Changes: It is believed that currents of injury produce the ST segment deviation. Two mechanisms have been shown to explain this phenomenon.

1. Injury current of rest–"Injured" muscle (as occurs in myocardial ischemia and myocardial infarction) is electrically negative in relation to normal resting muscle. (See Fig 10–1.)

This can be illustrated by observation of the events that occur in an injured muscle strip. The pattern overlying the injured area (right side of diagram) will be considered first. Diagram (1) represents a normal resting muscle; E is an electrode, and the straight and dotted line represents the base line of the ECG. Diagram (2) represents a muscle the right end of which has been injured. This area is now electrically negative. The overlying electrode will therefore record a depressed base line during the resting period. In (3) the left end of the muscle strip has been stimulated, initiating an advancing negative charge in front of which is a positive charge (see p 19). The electrode therefore records a positive deflection. At (4) the stimulus has reached the injured area. At this point there is no longer any difference of electrical potential between the 2 ends of the muscle strip, so the tracing returns to the

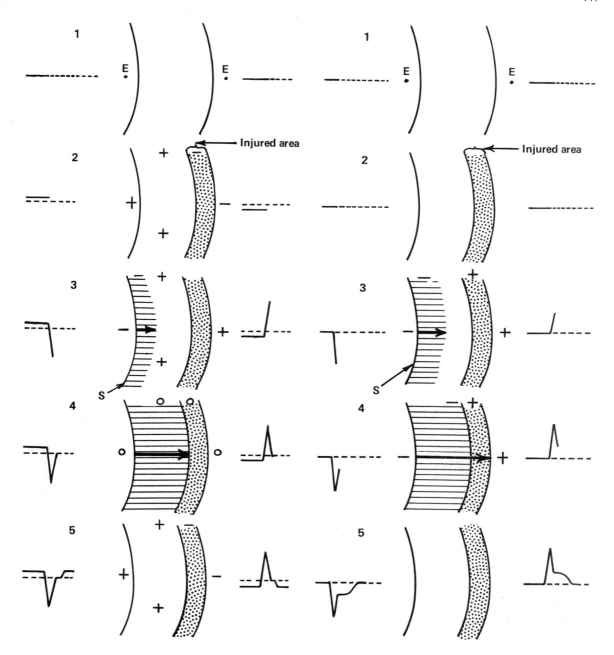

Figure 10–1. Injury current of rest. (The muscle strips are curved to simulate the wall of the myocardium.)

Figure 10–2. Injury current of activity. (The muscle strips are curved to simulate the wall of the myocardium.)

base line as in a normal resting muscle (1). This produces the appearance of ST segment elevation. The tracing remains at this level until the uninjured portion of the muscle returns to the resting state (5), at which time a difference of potential again exists (as in 2) and the tracing returns to the lower base line.

The reverse occurs when the electrode faces the uninjured side of the muscle strip (see complexes on left side of diagram). At (2) the electrode is facing a positive charge, and the base line is therefore elevated. At (3) the electrode is facing a negative charge resulting from the muscle stimulation, producing a downward deflection. At (4) there is again no difference in electrical potential, so the tracing returns to the base line corresponding to normal resting muscle. At (5) the electrical difference again occurs, and the tracing returns to the elevated base line. Thus, a pattern of ST depression results.

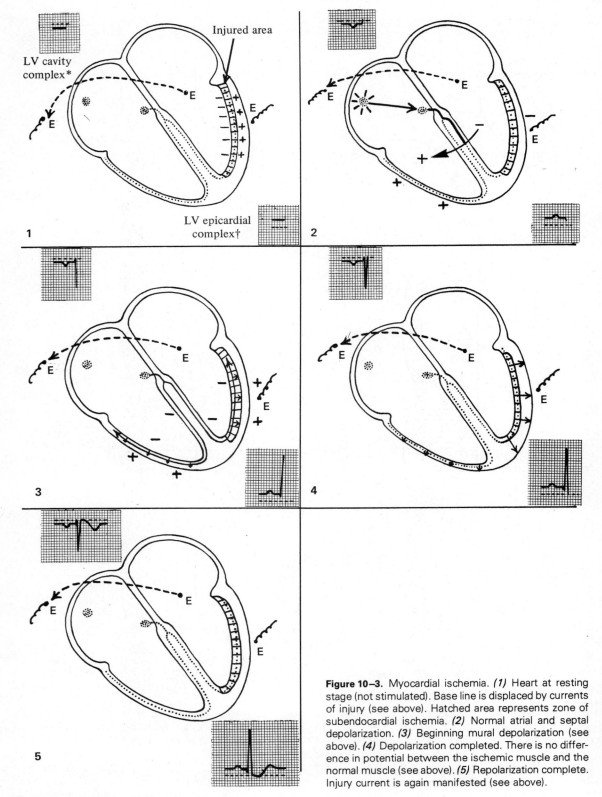

Figure 10–3. Myocardial ischemia. *(1)* Heart at resting stage (not stimulated). Base line is displaced by currents of injury (see above). Hatched area represents zone of subendocardial ischemia. *(2)* Normal atrial and septal depolarization. *(3)* Beginning mural depolarization (see above). *(4)* Depolarization completed. There is no difference in potential between the ischemic muscle and the normal muscle (see above). *(5)* Repolarization complete. Injury current is again manifested (see above).

*Lead aVR or aVL, depending on heart position.
†For example, V₅.

2. Injury current of activity—Experimental evidence indicates that injured muscle does not become as electrically negative as normal muscle when stimulated. Thus, the injured muscle during stimulation will have a lesser negative charge and hence a greater positive charge than normal stimulated muscle. An electrode directly overlying the injured end of the muscle will face this positive charge and result in an elevation of the ST segment. An electrode overlying the uninjured end will face a negative charge during stimulation and therefore record ST segment depression. (See Fig 10-2.)

As a practical rule, an electrocardiographic tracing taken directly over injured muscle will record ST segment elevation. If normal muscle lies between the injured muscle and the electrode, ST segment depression will result.

B. T Wave Changes: As a result of ST segment depression, the T wave may be "dragged" downward, producing the appearance of T wave inversion. In addition, true T wave inversion may occur in those leads that record ST segment depression. This T wave inversion is usually of slight to moderate degree. Occasionally, one may see very deep T wave inversion simulating that seen in myocardial infarction.

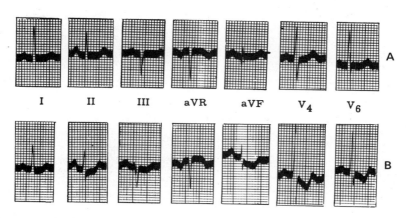

Figure 10-4. Spontaneous angina (coronary insufficiency, myocardial ischemia). *A:* Taken when patient was free of pain. Tracing is within normal limits. *B:* Taken during attack of angina. ST segment depression is most marked in leads II, aVF, V₄, and V₆. Depression is 2 mm in aVF and V₄. Slight ST elevation in aVR. *Clinical diagnosis:* Arteriosclerotic heart disease, anginal syndrome.

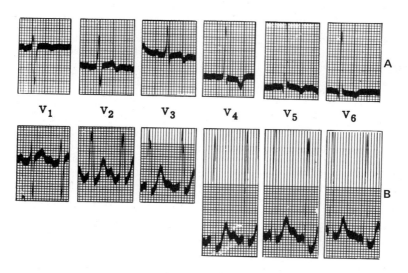

Figure 10-5. Spontaneous angina (coronary insufficiency). *A:* Taken when patient was free of pain. T waves are inverted in V₃₋₆; indicative of anterior wall damage; clinically, the result of an old anterior wall infarction. *B:* During episode of angina. ST segments are now depressed, but T waves are upright in V₂₋₆. This abrupt change from an inverted to an upright T is just as diagnostic of coronary insufficiency as the more usual reverse pattern. The pattern reverted to that seen in (A) a few minutes after the pain subsided.

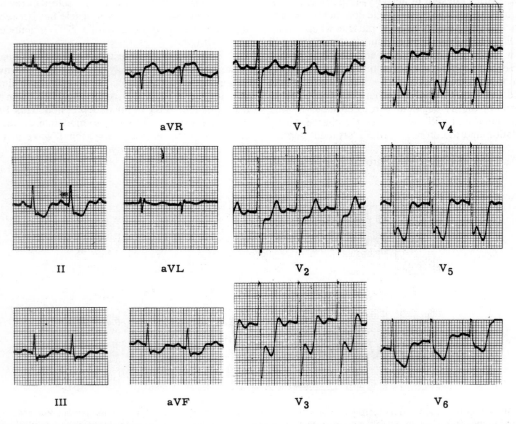

Figure 10–6. Tracing recorded during a spontaneous episode of anginal pain. The ECG was normal before and after. There is marked ST depression in leads I, II, III, aVF, and V_{2-6}. In leads V_{3-5}, the ST depression is 10 mm. This tremendous degree of ST depression is most consistent with triple vessel or left main coronary disease. Coronary arteriography revealed over 90% stenoses in the left main, left anterior descending, circumflex, and right coronary arteries.

ELECTROCARDIOGRAPHIC PATTERNS RESULTING FROM MYOCARDIAL ISCHEMIA

Spontaneous Angina Pectoris (Acute Coronary Insufficiency)

Frequently, the resting ECG is normal in patients who suffer with angina. However, if a tracing is taken during an attack of pain, one may see the pattern of myocardial ischemia. Typically, this produces ST segment depression and, at times, associated T wave inversion in leads that reflect the left ventricular epicardial potential. These are usually the left precordial leads V_{4-6} and leads I, aVL, or aVF, depending upon the heart position. These changes are thought to be due to subendocardial currents of injury. As in the muscle strip illustrations, a left precordial lead electrode records ST segment depression. A cavity lead (such as aVR or aVL, again depending upon heart position) directly faces the muscle area (subendocardial) that has the current of injury and records an ST segment elevation.

In the above circumstances, the ECG returns to normal in a matter of minutes after the anginal episode subsides.

A. Spontaneous Angina With T Wave Changes: If T wave changes do occur, the more common event is inversion of previously upright T waves in left precordial leads and corresponding frontal plane leads (I, aVL). Inverted T waves occasionally become upright during coronary insufficiency. This sudden change is just as indicative of further coronary insufficiency as the former pattern, even though the tracing has a more "normal" appearance.

B. Spontaneous Angina With ST Elevation: ST segment depression is the most typical pattern in the ECG. Less commonly, one may see ST segment elevation during angina. There is evidence that the ST elevation reflects severe transmural ischemia—in contrast to the more usual ST segment depression, which indicates subendocardial ischemia. Such an occurrence in association with major obstructive coronary artery disease has more serious prognostic significance and may predict acute myocardial infarction in the near future. Clinically, such patients commonly

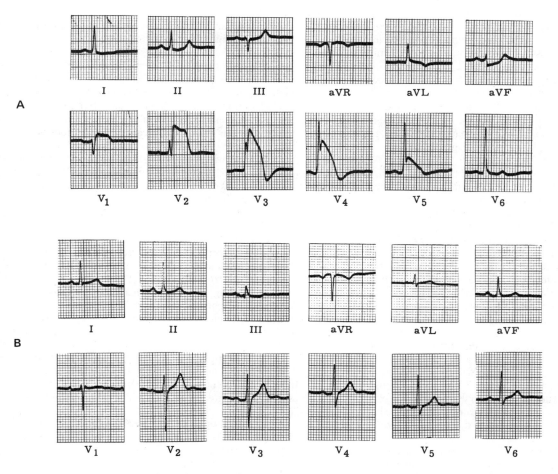

Figure 10–7. Spontaneous angina with ST elevation. *A:* Tracing taken during an episode of anginal pain that occurred while the patient was at bed rest in the hospital. There is marked ST elevation in leads V$_{2-5}$ with some ST depression in aVF. *B:* This tracing was taken 30 minutes after (A). The patient was pain-free and asymptomatic. The ST segments are isoelectric, and the ECG is normal. Subsequent clinical evaluation, including serial ECGs and enzyme determinations, revealed no evidence of acute myocardial infarction. Although tracing (A) is quite typical of early infarction, the rapid disappearance of the ST elevation and the absence of clinical and electrocardiographic evidence of infarction on subsequent examinations indicate that tracing (A) is representative of severe, acute, and reversible ischemia.

have rest angina. The underlying pathologic process may be atherosclerotic coronary artery disease, coronary artery spasm, or both (Fig 10–7). The above is often called the Prinzmetal syndrome or variant angina.

EXERCISE TESTS

Since the resting ECG is normal in 25–40% of patients with angina, exercise tests have been devised to produce myocardial ischemia. It is to be emphasized that the electrocardiographic findings must be used in conjunction with the clinical findings for proper evaluation of the patient.

Types of Exercise Tests

Graded exercise tests utilizing a treadmill or bicycle ergometer have largely replaced the former "two-step" (Master) test. A treadmill test, employing the Bruce protocol, has been extensively studied. A base-line 12-lead ECG is recorded, and the ECG utilizing the lead or leads for the exercise test is then recorded prior to exercise with the patient in the upright position. Since hyperventilation alone (see p 83) can produce ST changes that are indistinguishable from those of myocardial ischemia, a 60-second hyperventilation test is performed prior to exercise. If ST changes occur in association with hyperventilation, this will preclude an interpretation of a positive exercise test. Such changes with hyperventilation have also been reported in individuals with mitral valve prolapse syndrome.

After the patient has been informed of the test and what is expected, he begins walking on the treadmill. The first stage involves walking at 1.7 miles per hour (mph) (2.83 km) at a 10% grade. This is continued for 3 minutes. Unless chest pain or definite electrocardiographic changes (see below) appear, progressive exercise is continued for 3-minute periods at the following levels of exercise: stage 2 = 2.5 mph (4.17 km), 12% grade; stage 3 = 3.4 mph (5.7 km), 14% grade; stage 4 = 4.2 mph (7 km), 16% grade; stage 5 = 5 mph (8.3 km), 18% grade; stage 6 = 5.5 mph (9.12 km), 20% grade; stage 7 = 6 mph (10 km), 22% grade. It is uncommon for patients with coronary artery disease to exercise past stage 5.

The ECG is constantly monitored throughout the test. It has been common practice to record a single lead, usually V_5 (or a modified V_5). However, utilization of multiple leads (eg, V_2, V_5, and aVF) has increased the sensitivity of the test. A physician must be in attendance, and all resuscitation equipment must be available for immediate use. Although the risk of the test in carefully selected patients is small, one must be prepared to treat any untoward event (eg, ventricular fibrillation). In addition to continuous observation of the ECG, the physician instructs the patient to relate any symptoms, especially chest pain, and the physician monitors blood pressure and other physical signs as indicated. The test is continued through the stages mentioned above up to the point of the patient's maximal tolerance or until any of the following appear, in which case the test is discontinued.

(1) Chest pain consistent with angina.

(2) Electrocardiographic changes (see below): Some investigators advise continuation of the test in the absence of chest pain even if electrocardiographic changes (other than ventricular tachycardia) are observed. This author does not recommend this. It is safer to discontinue the test and reevaluate the situation. One can always repeat the test.

(3) Exhaustion, leg pain, or leg weakness which precludes further exercise.

(4) The recognition of other significant clinical signs, such as hypotension, the appearance of a third heart sound, or a new murmur (eg, mitral insufficiency).

Following termination of exercise, the ECG is monitored for at least 6 minutes, and longer if abnor-malities appear, in which case monitoring is continued until the changes have resolved.

Electrocardiographic Criteria (See Fig 10–8.)

A. ST Segment Depression: The most significant criterion for a positive test is ST segment depression of 1 mm or more at a point 0.08 s after the onset of the ST segment (J point). The character of the ST depression has major significance. The various types are as follows:

1. Downsloping ST segment–There is 1 mm or more ST depression at the J point, and the ST segment continues downward for 0.08 s or more. This finding yields the highest specificity for the recognition of myocardial ischemia (based on coronary arteriography as the index for diagnosis). The false-positive incidence is less than 1%.

2. Horizontal ST segment–There is 1 mm or more ST depression at the J point, and the ST segment continues horizontally for 0.08 s or more. Although such a finding has been considered diagnostic of myocardial ischemia, the incidence of false positives (based on the absence of clinical evidence of disease and normal coronary arteriography) is approximately 15%.

3. Slow upstroke of the ST segment–This is defined as ST depression of 1 mm or more at 0.08 s after the J point and an upward sloping of the ST segment not greater than 1 mV/s. The incidence of false positives exceeds 30%.

4. Rapid upstroke of the ST segment–There is 1 mm or more J point depression, but the ST segment is rapidly upward and the slope exceeds 1 mV/s. This is of no diagnostic significance (see below).

B. ST Segment Elevation: Uncommonly, ST segment elevation of more than 1 mm develops. This is evidence of more severe transmural ischemia and is similar to such spontaneous occurrence in Prinzmetal's angina (see p 145).

C. Ventricular Arrhythmias: In the absence of the above-mentioned ST changes, the appearance of occasional ventricular ectopic beats has no diagnostic significance. The appearance of ventricular bigeminy or runs of ventricular ectopic beats is correlated positively with the presence of significant coronary artery disease.

D. R Wave Voltage: In normal persons, the volt-

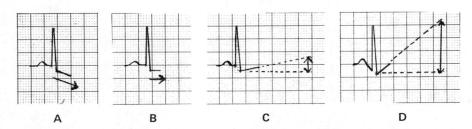

A   B   C   D

Figure 10–8. Diagrams of types of ST segment depressions. *A:* Downsloping. *B:* Horizontal. *C:* Slow upstroking. *D:* Rapid upstroking.

age of the R waves in the monitored leads is reduced or does not change with exercise. In most patients with significant coronary artery disease, the voltage of the R waves will increase in response to exercise. It is believed that this is the result of an increase in left ventricular volume or an alteration in ventricular conduction.

Prognostic Significance

(1) Negative test: An exercise test can be interpreted as negative (ie, none of the above changes appear) only if maximal or near-maximal exercise has been achieved. This is defined by the heart rate. A heart rate of 85% of maximal prediction is essential for such evaluation. A simple method of determining maximal predicted heart rate is 220 minus the patient's age. (***Example:*** For an individual at age 50, a heart rate = 85% [220 − 50] = 145 is a minimum requirement.)

A negative test does not exclude the diagnosis of coronary artery disease. The sensitivity of the test is 60–70%, indicating that 30–40% of patients with known coronary artery disease (based on coronary arteriography) will have a negative test. However, such is more commonly seen in patients with single vessel disease and indicates a relatively good prognosis.

(2) Time of appearance of the electrocardiographic changes: In many individuals, the ST changes will appear—or become more diagnostic—in the immediate postexercise (recovery) period. The earlier these changes appear, the more severe is the coronary artery disease. A positive test occurring during stage 1 or 2 is a more significant finding.

(3) Degree of ST depression: The appearance of 3 mm or more ST depression (downsloping or horizontal) is correlated positively with the presence of severe coronary artery disease, often triple vessel or main left coronary artery disease.

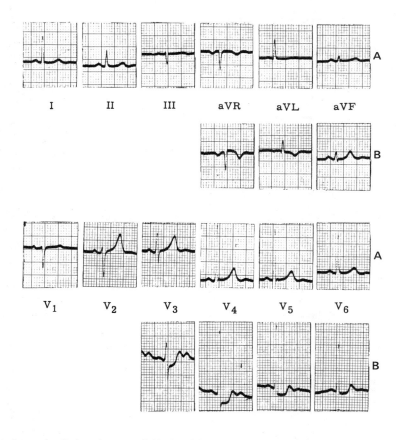

Figure 10–9. Effect of exercise (induced myocardial ischemia). *A:* Taken when patient was free of pain. The only suggestive abnormality is a flat T wave in aVL. *B:* Taken after a standard Master's exercise test. There is minimal ST elevation in aVR and slight ST depression with T wave inversion in aVL. The most striking changes are seen in the precordial leads: There is 2 mm ST depression in V$_3$ and V$_5$; 3.5 mm in V$_4$; 1 mm in V$_6$. *Clinical diagnosis:* Arteriosclerotic heart disease; anginal syndrome.

(4) Duration of ST depression: The duration of the abnormal ST changes during the recovery period is correlated positively with increasing severity of the coronary disease. Persistence for 8 minutes or longer is associated with double or triple vessel disease.

(5) Other significant findings in association with the exercise test are as follows:

(a) Appearance of anginal pain, which is of obvious clinical significance.

(b) Development of hypotension: This is of major significance and indicates abnormal ventricular function.

(c) The appearance of a third heart sound or murmur of mitral insufficiency is evidence of abnormal ventricular function.

Computer Analysis

Computers are commonly used to accurately measure the amount of ST depression and the slope of the ST segment. This is often more accurate than the visual interpretation of the record, since many artifacts can be eliminated and the measurements are made by averaging long periods of recording. Newer computer programs are being developed which, in addition to the above, calculate the area of ST depression in multiple leads and integrate R voltage changes, stage of exercise, and heart rate at which abnormalities appear and the duration of such changes. These techniques improve the sensitivity and specificity of the electrocardiographic stress test.

Atrial Pacing

Atrial pacing is commonly performed in the cardiac catheterization laboratory. It is an excellent method of evaluating ventricular function (by lactate measurements) but is of less value than an exercise test for electrocardiographic evaluation of myocardial ischemia. The latter stimulates catecholamine release, with its attendant cardiac effects; this does not occur with atrial pacing.

Indications for the Exercise Test

The following are the usual circumstances in which an exercise test is indicated:

(1) When the physician is uncertain of the diagnosis of coronary artery disease (eg, atypical chest pain) and the resting ECG is normal.

(2) When the diagnosis of coronary artery disease is known (eg, the patient with stable angina) and the test is done to evaluate the severity of the disease.

(3) When serial exercise tests are done before and after a specific therapeutic regimen (eg, surgery) in order to obtain objective data regarding the efficacy of such treatment.

(4) In the evaluation of suspected normal variants in the ECG (see p 81).

(5) In the evaluation of the patient following myocardial infarction. ECGs are recorded before and after specific amounts of physical activity the physician instructs the patient to perform.

Contraindications to the Exercise Test

An exercise test should not be done in the following circumstances:

(1) When acute myocardial infarction is suspected.

(2) When the clinical manifestations are consistent with crescendo angina or rest angina. Some exceptions may be made, depending on clinical judgment.

(3) When the patient is on digitalis therapy or is hypokalemic. Under these conditions, the appearance of the ST changes after exercise described above is not necessarily indicative of myocardial ischemia.

(4) When the ECG demonstrates ventricular hypertrophy. Diagnostic changes may appear that indicate myocardial ischemia but do not prove the existence of coronary artery disease.

(5) When a WPW rhythm is present (see p 272). Clinically normal individuals with this electrocardiographic finding may develop, after exercise, significant ST depression that is not indicative of myocardial ischemia.

PSEUDODEPRESSION VERSUS ISCHEMIC ST DEPRESSION

Some normal individuals will show apparent ST segment depression in either a resting or postexercise ECG. This is usually associated with tachycardia or anxiety (see p 83). The presence of a prominent T_a wave explains this electrocardiographic finding. The T_a wave persists through ventricular depolarization and is still evident after the QRS complex, thereby producing pseudodepression of the ST segment. This latter pattern can be distinguished from true ST segment depression by the contour of the ST segment and associated downsloping of the PR segment. In pseudodepression associated with tachycardia and an exaggerated T_a wave, the ST segment displays a continuous ascent with upward concavity. In true ST segment depression associated with myocardial ischemia, the ST segment assumes a horizontal or sagging depression. (See Fig 10–10.)

ANEMIA

Any anemia (pernicious anemia, anemia resulting from gastrointestinal hemorrhage, etc) can result in an electrocardiographic pattern of myocardial ischemia, but this usually does not occur in a "normal" heart subjected to anemia. When it is seen in the absence of clinical evidence of heart disease, it usually indicates that there is some degree of subclinical heart disease. In such instances, the ECG becomes normal when the anemia is corrected. (See Figs 10–11 and 10–12.)

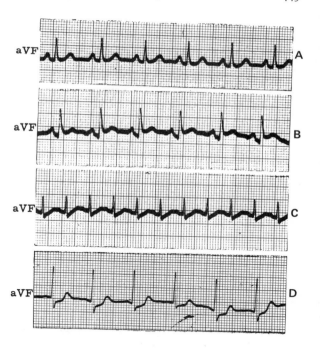

Figure 10–10. Pseudodepression versus coronary type of ST segment depression. *A:* Normal tracing; rate = 92; ST segment isoelectric. *B:* Prominent T_a waves; rate = 100; ST segment is isoelectric, being on the same level as the T–P segment. The PR segment is downsloping. *C:* Sinus tachycardia; rate = 168. ST segments appear depressed, but the ST segment displays a continuous ascent with upward concavity. This is typical of the pseudodepression associated with tachycardia and an exaggerated T_a wave. *D:* True ST segment depression associated with myocardial ischemia (postexercise record); the contour of the ST segment is that of horizontal depression.

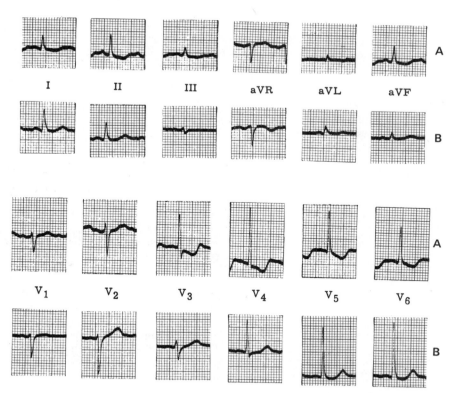

Figure 10–11. Anemia. *A:* Tracing of a 50-year-old man with massive gastrointestinal hemorrhage from a bleeding duodenal ulcer. Red blood count = 1.2 million. There is ST depression in leads aVF and V_{3-6}. Such a pattern is consistent with but by no means diagnostic of myocardial ischemia, since other conditions can produce a similar pattern. Clinically, there was no evidence of heart disease. The patient was not in shock at the time of this record. *B:* Taken 3 days after (A); patient had received blood transfusions; red blood count = 3.5 million. Slight ST depression persists in V_{4-6}, but marked improvement has occurred.

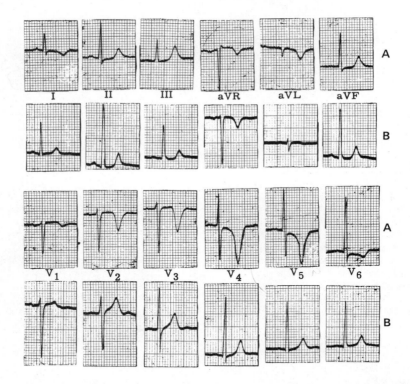

Figure 10–12. Anemia. *A:* Tracing of a 55-year-old man with pernicious anemia; red blood count = 1 million. Note the very deep and symmetrically inverted T waves in the precordial leads with a lesser degree of T wave inversion in leads I and aVL. This pattern is quite consistent with myocardial infarction (? subendocardial). Clinically, however, this patient had no evidence of heart disease. *B:* Taken 10 days after (A). The patient had received blood transfusions and vitamin B_{12}; red blood count = 4 million. The present tracing is within normal limits. Several subsequent tracings remained normal. ¶The pattern in (A) is an extreme and unusual pattern of myocardial ischemia. Actual myocardial infarction was initially suspected, but the lack of clinical evidence of heart disease and the reversal to a normal pattern in 10 days favored a diagnosis of myocardial ischemia.

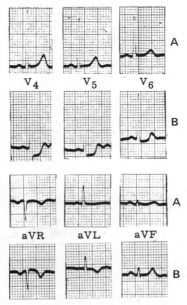

Figure 10–13. Myocardial ischemia. *A:* Resting ECG. *B:* During spontaneous angina or after exercise.

SUMMARY OF ELECTROCARDIOGRAPHIC CRITERIA OF MYOCARDIAL ISCHEMIA

(1) Precordial leads: ST segment depression or T wave inversion (or both) in precordial leads V_{2-6}.

(2) Extremity leads: Changes similar to those described in precordial leads are seen in aVL or aVF (depending upon the direction of the frontal plane vector). Reciprocal ST segment elevation may be seen in aVR.

(3) Standard leads (not shown at the left): These will reflect the pattern present in the extremity leads. If the changes noted above are seen in aVL, they will be present in I; if seen in aVF, they will be present in III.

The above changes seen in any single ECG are not diagnostic of coronary insufficiency. The sudden change from a normal tracing to the above pattern (or the reverse) in association with clinical evidence of angina is necessary for correct evaluation.

Myocardial infarction is characterized by the necrosis of a portion of the myocardium resulting from a lack of sufficient blood supply to keep the muscle viable.

Etiology & Incidence

The same conditions that produce coronary insufficiency (myocardial ischemia) can produce myocardial infarction. The most common cause is complete occlusion of a coronary artery by arteriosclerotic coronary thrombosis. However, infarction may result from incomplete occlusion of a coronary artery if this latter process sufficiently reduces the blood supply to that portion of the myocardium and if collateral circulation is insufficient. Furthermore, complete thrombosis of a coronary artery can occur without myocardial infarction if a sufficient collateral circulation already exists. Hence, the terms myocardial infarction and coronary thrombosis are not synonymous. The left ventricle is involved in practically all instances of myocardial infarction. The right ventricle may become infarcted in association with left ventricular infarction. This most commonly occurs in association with inferior wall infarction and is manifested clinically by evidence of right ventricular failure in the absence of left ventricular failure.

Differential Diagnosis

The electrocardiographic differential diagnosis is discussed on pp 189–192. Clinically, the diagnosis of myocardial infarction must be differentiated from many disease processes that occur within the thorax and abdomen, eg, pulmonary embolism, hiatal hernia, dissecting aneurysm, thoracic radiculitis, and diseases of the biliary tract, upper gastrointestinal tract, and pancreas.

Clinical Significance

The diagnosis of myocardial infarction must never rest solely upon electrocardiographic findings. The ECG may actually be normal in myocardial infarction or may merely show nonspecific changes that are not diagnostic of infarction. It is frequently necessary to take serial ECGs to show progressive changes.

Of the greatest importance is the fact that the ECG must be used in conjunction with the clinical findings. If the history, physical examination, and other labora-

tory data (white blood cell count, sedimentation rate, serum enzymes) strongly indicate myocardial infarction, the diagnosis must not be discarded merely because the infarct cannot be diagnosed by the ECG.

Prognosis

In general, an uncomplicated inferior (or posterior) wall infarction has a less serious immediate prognosis than an anterior wall infarction. However, the location and "size" of the infarct as interpreted from the ECG must not be used alone in evaluating the immediate prognosis. A "small" infarct can be fatal, and a patient with a "large" infarct may have an entirely uneventful course.

In the long-term follow-up of the patient, the ECG should not be relied upon as the sole method of evaluation. Naturally, a stable ECG is a favorable sign. However, even if the ECG reverts to normal, neither the physician nor the patient should be lulled into believing that the heart is "normal."

A sudden change of previously inverted T waves to more "normally" upright T waves usually means further coronary insufficiency rather than improvement (Fig 11–68).

MECHANISM OF THE ELECTROCARDIOGRAPHIC PATTERN

THE ABNORMAL Q WAVE & THE QS COMPLEX

The most diagnostic electrocardiographic finding in myocardial infarction is an abnormal Q wave (or QS complex). In order to understand the significance and genesis of this Q wave, it is essential to emphasize the following:

(1) Small q waves are normal in many leads (see Chapter 5). They are commonly recorded in leads I, aVF, and V_{4-6}, are not over 0.02 s in duration, and the Q:R ratio is less than 25%.

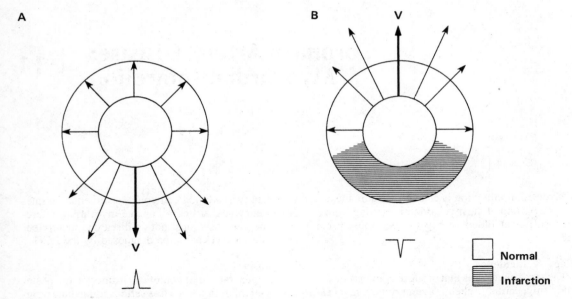

Figure 11–1. *A:* Cross section of the left ventricle. The arrows pointing from the endocardium to the epicardial surface represent normal depolarization. In this illustration (eg, the initial 0.04 s of ventricular depolarization), there are greater forces directed downward, resulting in a mean force in that direction (heavy arrow, V). An electrode overlying this area will record an upright deflection. *B:* An area of myocardial infarction in the area of myocardium that had previously resulted in the major and mean forces (see [A] at left). Therefore, there will be a loss of such forces, resulting in a mean force now oriented in an opposite direction (heavy arrow, V). An electrode overlying this area will record a negative deflection (abnormal Q wave or QS complex).

(2) The electrocardiographic recording at any given moment in time represents the mean of electrical forces going in many spatial directions. Because of this, approximately 90% of such forces are canceled, leaving only 10% to be recorded (Fig 11–1, at left). When myocardial infarction of significant extent occurs, the forces of depolarization from that area will be lost. The result will be a change in direction of the mean forces which will now be directed away from the site of infarction (Fig 11–1, at right). This is most significant during the initial 0.04–0.05 s of ventricular depolarization and results in the abnormal Q wave (or QS complex) in leads overlying the infarct zone. A smaller area of infarction may be insufficient to alter the mean forces to a sufficient degree to produce the above but may merely reduce the magnitude of the normal mean force. This will result in a reduction in R wave voltage. Such a finding, however, has less diagnostic significance than the recording of an abnormal Q wave. The emphasis, as stated above, is on the initial 0.04–0.05 s of ventricular depolarization. There are undoubtedly abnormalities occurring in the late period of ventricular depolarization, but these do not result in any definite electrocardiographic changes of diagnostic significance in clinical electrocardiographic interpretation.

An abnormal Q wave is defined by the following criteria:

(1) Q duration of 0.04 s or greater.
(2) Q:R ratio = 25% or greater.

Major exceptions to the above are the following:

(1) Above criteria in lead III alone: It is common for lead III to record Q waves of 0.04 s duration and a Q:R ratio greater than 25%. This is especially so in normals with mean frontal plane QRS axes of +30 degrees to 0 degrees (horizontal heart position). When such is seen as a normal finding, lead aVF will not record an abnormal Q wave. Therefore, the diagnosis of infarction (inferior wall) must never be made on the basis of lead III alone.

(2) Above criteria in aVL alone: In normal persons, especially those with frontal plane QRS axes of +60 degrees to +90 degrees (vertical heart position), lead aVL may record the above criteria. However, in the absence of significant abnormalities in lead I or precordial leads, this finding in aVL alone is a very unreliable sign of myocardial infarction. It has been suggested that such is an indication of a "high-lateral myocardial infarction" and that third interspace precordial leads would offer useful information when the conventional precordial leads are normal. However, in this author's opinion, the latter will result in an unacceptable number of incorrect diagnoses of infarction.

(3) Any q wave in V_2: This is defined as a q wave followed by an R wave (a qR or qrS complex, but not a QS complex). It is abnormal in over 95% but is not pathognomonic of myocardial infarction (anteroseptal), since other conditions that mimic infarction can produce this (see p 190).

Vector Analysis

The alterations in the QRS vector resulting from transmural infarction are as follows:

(1) The QRS vector, and especially the initial 0.04 s, is abnormally directed, pointing away from the zone of infarction. Thus, in anterior wall infarction the vector is directed posteriorly; in posterior wall infarction it is directed anteriorly; in inferior wall infarction it is directed superiorly; and in lateral (left) wall infarction it is directed to the right. This produces the abnormal Q wave or QS complex in the ECG.

(2) This abnormally directed QRS vector is at least 0.04 s in duration; for this reason the abnormal Q wave is similarly at least 0.04 s in duration.

THE ST SEGMENT CHANGES

Most frequently, the first electrocardiographic finding in myocardial infarction is ST segment elevation in a lead overlying the area of infarction. The ST segment characteristically has a convex upward curvature.

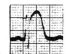

**Epicardial lead
directly over infarct**

Cavity leads and leads that are placed approximately 180 degrees from the area of infarction show reciprocal ST segment depression. These changes are analogous to those described for injury currents in the isolated muscle strip. (See p 140.)

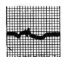

Cavity lead

It is believed that completely dead muscle cannot produce ST segment changes. Therefore, the occurrence of these changes early in infarction indicates the presence of some viable muscle in the epicardial region.

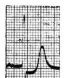

**Epicardial lead
180 degrees from infarct**

THE T WAVE CHANGES

Within the first few hours of infarction, "giant" upright T waves may be seen in leads overlying the infarct. The exact cause is not known but, in part, may be due to leakage of intracellular potassium from the damaged muscle cells into the extracellular spaces.

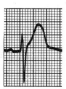

Over infarct

After a period of hours or days (up to 2 weeks), the ST segment returns to the isoelectric line and T wave changes occur. The T wave changes may begin to develop while the ST segments are still deviated. The T waves begin to invert in those leads that showed ST segment elevation.

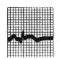

Over infarct

The typical infarction T wave is inverted and abnormally symmetric, ie, the peak of the T is midway between the beginning and the end.

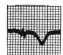

Over infarct

In leads that showed ST segment depression, the T waves become tall and are likewise symmetric.

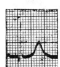

180 degrees from infarct

The "coronary T" or "Pardee T" refers to an inverted T wave in which the ST segment is isoelectric but shows an upward convexity.

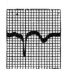

The "cove-plane T" refers to an elevated ST segment with upward convexity followed by an inverted T.

The T waves may remain inverted for the remainder of the patient's life; or, after many months, the T waves may gradually revert to normal.

The abnormal Q waves may appear very early or late. They are usually not seen within the first few hours following an infarction. They may appear at any time thereafter, being seen while the ST segment changes are present or appearing after the ST segment has become isoelectric. They usually appear before marked T wave changes occur, but this is not invariable. As stated above, abnormal Q waves may never appear; instead, there may be reduced voltage of the R wave.

LOCALIZATION OF MYOCARDIAL INFARCTION BY ELECTROCARDIOGRAPHIC PATTERNS

By observing the above infarct patterns in specific leads of the ECG, one can localize anatomically the site of the infarction. In order to have a clearer understanding of this, it will be wise to review briefly the anatomy of the coronary circulation.

The blood supply to the heart is derived from the left and right coronary arteries, which arise from the left and right aortic sinuses, respectively. Shortly after its origin, the left coronary artery divides into the left anterior descending and the left circumflex arteries. The former supplies the anterior surface of the left ventricle, the medial portion of the anterior surface of the right ventricle, and the lower third of the posterior surface of the right ventricle. The remainder of the right ventricle is supplied by the right coronary artery. The left circumflex artery supplies the lateral wall and the lower (apical) half of the posterior wall of the left ventricle. The upper (basal) half of the posterior wall and the inferior wall of the left ventricle are supplied by the right coronary artery. There will be some variations of the above in normal individuals, depending upon the dominance of the right or left coronary systems. In disease states, the blood supply to myocardial areas will vary, depending upon the sites of coronary artery

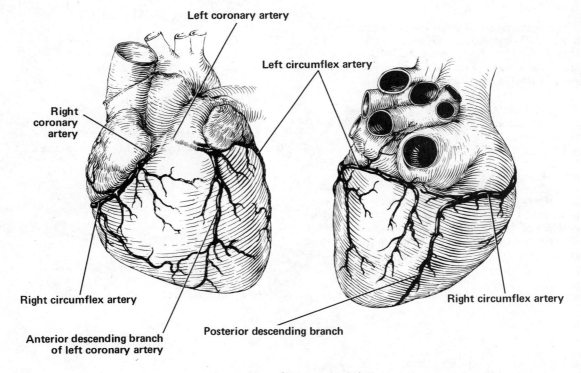

Figure 11–2. Coronary circulation.

disease and the presence or absence of collateral circulation.

The SA node has a dual blood supply from branches of the right coronary and the left circumflex arteries. The AV node receives its major supply from a branch of the right coronary artery. The His bundle is supplied by the above AV nodal artery and a septal branch of the left anterior descending artery. The proximal right bundle branch is supplied by both the AV nodal artery and by septal branches of the left anterior descending artery. The left anterior fascicle receives its major supply from septal branches of the left anterior descending artery. The left posterior fascicle has a dual supply from the posterior descending branch of the right coronary artery and septal branches of the left anterior descending artery.

By applying the criteria for recognition of infarction to specific leads, one can determine the site of infarction.

Site of Infarct	Leads That Reflect the Infarct
Anterior	V_{2-6}
Inferior	aVF (and II, III)
Lateral (left ventricle)	I, aVL, V_6
Posterior	V_{1-2} (esophageal leads)

Infarction of the interventricular septum can be suspected if there is a new bundle branch block. There are no reliable electrocardiographic criteria for the recognition of right ventricular infarction.

initial vector is oriented to the right, an abnormal Q wave will be seen in lead I. In the early stage of infarction, the ST vector is oriented anteriorly (and to the left), resulting in ST segment elevation in left precordial leads (and lead I). In the later stage, the T vector is oriented posteriorly (and to the right), producing inverted T waves in left precordial leads (and lead I).

Some investigators have attributed the pattern of inferior wall infarction to associated anterior infarction. It is postulated that the heart is in such a position that the anterior wall overlies the diaphragm and hence the anterior infarction is reflected into leads II, III, and aVF. The absence of infarction in esophageal leads was used to exclude posterior infarction. The last statement is true, but it does not exclude inferior infarction. Such records are most often indicative of anterior and inferior infarction, but the remote possibility of only anterior infarction exists.

[Text cont'd on p 164.]

ANTERIOR WALL INFARCTION

Early & Late Anterior Wall Infarction

The precordial leads best reflect infarction of the anterior wall. In frontal plane leads, I and aVL will usually show the infarction pattern. The characteristic findings in transmural infarction involving the entire thickness of the anterior wall will be the following:

A. Standard Leads: Epicardial infarction pattern (ST elevation → abnormal Q wave and T wave inversion) in I. Lead III may show reciprocal change, most characteristically ST depression.

B. Extremity Leads: The heart position is usually horizontal, and the left ventricular epicardial pattern will therefore be seen in aVL. Lead aVF may show reciprocal ST segment depression and, later, tall T waves.

C. Precordial Leads: Depending upon the extent of the anterior wall infarct, precordial leads from V_{1-7} will show the infarct.

D. Vector Analysis: The initial 0.04 s QRS vector is directed posteriorly, resulting in abnormal Q waves or QS complexes in precordial leads. If this

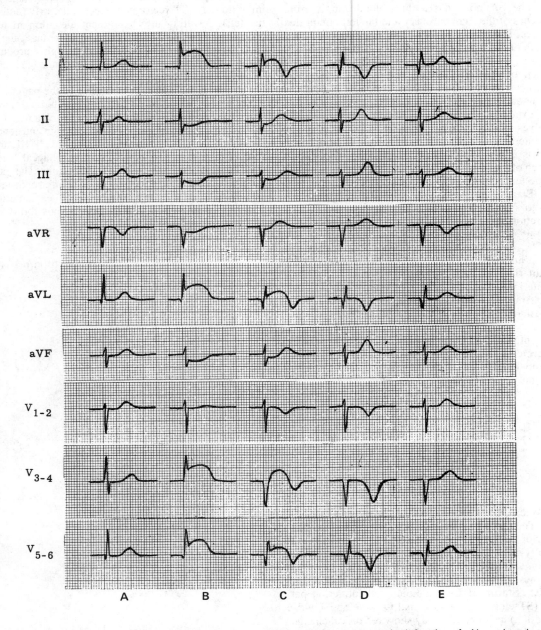

Figure 11–3. Diagrammatic illustration of serial electrocardiographic patterns in anterior infarction. *A:* Normal tracing. *B:* Very early pattern (hours after infarction): ST segment elevation in I, aVL, and V_{3-6}; reciprocal ST depression in II, III, and aVF. *C:* Later pattern (many hours to a few days): Q waves have appeared in I, aVL, and V_{5-6}. QS complexes are present in V_{3-4}. This indicates that the major transmural infarction is underlying the area recorded by V_{3-4}; ST segment changes persist but are of lesser degree, and the T waves are beginning to invert in those leads in which the ST segments are elevated. *D:* Late established pattern (many days to weeks): The Q waves and QS complexes persist; the ST segments are isoelectric; the T waves are symmetric and deeply inverted in leads that had ST elevation and tall in leads that had ST depression. This pattern may persist for the remainder of the patient's life. *E:* Very late pattern: This may occur many months to years after the infarct. The abnormal Q waves and QS complexes persist. The T waves have gradually returned to normal.

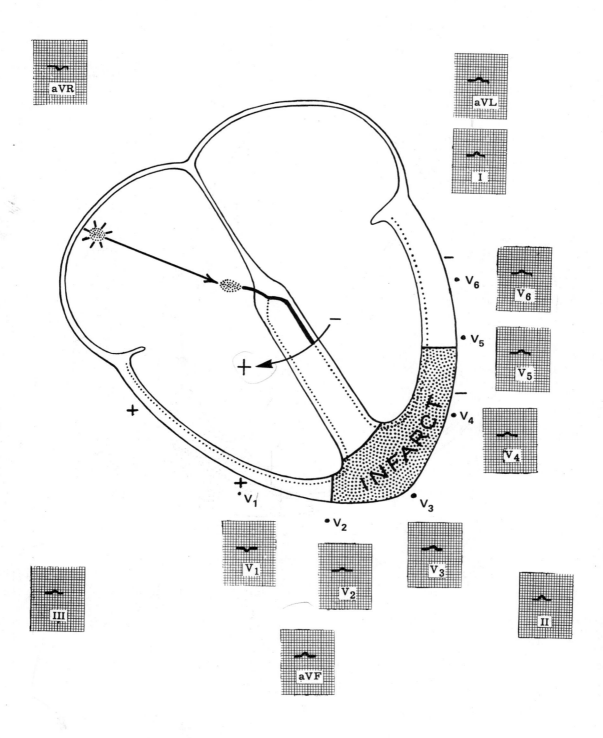

Figure 11—4. Sequence of anterior wall infarction. Atrial and interventricular septal activation.

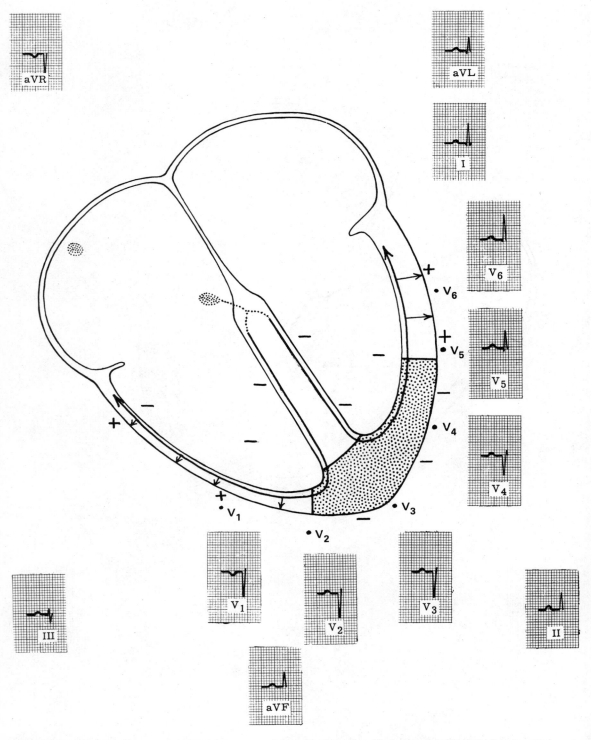

Figure 11–5. Sequence of anterior wall infarction. Ventricular depolarization. The pattern as illustrated demonstrates an infarct of several days' duration, thus accounting for abnormal Q waves and ST segment and T wave changes. The initial 0.04 s Q vector is oriented posteriorly (as a result of the anterior wall infarct), producing the abnormal Q waves in V_{2-4}.

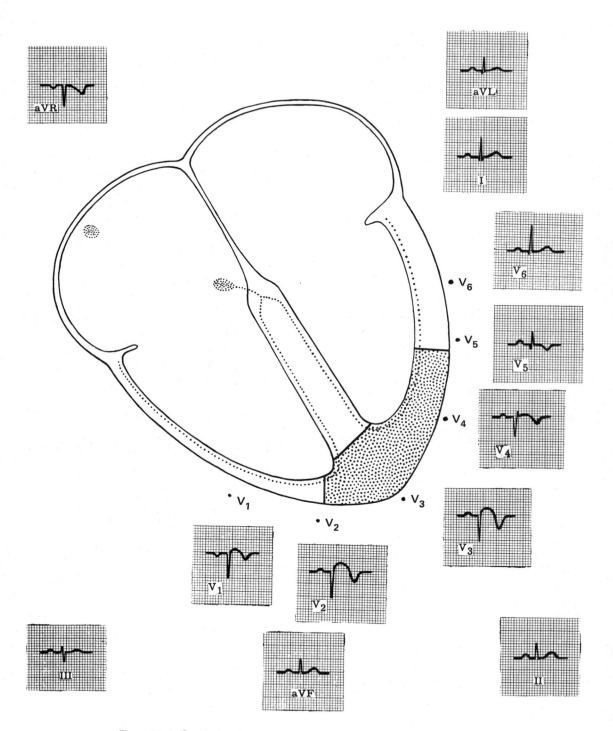

Figure 11–6. Sequence of anterior wall infarction. Ventricular repolarization.

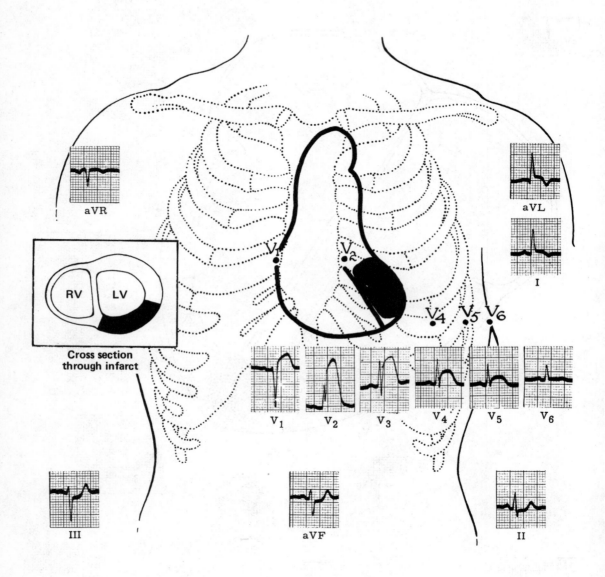

Figure 11–7. Early anterior wall infarction. Note the marked convex ST segment elevation in leads V₂₋₅; the lesser degree of ST elevation with T wave inversion in I and aVL; the reciprocal ST depression in II, III, and aVF. *Clinical diagnosis:* Recent (6 hours) myocardial infarction.

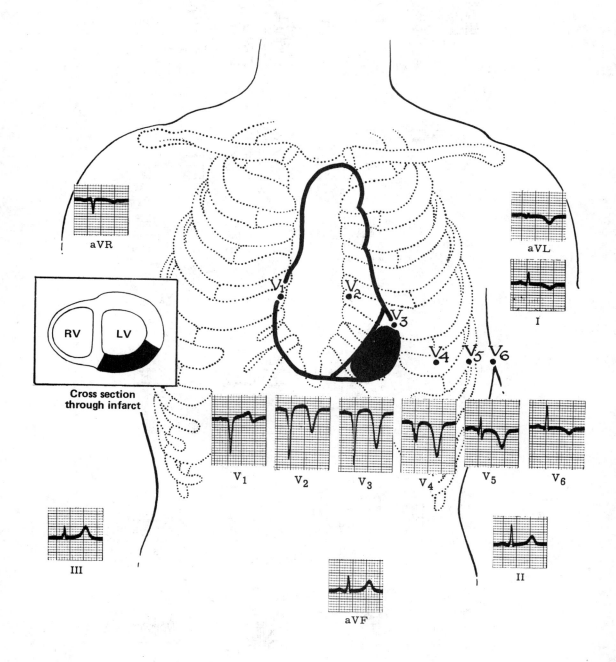

Figure 11–8. Late pattern of anterior wall infarction. QS complexes are present in V_{1-4}. The T waves are deeply and symmetrically inverted in I, aVL, and V_{2-6}. *Clinical diagnosis:* Myocardial infarction, 6 months old.

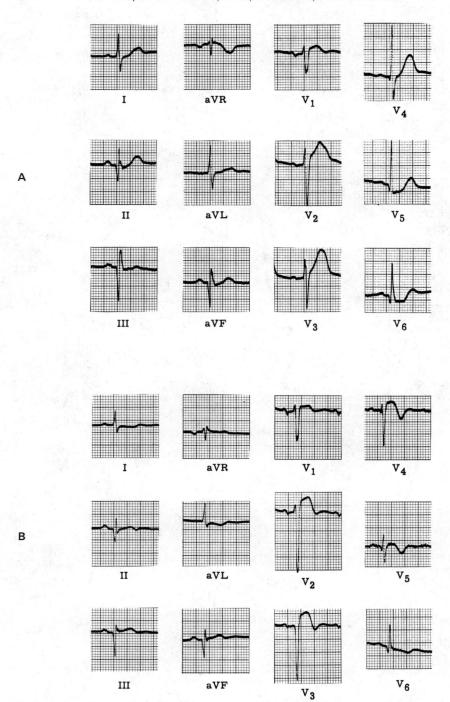

Figure 11–9. Acute anterior infarction (and old inferior infarction). *A:* There is ST elevation in V_{1-3} and ST depression in V_{4-6}. There are large, broad, upright T waves in I, II, and V_{2-4}. The above are consistent with recent anterior infarction. In addition, the Q waves in II, III, and aVF are indicative of inferior wall infarction (see p 169) and the S in I and R in aVF are evidence of associated left posterior fascicular block (see p 205). Clinically, this record was taken 1 hour after the onset of severe, crushing substernal pain. The patient had a documented inferior wall infarction 1 year previously. *B:* One day after the above: The giant T waves are no longer present. The T waves have become inverted in I, II, and precordial leads. A QS complex has appeared in V_3. The above is evidence of recent anterior wall infarction.

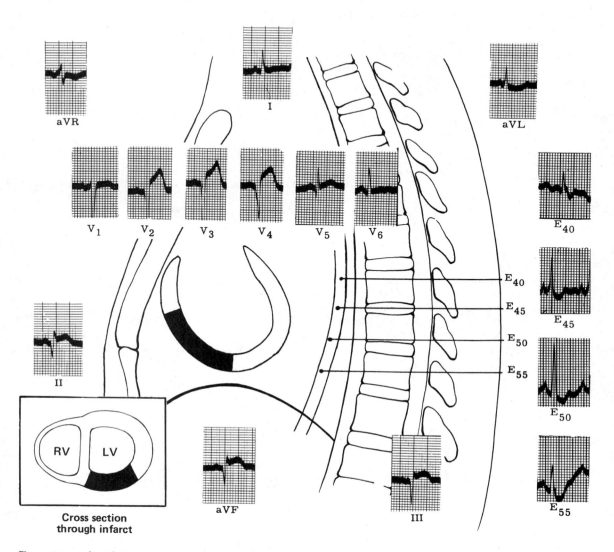

Figure 11–10. Anterior wall infarction pattern "reflected into lead aVF." *Standard leads:* There are deep, wide Q waves (producing Qr complexes) with elevated ST segments in II and III. *Extremity leads:* Deep, wide Q with elevated ST in aVF. The pattern in standard and extremity leads is typical of recent inferior wall infarction. *Precordial leads:* Normal r in V$_1$; small r in V$_2$; QS complexes in V$_{3-4}$; qR pattern in V$_5$. The ST segments are elevated in V$_{2-5}$. The T waves in these leads are still upright. This pattern definitely indicates recent anterior wall infarction. The above tracing indicates early infarction of the anterior and inferior walls of the left ventricle. *Esophageal leads:* To further investigate the latter diagnosis, esophageal leads were done. Leads E$_{40-55}$ show no abnormal Q waves. This definitely indicates the absence of true posterior wall infarction but does not exclude inferior infarction. *Clinical diagnosis:* Recent myocardial infarction (2 days old). *Autopsy diagnosis:* Recent infarction of anteroseptal and anteroapical surfaces of the left ventricle; occlusion of left anterior descending coronary artery; no infarction present on inferior or posterior walls. Thus, the patterns in leads II, III, and aVF are a reflection of the anterior wall infarct, probably as a result of backward displacement of the apex allowing the anterior wall to overlie the left diaphragm.

Anterior Wall Infarction Involving Limited Areas

Anterior wall infarction can be further subdivided into the following categories:

A. Anteroseptal Infarction: The infarct pattern will be seen in precordial leads V_{1-3}. Since the infarction does not extend to the lateral wall of the left ventricle, it will not be reflected into leads I and aVL; hence, the extremity leads and standard leads will not show the infarct pattern.

B. Anteroapical Infarction: Precordial leads V_{3-5} will show the infarct pattern. Again, this may not be seen in extremity and standard leads.

C. Anterolateral Infarction: The pattern is seen in precordial leads V_{4-7}. It is reflected into leads aVL and I.

In high anterolateral wall infarction, the usual precordial leads may not show the typical patterns. However, lead aVL usually will reflect the infarct pattern. In such an instance, it may be of value to take higher precordial leads (such as third interspace leads) to evaluate the pattern seen in aVL. Caution must be used in the interpretation of such high precordial leads. In some normal individuals, QS complexes can be seen in the V_{1-3} position in the third intercostal space. Therefore, this, as an isolated finding, must not be used for the diagnosis of myocardial infarction.

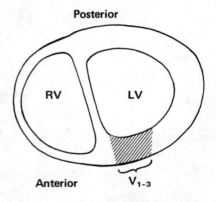

Figure 11–11. Anteroseptal infarction.

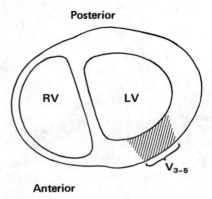

Figure 11–12. Anteroapical infarction.

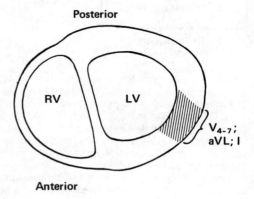

Figure 11–13. Anterolateral infarction.

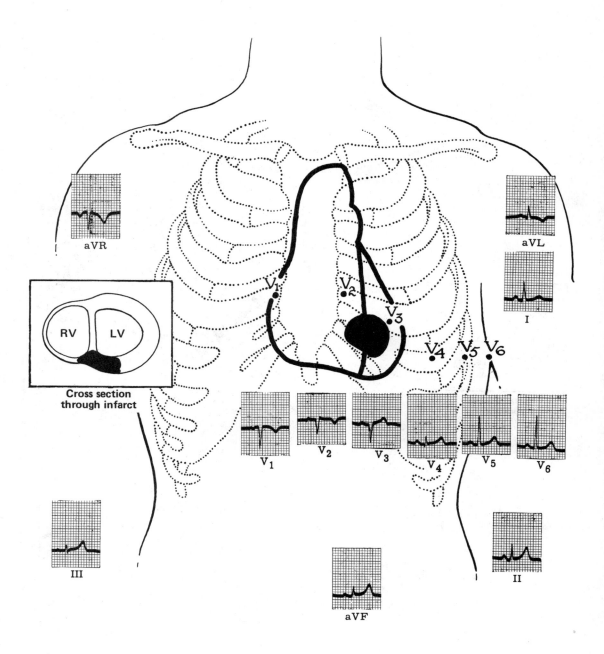

Figure 11–14. Anteroseptal infarction (late pattern). QS complexes are present in V_{2-3}. The T is inverted in V_{1-2} and aVL. *Clinical and autopsy diagnosis:* Anteroseptal infarction, 6 months old.

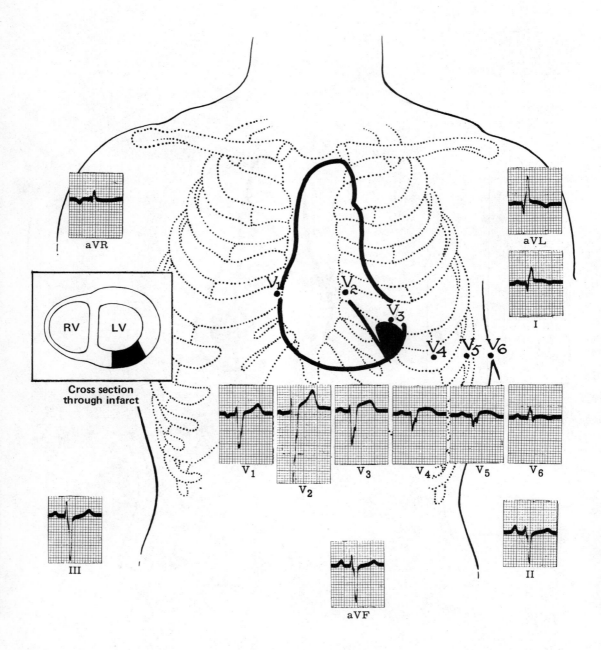

Figure 11–15. Anteroapical myocardial infarction. Wide Q waves are present in I and aVL; minute r waves are seen in V₄₋₅; the T waves are inverted in I, aVL, and V₆; the ST segments are elevated in I, aVL, and V₂₋₅. The frontal plane QRS axis = −75 degrees, indicating a left anterior fascicular block. *Clinical diagnosis:* Myocardial infarction, 2 weeks old.

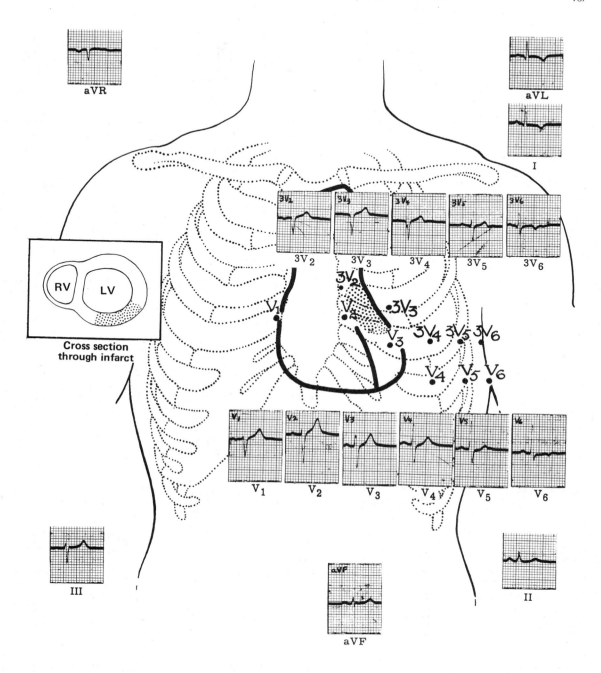

Figure 11–16. High anterior and lateral wall infarction. The above illustration shows the value of third interspace leads. A small but wide q wave is present in I and aVL. The T waves are inverted in V_6, aVL, and I. The precordial leads are not indicative of infarction. In view of the suspicious pattern in aVL, third interspace leads were taken, revealing QS complexes in $3V_{2-4}$. *Clinical diagnosis:* Arteriosclerotic heart disease; history of myocardial infarction 1 year previously.

SUMMARY OF ELECTROCARDIOGRAPHIC CRITERIA OF ANTERIOR MYOCARDIAL INFARCTION

A. Precordial Leads:

1. Convex ST segment elevation in more than one lead from V_{3-6} (early).

2. QS complexes or abnormal Q waves (ie, Q waves of 0.04 s or more in width or 25% or more of the voltage of the R wave in the same lead [or both]) in more than one lead from V_{3-6} (late).

3. T wave inversion (typically deep, symmetric inversion) in more than one lead from V_{3-6} (late).

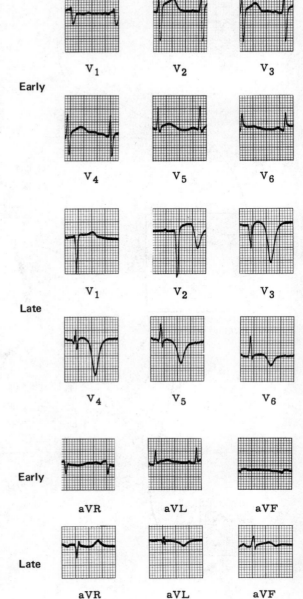

B. Extremity Leads:
The pattern described in precordial leads may be seen in aVL if the infarction involves the anterolateral wall (eg, seen in V_{6-7}).

A QS complex (vertical heart position) or a QR complex may normally be seen in aVL. In these circumstances, the P is inverted. The presence of an upright P with a QS or QR complex in aVL, and the presence of normal precordial leads or precordial leads that are not diagnostic of infarction, should make one suspicious of a high anterolateral wall infarction. In this circumstance, third interspace precordial leads may be of value.

C. Standard Leads:
With anterolateral wall infarction, the infarct pattern will be reflected in lead I.

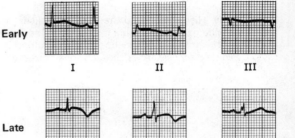

INFERIOR–POSTERIOR WALL INFARCTION

In electrocardiography the term posterior wall infarction has been used to describe an infarction that anatomically involves the inferior (diaphragmatic) wall or the true posterior wall of the left ventricle. It is preferable to separate these 2 entities since the resulting electrocardiographic patterns are different.

Inferior (Diaphragmatic) Wall Infarction

Since this area of infarction overlies the left diaphragm, the pattern will be seen in leads aVF, II, and III. The characteristic findings of transmural infarction in this area will be the following:

A. Standard Leads: Infarct pattern in leads II and III. At the time of ST segment elevation in leads II and III, reciprocal ST depression will be seen in lead I. Later, with deep T wave inversion in II and III, the T will become tall in I.

B. Extremity Leads: Infarct pattern in aVF. Similar reciprocal changes in aVL, as seen in lead I.

C. Precordial Leads: Usually the precordial leads are not abnormal. At times, they may show reciprocal changes with early ST segment depression and, later, abnormally tall, symmetric T waves in leads V_{1-3} as evidence of true posterior wall infarction.

D. Vector Analysis: The initial 0.04 s QRS vector is directed superiorly, thus producing the abnormal Q wave in leads aVF, II, and III. In the early stage of infarction, the ST vector is directed inferiorly, producing ST segment elevation in these leads. In the later stage, the T vector is oriented superiorly, resulting in inverted T waves in aVF, II, and III.

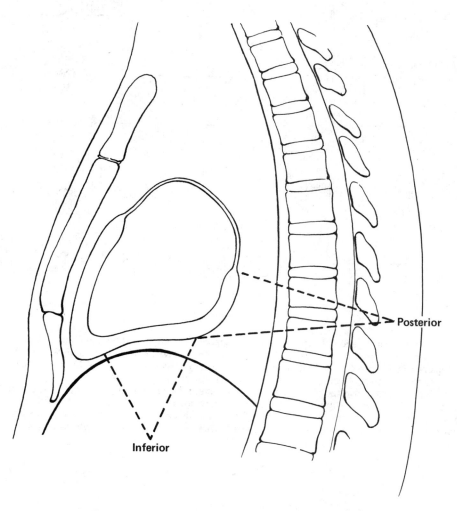

Figure 11–17. Inferior (diaphragmatic) and posterior locations.

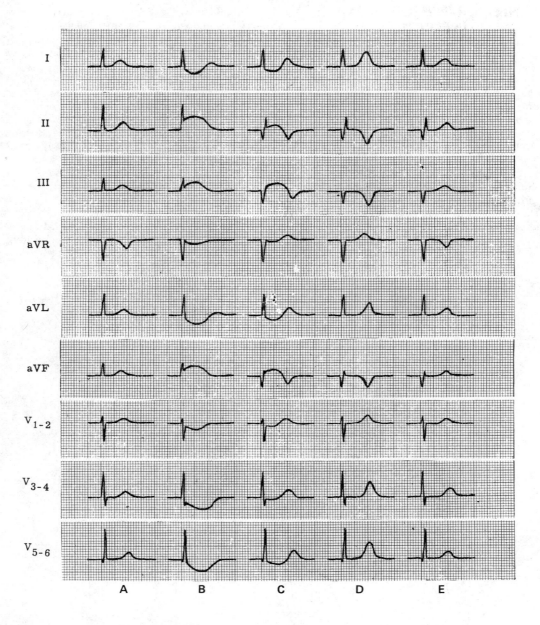

Figure 11–18. Diagrammatic illustration of serial electrocardiographic pattern in inferior (and posterior) wall infarction. *A:* Normal tracing. *B:* Very early pattern (hours after infarction): ST segment elevation in II, III, and aVF; ST segment depression in I, aVR, aVL, and precordial leads. *C:* Later pattern (many hours to a few days): Abnormal Q waves have appeared in II, III, and aVF. There is less ST segment elevation in these leads and less reciprocal ST segment depression in the leads shown in (B). The T waves are becoming inverted in II, III, and aVF. *D:* Late established pattern (many days to weeks): The ST segments are now isoelectric. Deep symmetrically inverted T waves are seen in II, III, and aVF. This is evidence of inferior wall infarction. The T waves are abnormally tall and symmetric in I, aVL, and precordial leads. These are the reciprocal results of true posterior wall infarction. *E:* Very late pattern (many months to years): The abnormal Q waves persist, but the T waves have become normal.

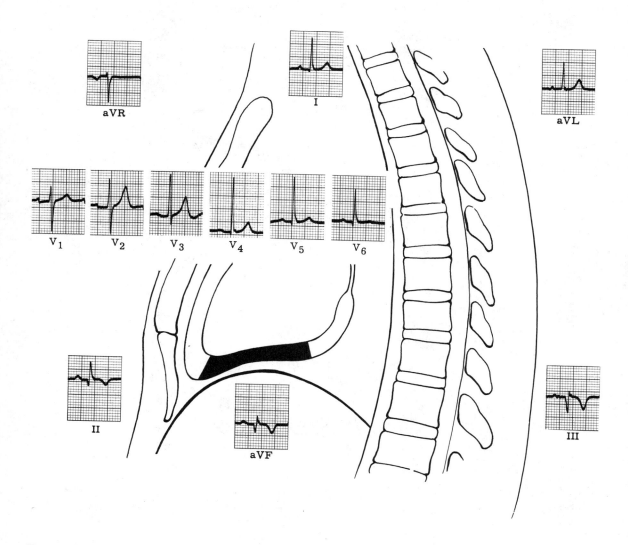

Figure 11–19. Inferior wall infarction. Deep and wide Q waves are present in leads II, III, and aVF. The T waves are deeply and symmetrically inverted in these leads. *Clinical diagnosis:* Myocardial infarction, 2 weeks old.

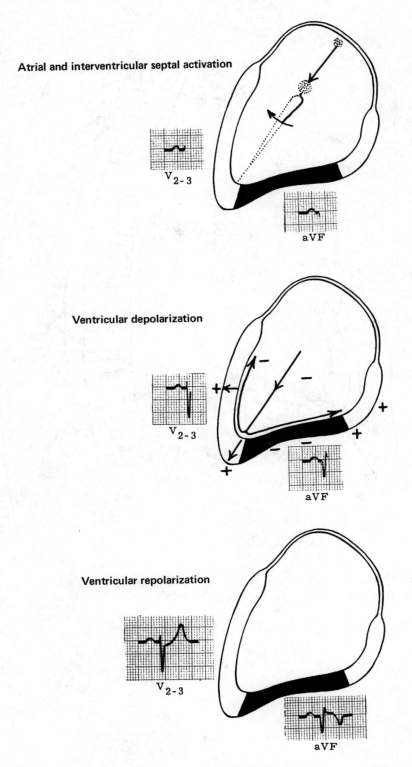

Figure 11–20. Inferior wall infarction. The pattern as illustrated demonstrates an infarct of several days' duration, thus accounting for the abnormal Q waves and ST segment and T wave changes. The initial 0.04 s QRS vector is oriented superiorly (Q in aVF), the ST vector is oriented inferiorly (ST elevation in aVF) and posteriorly (ST depression in V_{2-3}), and the T vector is oriented superiorly (inverted T in aVF) and anteriorly (abnormally tall T in V_{2-3}).

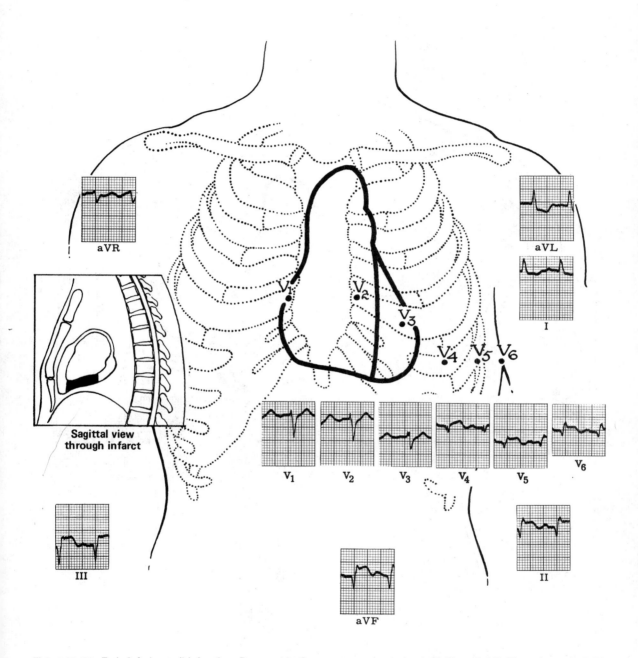

Figure 11–21. Early inferior wall infarction. Deep, wide Q waves are seen in leads II, III, and aVF. There is marked ST elevation in these leads which is typical of recent inferior wall infarction. Similar changes are seen in V₄₋₆, indicating additional anterolateral wall infarction. Reciprocal ST depression is seen in leads I, aVL, and V₁₋₃. *Clinical diagnosis:* Myocardial infarction, 24 hours old.

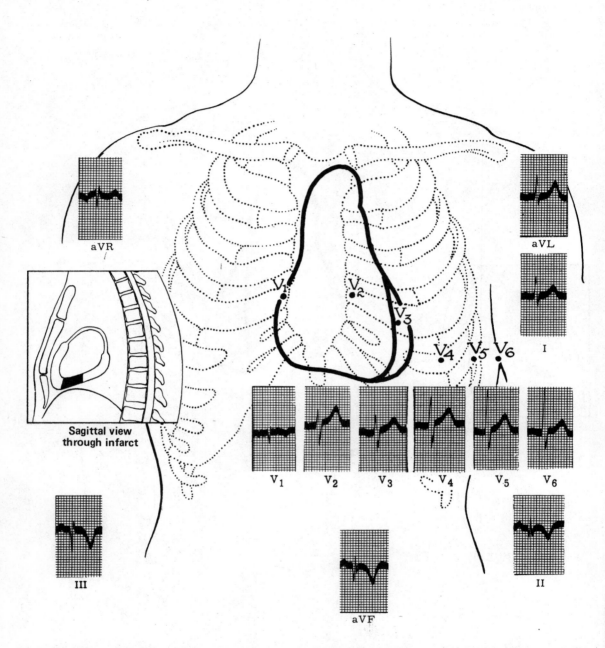

Figure 11–22. Late inferior wall infarction. Wide Q waves with deeply inverted T waves are present in II, III, and aVF. The precordial leads are normal. The ST segments are isoelectric. *Clinical diagnosis:* Myocardial infarction, 4 weeks old.

True Posterior Wall Infarction

In this instance, the infarct is not overlying the diaphragm and hence is not reflected into aVF. Therefore, the usual leads (I–III, aVR, aVL, aVF, V_{1-6}) will not show a typical infarct pattern. As a result of posterior infarction, the initial 0.04 s of the QRS will be directed anteriorly. This will result in abnormally tall R waves in V_1 and V_2 (the reciprocal of Q waves which would be recorded over the posterior wall with esophageal leads). ST depression in V_1 and V_2 will be seen in early posterior infarction and tall symmetric T waves will appear in these leads as a later event.

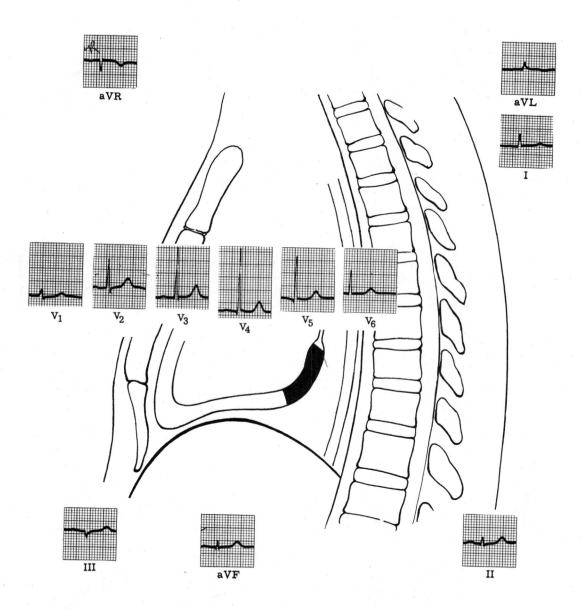

Figure 11–23. Posterior wall infarction. There are abnormally tall R waves in leads V_{1-2}. The R:S ratio in V_1 = 3 (normal = less than 1). The T waves are also upright in V_{1-2}. The above indicates abnormally prominent anterior QRS forces along with an anteriorly oriented T vector. The tall R waves in V_{1-2} are not due to right ventricular hypertrophy since there are no other criteria for the latter, ie, no right axis deviation, no abnormal P waves, and the T waves are not inverted in right precordial leads. *Clinical diagnosis:* Myocardial infarction, 1 month old.

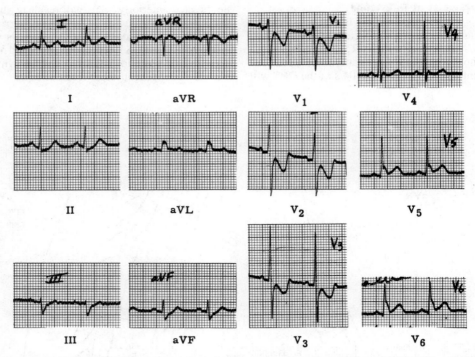

Figure 11–24. Acute posterior wall infarction. There is marked ST segment depression in leads V_{1-3}. This could represent anterior wall subendocardial ischemia or an acute posterior wall current of injury resulting from transmural ischemia or infarction. There is notching of the terminal portion of the R wave in leads I and V_{5-6}, indicating a distal left ventricular conduction delay. (See Fig 11–25.)

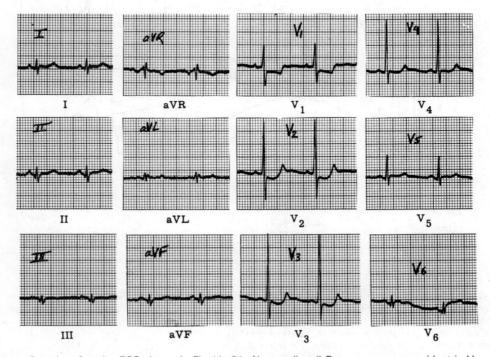

Figure 11–25. One day after the ECG shown in Fig 11–24. Abnormally tall R waves are now evident in V_{1-2}. The ST segments are less depressed and the T waves upright in V_{1-3}. All of the above are diagnostic of acute posterior wall infarction. Small but new q waves in aVF and new s waves in leads I and V_{5-6} are consistent with additional inferior and lateral infarction.

Posterior-Inferior Wall Infarction

The ECG will show evidence of posterior infarction, ie, tall R waves and tall T waves in V_1 and V_2, plus inferior infarction, ie, abnormal Q waves with T wave inversion in II, III, and aVF.

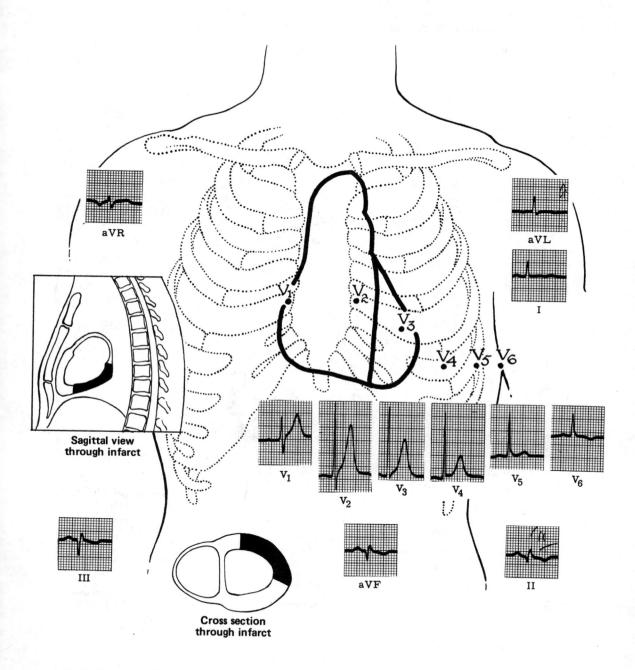

Figure 11–26. Posterior-inferior wall infarction. There are abnormally tall R waves in V_{1-2}. The R:S ratio in V_1 = 2. The T waves are abnormally tall in V_{1-2}. The above is indicative of posterior wall infarction. The wide Q waves and inverted T waves in II, III, and aVF indicate inferior wall infarction. *Clinical diagnosis:* Myocardial infarction, 3 weeks old.

Inferior-Posterior & Lateral Wall Infarction

The ECG will show evidence of infarction of all 3 sites. The inferior wall infarction will be evidenced by abnormal Q waves and T wave inversion in leads II, III, and aVF. The posterior wall infarction will produce abnormally tall R waves with upright T waves in V_1 and V_2. The lateral wall infarction will produce abnormal Q waves and inverted T waves in I and V_{5-7}. By vector analysis, it can be appreciated that the initial 0.04 s QRS vector is oriented to the right (lateral infarction), superiorly (inferior infarction), and anteriorly (posterior infarction).

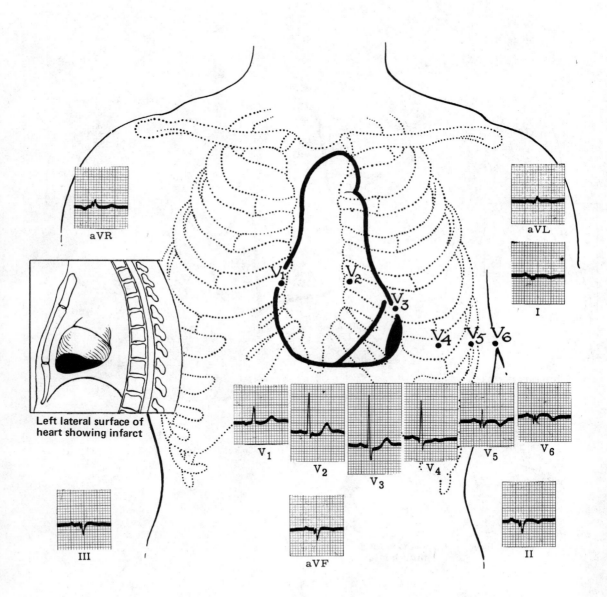

Figure 11–27. Inferior, posterior, and lateral wall infarction with tall R in right precordial leads. Note the infarction pattern in leads I, II, aVF, and V_6 (QS complexes with inverted T waves); tall R waves with ST depression are seen in V_{1-3}; a notched R wave is seen in aVR. The latter findings are a result of posterior wall infarction and do not indicate right ventricular hypertrophy. *Clinical diagnosis:* Recent myocardial infarction; no clinical evidence to suggest right ventricular hypertrophy. *Autopsy diagnosis:* Inferior, posterior, and lateral wall infarction; normal size right ventricle; occlusion of the left circumflex coronary artery.

SUMMARY OF ELECTROCARDIOGRAPHIC CRITERIA OF INFERIOR & POSTERIOR WALL INFARCTION

A. Extremity Leads: Lead aVF is the best lead for determining the presence of inferior wall infarction.

1. Convex ST segment elevation (early).

2. The presence of a QS complex or an abnormal Q wave (ie, a Q wave of 0.04 s or more in width or 25% or more of the voltage of the R wave in aVF [or both], assuming R = 5 mm or more). It must be remembered that a QS complex may be a normal finding in aVF in a horizontal heart. In this instance, there must be ST segment and T wave changes in addition to the QS complex in order to interpret the record as that of inferior wall infarction.

3. T wave inversion occurs later (typically deep and symmetric inversion).

B. Standard Leads: The pattern similar to aVF is recorded in II and III.

C. Precordial Leads: Usually normal in inferior wall infarction.

D. Posterior Infarction: Precordial leads V_{1-3} will show ST depression initially. Later, abnormally tall R waves and T waves will be evident.

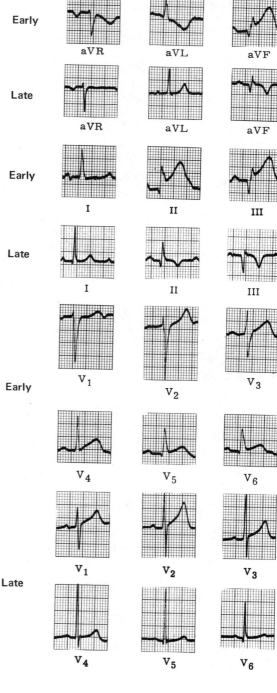

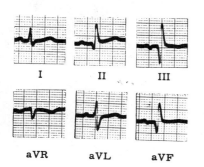

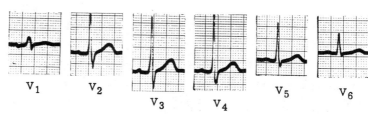

SUBENDOCARDIAL INFARCTION

For many years the ECG has been used to differentiate transmural from subendocardial (nontransmural) infarction. It had been considered that the subendocardial portion of the myocardium was "electrically silent" during depolarization and that infarction occurring in this area would therefore not be associated with an abnormal Q wave. However, the basic concept is not valid, and correlations of electrocardiographic and autopsy findings have clearly documented the unreliability of the ECG in establishing an accurate differential. Therefore, although many transmural infarctions are manifested by abnormal Q waves, it must be appreciated that a significant number are not so manifested. Many nontransmural infarctions, as documented by autopsy, will demonstrate the abnormal Q wave. This inability to distinguish clearly between transmural and nontransmural infarction probably explains the absence of prognostic significance of the diagnostic criteria formerly used.

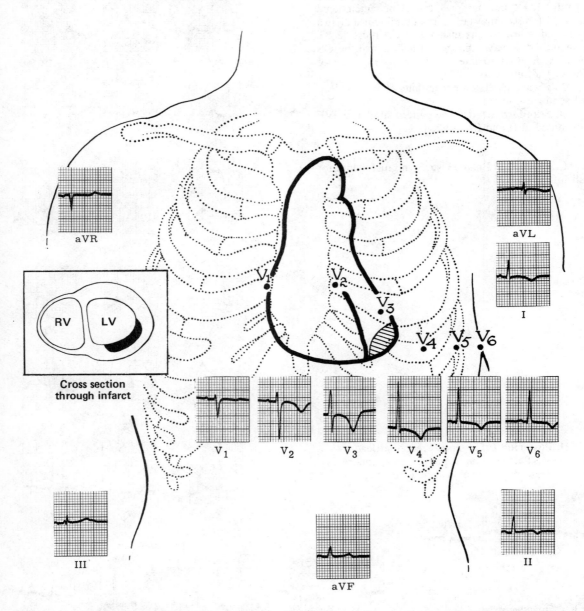

Figure 11–28. Subendocardial infarction. There are symmetrically inverted T waves in leads I, II, aVL, and V_{2-6}. No abnormal Q waves are present. Clinically, the patient had sustained an acute myocardial infarction, and this tracing is representative of several taken over the course of 1 week. The patient died from massive variceal bleeding. Autopsy revealed extensive anterior and lateral subendocardial infarction.

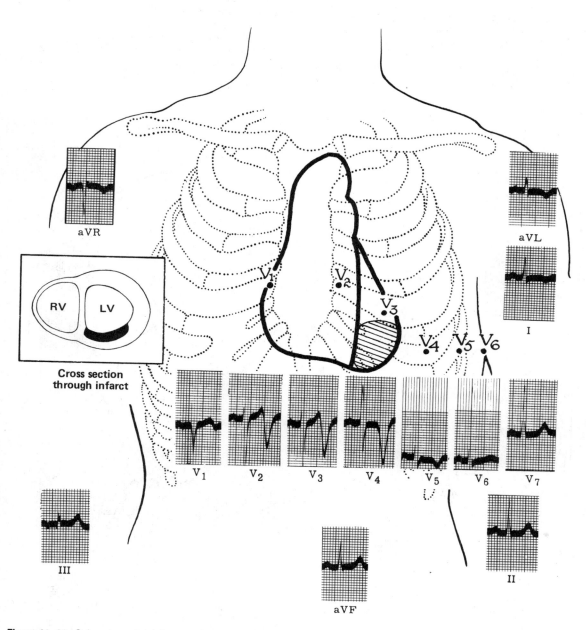

Figure 11–29. Subendocardial infarction. Tracing of a 60-year-old man 3 weeks after a clinical episode of myocardial infarction. Note the very deep and symmetrically inverted T waves in V_{2-4}, with lesser T wave inversion in V_5, I, and aVL. The above pattern, in conjunction with the clinical history, is consistent with a diagnosis of subendocardial infarction involving the anterior myocardium, with the major area of infarction in the anteroseptal region. *Autopsy diagnosis:* Anterior wall infarction; the infarction is not transmural but involves the endocardial half of the myocardium. The major area of infarction is anteroseptal. ¶Although this ECG and Fig 11–28 do show a correlation between the absence of Q waves and nontransmural infarction, it must be appreciated that this correlation is by no means an absolute one.

MULTIPLE INFARCTS

If the ECG reverts to normal after the initial infarction, a second infarct will produce a pattern as would be expected with initial infarction.

The abnormal Q waves which may persist following the initial infarct (eg, precordial leads in anterior wall infarction) may not be altered by a second infarct involving the opposite wall (eg, inferior wall infarction). However, the ST segment elevations that will occur with the second infarct (eg, in lead aVF in inferior wall infarction) will cause ST segment depression in the area of the initial infarct (eg, precordial leads in anterior wall infarction). The development of inverted T waves (eg, in aVF) as a result of the second infarct can cause the previously inverted T waves resulting from the initial infarct (precordial leads) to become upright.

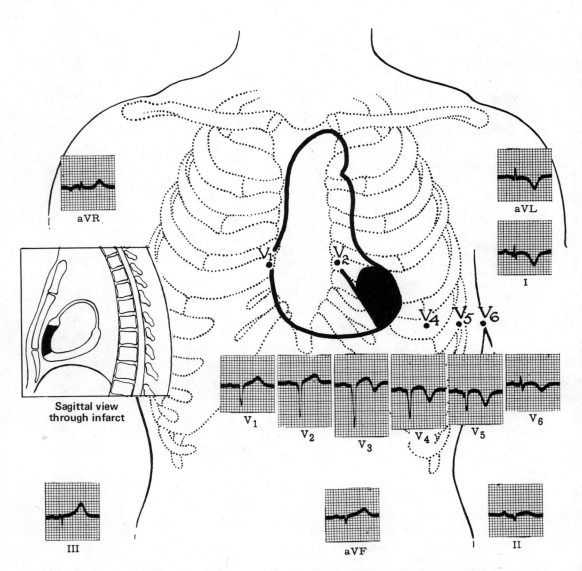

Figure 11–30. Initial infarction of multiple myocardial infarctions. There are QS complexes present from V_{1-5}. The T waves are inverted from V_{3-6}, I, and aVL. The pattern is indicative of anterior wall infarction. This electrocardiographic pattern was stable for several weeks after the episode of infarction. (See Fig 11–31.)

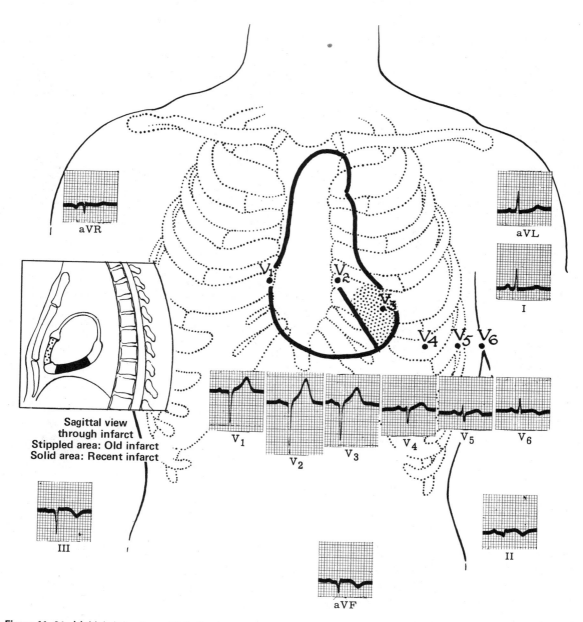

Figure 11–31. Multiple infarctions. Clinically, the patient suffered a second myocardial infarction 1 month after the tracing in Fig 11–30 was taken. A deep Q with inverted T has now appeared in aVF, indicating inferior wall infarction. As a result of this, the previously inverted T waves have now become upright in I, aVL, and V$_{3-5}$.

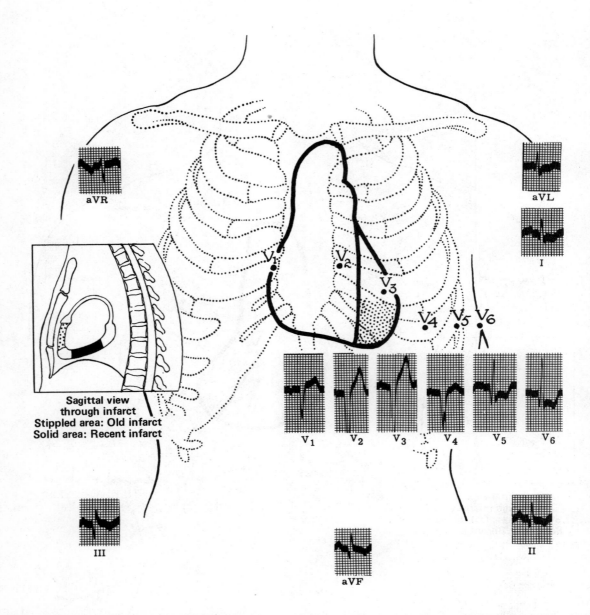

Figure 11–32. Multiple myocardial infarctions. The pattern in standard and extremity leads is typical of inferior wall infarction (abnormal Q and T wave inversion in II, III, and aVF). Precordial leads (and I, aVL) indicate anterior wall infarction (QS complexes in V_{2-4}, abnormal Q waves in V_{5-6}, aVL, and I). *Clinical diagnosis:* Recent myocardial infarction; old myocardial infarction (by history, 10 months previously). *Autopsy diagnosis:* Old anterior wall infarction; recent inferior wall infarction; occlusion of left anterior descending and left circumflex arteries.

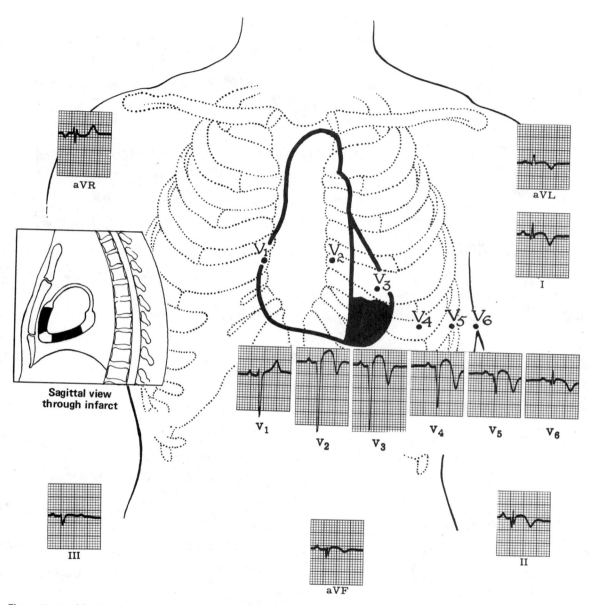

Figure 11–33. Multiple sites of acute infarction. There are abnormal Q waves in I, II, aVF, and V₆; QS complexes are present in V₂₋₅. The ST segments are elevated and the T waves inverted in these leads. The tracing is indicative of recent anterior, lateral, and inferior myocardial infarction.

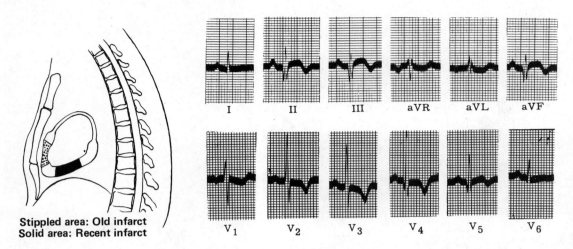

Stippled area: Old infarct
Solid area: Recent infarct

Figure 11–34. Multiple myocardial infarctions. The elevated ST segments and inverted T waves in standard and extremity leads (II, III, aVF) are indicative of recent inferior wall infarction. The inverted T waves in V_{2-5} in the precordial leads are indicative of anterior wall infarction; the isoelectric ST segments indicate that this is not as recent as the inferior infarct. *Clinical diagnosis:* Recent myocardial infarction; old myocardial infarction (by history, 1 year previously).

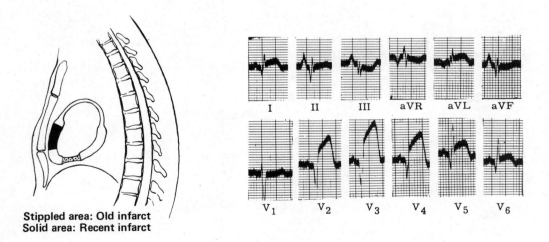

Stippled area: Old infarct
Solid area: Recent infarct

Figure 11–35. Multiple myocardial infarction. The QS complexes and elevated ST segments in the precordial leads and the qr complexes with elevated ST segments in leads I and aVL are indicative of recent anterior wall infarction. Abnormal Q waves in II, III, and aVF are indicative of inferior wall infarction; since the ST segments are isoelectric, this is not as recent as the anterior infarct. *Clinical and autopsy diagnosis:* Recent anterior wall infarction; old inferior wall infarction; occlusion of left anterior descending and left circumflex arteries.

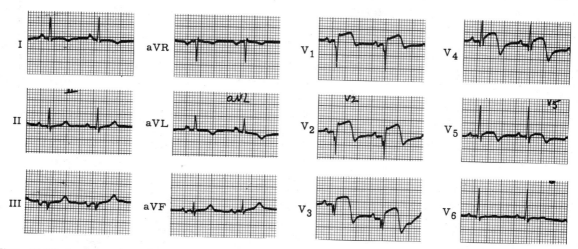

Figure 11–36. Acute anterior wall infarction. The patient had onset of symptoms of myocardial infarction 1 day prior to this record. It reveals deep Q waves in leads V_{1-3} with ST segment elevation in leads V_{1-5} and T wave inversion in leads I, aVL, and V_{1-5}. All the above is typical of acute anterior myocardial infarction. (See Figs 11–37 and 11–38.)

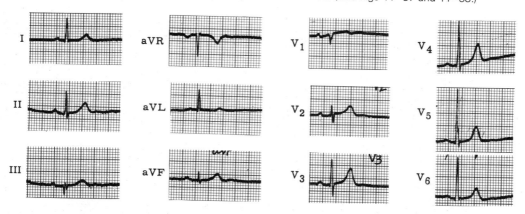

Figure 11–37. Recovery. This ECG was recorded 10 months after Fig 11–36. The patient had been asymptomatic in the interval. The only suspicious abnormality is the small q wave in V_2. This record could be interpreted as normal.

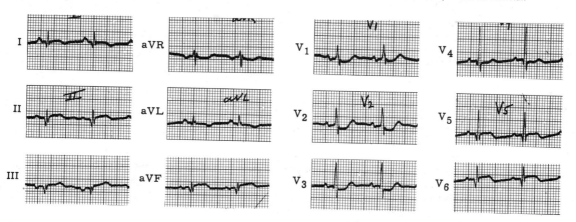

Figure 11–38. Second acute myocardial infarction. This ECG was recorded 8 months after Fig 11–37. The patient was having recurrent severe chest pain over many hours. In comparison with the previous record, there are new and significant Q waves in leads I, II, aVF, and V_{5-6}, and the ST segments are elevated in these leads. Abnormally tall R waves are evident in V_{1-2}, with ST segment depression in these leads. The above is typical of acute inferior-posterior-lateral myocardial infarction.

VENTRICULAR ANEURYSM

An aneurysm of the left ventricular myocardium may result following an episode of myocardial infarction. The most consistent electrocardiographic finding is the persistence of ST segment elevation in the epicardial leads reflecting the area of infarction for a period of months or years. The absence of persistent ST segment elevation does not necessarily indicate the absence of an aneurysm, since this pattern is seen in only approximately 50% of proved cases.

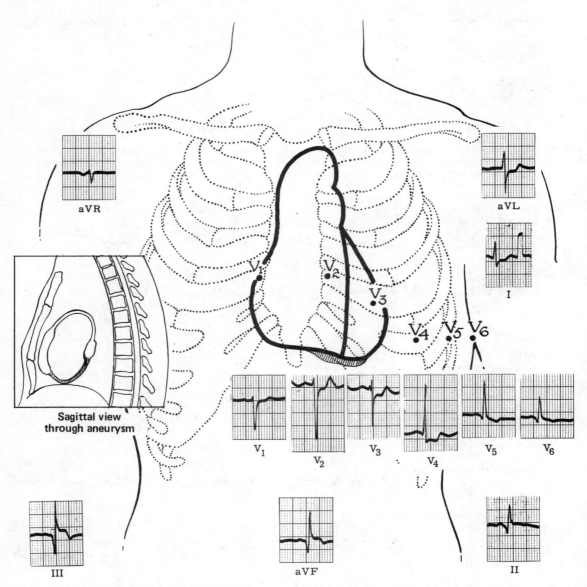

Figure 11–39. Ventricular aneurysm. Deep, wide Q waves with T wave inversions are present in II, III, and aVF as evidence of inferior wall infarction. There is ST elevation in the above leads and reciprocal depression in I, aVL, and precordial leads. This is consistent with recent inferior wall infarction, but this electrocardiographic pattern had been unchanged for 1 year following a clinical episode of infarction. An inferior wall ventricular aneurysm was confirmed by cineangiography and surgery.

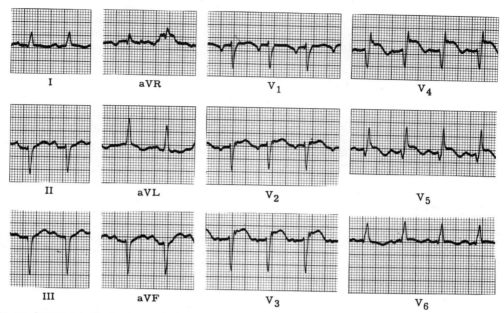

Figure 11–40. Anterior ventricular aneurysm. The frontal plane axis = −60 degrees, indicating a left anterior fascicular block. There are small q waves in V_1 and V_2, a diminutive r in V_3, and wide Q waves in V_{5-6}. The ST segments are elevated in V_{3-5}. This is consistent with acute anterior myocardial infarction. Clinically, the infarction had occurred 1 year previously and serial ECGs had shown no change. A large anterior ventricular aneurysm was documented by left ventricular angiography.

DIFFERENTIAL DIAGNOSIS OF MYOCARDIAL INFARCTION

Normal

The usual criteria for an abnormal Q wave as evidence of myocardial infarction are a Q duration of 0.04 s or a Q:R ratio of 25% (or both). These criteria are not valid for the diagnosis of infarction when present in lead III alone. A Q wave of 0.04 s in lead III is found in 35% of normal individuals and a Q:R ratio of 25% is found in 40% of normal individuals. The additional finding of an inverted T wave in lead III is of no diagnostic value. Therefore, the diagnosis of inferior wall infarction is dependent upon the findings in lead aVF, not III. The recording of lead III in deep inspiration has been advised as a means of differentiating normal from abnormal in lead III. The depth of inspiration is not standardized and there are no reliable data on large and clearly defined samples to indicate the value of such. It is, therefore, not recommended.

QS complexes may normally be seen in V_1 and V_2, especially with clockwise rotation.

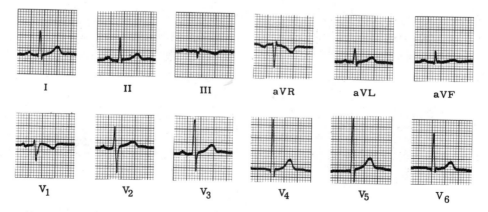

Figure 11–41. Normal pattern with Q and T inversion in III. A q wave of 0.04 s duration, a Q:R ratio of over 100%, and an inverted T wave are seen in lead III. However, aVF and the remainder of the tracing are normal. Such a record must not be interpreted as inferior wall infarction.

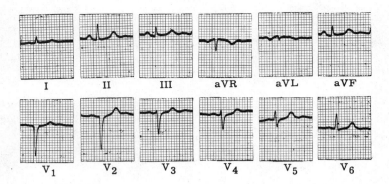

Figure 11–42. Normal pattern with QS in V_{1-2}. QS complexes are seen in V_{1-2}. The R waves progressively increase in height from V_{3-6}. There are no ST–T abnormalities. Such a pattern can be entirely normal. However, it could represent an old localized anteroseptal infarct. The differential diagnosis will depend upon the clinical picture. Third interspace leads may be of value. They were normal in this instance, but if QS complexes were seen in the $3V_{3-4}$ positions it could be indicative of a high anterior wall infarct. *Clinical diagnosis:* No evidence of heart disease. *Autopsy diagnosis:* No heart disease; death due to carcinoma.

Left Ventricular Hypertrophy

In this condition, QS complexes may be seen in V_1 and V_2. On rare occasions, QS complexes may extend from V_{1-4}. Therefore, in the presence of left ventricular hypertrophy, such QS complexes are not necessarily diagnostic of anterior wall infarction.

These QS complexes are seen especially in patients with hypertrophic cardiomyopathy (asymmetric septal hypertrophy, idiopathic subaortic stenosis). Because of the marked septal hypertrophy the forces of septal depolarization are markedly increased, producing large Q waves which mimic myocardial infarction.

Chronic Lung Disease & Right Ventricular Hypertrophy

In association with chronic lung disease and hyperinflation of the lungs, changes occur in the ECG which mimic myocardial infarction. Most commonly, there is a marked reduction or total absence of anterior QRS forces. This results in small r waves or QS complexes in precordial leads V_{1-3} (or V_4) that mimic anterior wall infarction. If there is additional right ventricular hypertrophy, the T waves may be inverted in these same leads, making the differential diagnosis even more difficult.

Pulmonary emphysema can distort the electrical forces in the frontal plane, resulting in an abnormal superior (left) frontal plane QRS axis. This will simulate left anterior hemiblock. In addition, abnormal Q waves or QS complexes can be recorded in aVF that mimic inferior wall infarction. The one clue that suggests pulmonary emphysema is low voltage, but clinical evaluation is essential in the differential diagnosis.

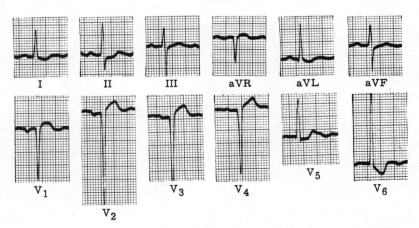

Figure 11–43. Left ventricular hypertrophy. $SV_1 + RV_6 = 47$ mm; R = 13 mm in aVL; there is ST depression in I, aVL, and V_6. The above criteria are indicative of left ventricular hypertrophy. In addition, QS complexes are present in leads V_{1-4}. This is consistent with anterior wall infarction. *Clinical and autopsy diagnosis:* Left ventricular hypertrophy secondary to syphilitic aortitis with aortic insufficiency; no evidence of myocardial infarction.

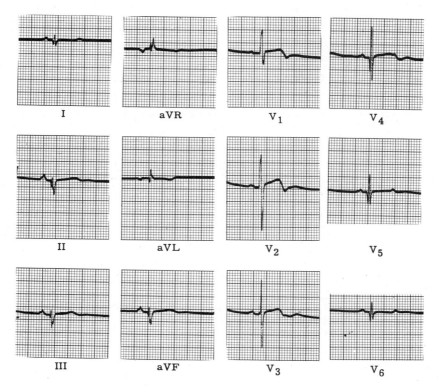

Figure 11–44. Hypertrophic cardiomyopathy. There are deep but narrow Q waves in leads I and V_{4-6}. The R:S ratio in V_1 is greater than 1. There is late T inversion in V_{1-2}. These findings are consistent with posterolateral infarction. Clinical evaluation, echocardiography, and cardiac catheterization indicated the presence of hypertrophic cardiomyopathy without outflow obstruction. Coronary angiograms were normal.

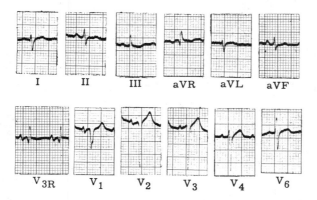

Figure 11–45. Right ventricular hypertrophy. QS complexes with upright T waves are seen in V_{1-3}. This could represent an old anteroseptal infarction. However, there is marked clockwise rotation, as evidenced by a deep S in V_6. Lead V_{3R} shows the typical pattern of right ventricular hypertrophy. Therefore the QS complexes in V_{1-3} are a reflection of a dilated right ventricle and do not represent infarction. *Clinical and autopsy diagnosis:* Right ventricular hypertrophy secondary to chronic pulmonary disease; no evidence of infarction.

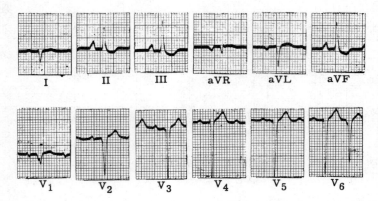

Figure 11–46. Right ventricular hypertrophy. QS complexes are present in leads V_{1-3}. In view of the marked clockwise rotation (rS complexes in leads V_{4-6}), this is not necessarily indicative of infarction but probably represents leads taken over a greatly dilated right ventricle. The tall P waves in II, III, and aVF, the right axis deviation (+115 degrees), and the ST–T changes in II, III, and aVF are consistent with right atrial and right ventricular hypertrophy. *Clinical and autopsy diagnosis:* Right atrial and ventricular hypertrophy and dilatation due to chronic pulmonary disease; no infarction present.

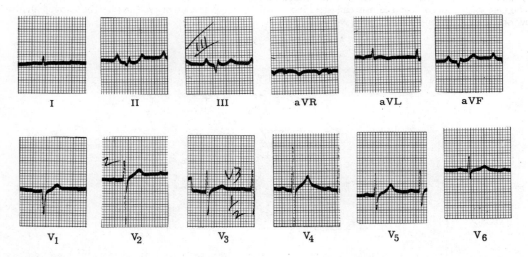

Figure 11–47. Right ventricular hypertrophy. The QRS complexes are of low voltage in frontal plane leads. Wide Q waves are present in II, III, and aVF, which are consistent with inferior wall infarction. The P waves are peaked in the latter leads, indicating right atrial overload. The precordial leads show clockwise rotation (V_3 is half-standardized). *Clinical and autopsy diagnosis:* Right ventricular hypertrophy secondary to pulmonary disease; no infarction.

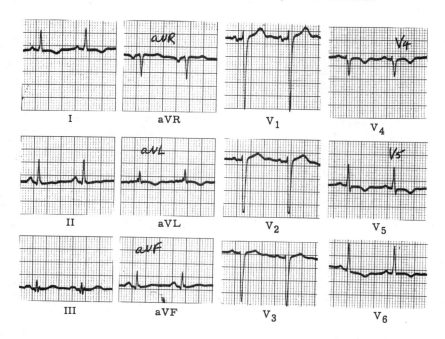

Figure 11–48. Anterior-lateral myocardial infarction. This ECG is representative of many taken over the past year. The patient had had a myocardial infarction 3 years previously. There are small r waves in V_3 and V_4 with T wave inversion in leads I, aVL, and V_{4-6}, consistent with old anterior and lateral infarction. (See Fig 11 –49.)

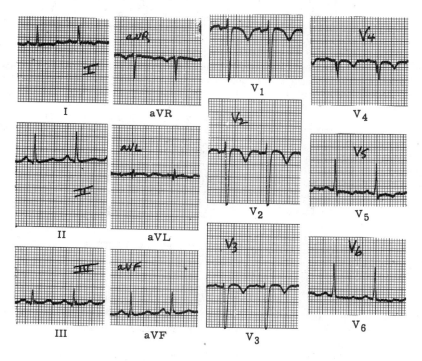

Figure 11–49. Right ventricular overload. The patient (same as in Fig 11 –48) had an aorta–femoral artery bypass procedure. On the third postoperative day, he had an episode of chest pain lasting 1 hour which he stated was "exactly like the pain I had with my prior heart attack." The ECG now reveals new, deep T wave inversion in leads V_{1-3}. This was initially interpreted as representing acute anterior wall ischemia or infarction. This pattern persisted for several days in spite of no further chest pain and no elevation of the cardiac enzymes. A lung scan revealed a large wedge-shaped defect in the right upper lobe in the presence of a normal chest x-ray. Therefore, these T wave changes in leads V_{1-3} indicated an acute right ventricular overload in spite of the absence of a significant frontal plane axis shift or a change in P wave morphology.

INFARCTION ASSOCIATED WITH BUNDLE BRANCH BLOCK

As a general rule, a right bundle branch block does not obscure the pattern of infarction, whereas a left bundle branch block does. The most diagnostic feature of infarction is the abnormal direction of the initial 0.04 s QRS vector (ie, the abnormal Q wave). Since the initial 0.04 s QRS vector in uncomplicated right bundle branch is normal, the presence of superimposed infarction can be detected here when it occurs. However, since the initial QRS vector is abnormally directed in left bundle branch block, it will obscure the infarction vector, and the abnormal Q wave will not appear.

Infarction Associated With Right Bundle Branch Block

The simultaneous occurrence of a right bundle branch block in association with an infarction pattern indicates infarction of the septum. Anterior wall infarction in association with a right bundle branch block will result in disappearance of the initial r wave (rSR′ of right bundle branch block) in right ventricular epicardial leads, resulting in QR complexes.

Posterior Infarction Associated With Right Bundle Branch Block

A right bundle branch block alters the late forces of ventricular depolarization. Posterior wall infarction alters the initial vector forces in an abnormal anterior direction. This will be evident in the right precordial

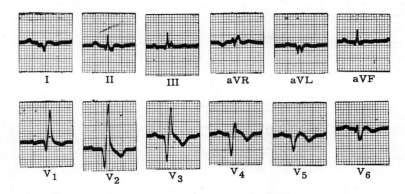

Figure 11–50. Anterior wall infarction in association with right bundle branch block. The QRS interval = 0.14 s; VAT in V₁₋₂ = 0.1 s. The initial r waves of an uncomplicated right bundle branch block normally seen in right precordial leads are not present; deep, wide Q waves indicative of anterior wall infarction are present instead.

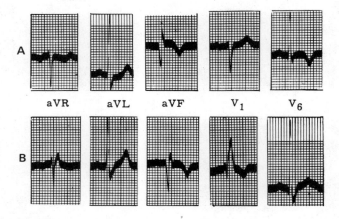

Figure 11–51. Inferior wall infarction in association with right bundle branch block. Leads aVR, aVL, aVF, and V₁ and V₆ are illustrated. **A:** There is a deep, wide Q with elevated ST segment and inverted T in aVF. This is indicative of recent inferior wall infarction. A 22 mm R is seen in aVL; this is evidence of left ventricular hypertrophy. The pattern in V₁ is normal. The T is inverted in V₆, probably as a result of partial lateral wall infarction. **B:** Three weeks after (A). The QRS interval has increased from 0.08 s in (A) to 0.14 s in (B). The VAT in V₁ has increased from 0.02 s in (A) to 0.11 s in (B). Wide R′ waves are seen in aVR and V₁; wide S waves are seen in aVL and V₆. The pattern of inferior wall infarction in aVF is not altered by the development of the right bundle branch block. This patient recovered. It is reasonable to assume that the right bundle branch block resulted from further infarction involving the interventricular septum.

leads. In addition to the late R' waves indicative of right bundle branch block, the initial portion of the QRS complex will reveal an abnormally tall R wave (see p 178). Thus, right precordial leads will reveal a tall, slurred R wave or rR' complex. A similar pattern may be seen in right ventricular hypertrophy associated with a right bundle branch block. There is autopsy evidence that the same pattern can occur in the absence of either posterior wall infarction or right ventricular hypertrophy and is therefore assumed to be the manifestation of a right bundle branch block alone. The reason for this is not known. The ST segments will be depressed in the early stage of infarction and the T waves upright and tall in the late stage of infarction in the same leads.

Infarction Associated With Left Bundle Branch Block

A left bundle branch block may result from myocardial infarction, but one cannot diagnose the latter in the presence of the former. One may be suspicious of infarction if marked ST segment elevation appears in leads that formerly showed the typical left bundle branch pattern (Fig 11–53). Rarely, one may see Q waves in association with a left bundle branch

block. This is said to be due to associated infarction of the septum, which allows the initial negativity of the right ventricular cavity to be transmitted into the left cavity and hence into a left ventricular epicardial lead. However, there is little pathologic evidence to support this view; a more likely explanation is the presence of infarction plus a conduction defect in the left ventricle distal to the left bundle (hence not a true left bundle branch block).

Given a left bundle branch electrocardiographic pattern prior to the onset of clinical myocardial infarction, a marked reduction in the voltage of the QRS complexes may offer a clue to the presence of infarction.

Right Bundle Branch Block With Left Anterior Fascicular Block

In this type of bilateral bundle branch block (see p 134), q waves may be seen in leads V_{1-3} that do not indicate anterior wall infarction. Because of the block in the left anterior fascicle, there is loss of the normal depolarization of the anterior portion of the interventricular septum. The posterior septum is activated early, producing an initial posterior force that results in the above q waves. (See Fig 11–57.)

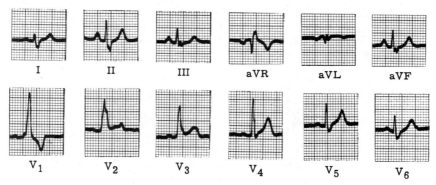

Figure 11–52. Posterior infarction plus right bundle branch block. The QRS interval is 0.12 s. The wide s waves in leads I, II, III, aVF, V_{5-6}, and the late portion of the R waves in V_{1-3} are indicative of right bundle branch block. The initial tall R deflection in V_{1-3} is consistent with associated posterior wall infarction. *Autopsy diagnosis:* Posterior and septal infarction. It is assumed that the septal infarction produced the right bundle branch block.

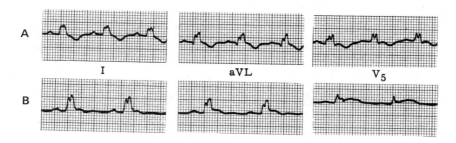

Figure 11–53. Infarction associated with left bundle branch block. *A:* Typical left bundle branch block. The patient had sustained a myocardial infarct 7 years previously, but such cannot be diagnosed in the presence of the left bundle branch block. *B:* Recorded during an episode of prolonged chest pain. The ST segments are now elevated in leads I, aVL, and V_5. This is indicative of an acute current of injury and, combined with marked elevation of specific cardiac enzymes, is evidence of acute myocardial infarction in the presence of left bundle branch block.

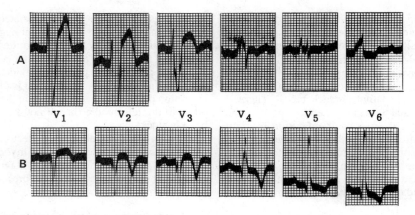

Figure 11–54. Anterior wall infarction in association with left bundle branch block. Only the precordial leads are illustrated. *A:* The patient had suffered an acute myocardial infarction 2 days previously. A typical left bundle branch block pattern is seen in leads V_{5-6}. Although there is ST segment elevation in leads V_{1-3} and coving of the T in V_{2-3}, it would be hazardous to make an electrocardiographic diagnosis of infarction on this basis in the presence of a left bundle branch block. *B:* One week after first tracing. The left bundle branch block pattern has disappeared and the pattern of anterior wall infarction has become evident.

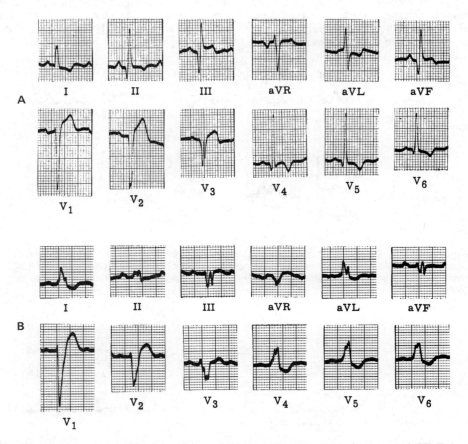

Figure 11–55. Infarction associated with left bundle branch block. *A:* The deep, wide Q waves with ST–T changes in II, III, and aVF are indicative of inferior wall infarction. The QS complexes in V_{2-3} and abnormal q waves with T inversion in V_{4-6} are indicative of anterior wall infarction. $SV_1 + RV_5 = 40$ mm and is consistent with left ventricular hypertrophy. Clinically, the patient had suffered 2 episodes of myocardial infarction. *B:* Following a third clinical episode of myocardial infarction, the ECG now demonstrates a left bundle branch block and the previous signs of infarction and hypertrophy are gone. *Autopsy diagnosis:* Left ventricular hypertrophy, old infarction involving anterior and inferior portions of the left ventricle; recent septal infarction. The latter probably explains the left bundle branch block.

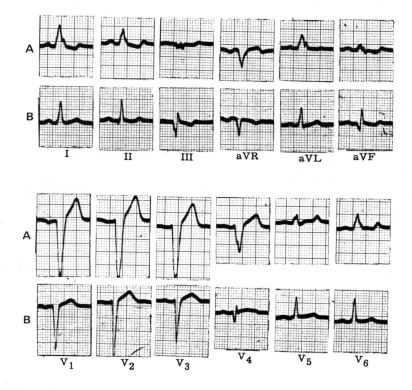

Figure 11–56. Inferior wall infarction in association with left bundle branch block. *A:* The patient had suffered an acute myocardial infarction 1 day previously. The electrocardiographic pattern is that of a left bundle branch block. *B:* Seven days after (A) there was no clinical evidence of further coronary insufficiency or infarction. The left bundle branch pattern has disappeared, uncovering a definite pattern of inferior wall infarction as evidenced by the deep, wide Q in aVF (also II and III). It is likely that the left bundle branch block in (A) was due to temporary coronary insufficiency in the region of the left bundle branch.

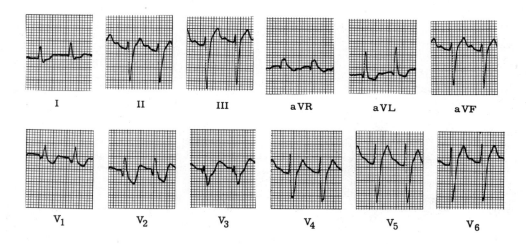

Figure 11–57. Right bundle branch block plus left anterior fascicular block. The mean vector of the initial 0.05 s QRS in the frontal plane = −60 degrees, indicating a left anterior fascicular block. The wide S waves in I and the wide R waves in V_{1-2}, with a QRS interval = 0.12 s, are evidence of right bundle branch block. The q waves in V_{1-3} could indicate associated anterior wall infarction but, in view of the bilateral bundle branch block, are not diagnostic of infarction and could result from the block alone. *Autopsy findings:* Fibrosis and calcification involving the bundle branches; no myocardial infarction; death due to carcinoma.

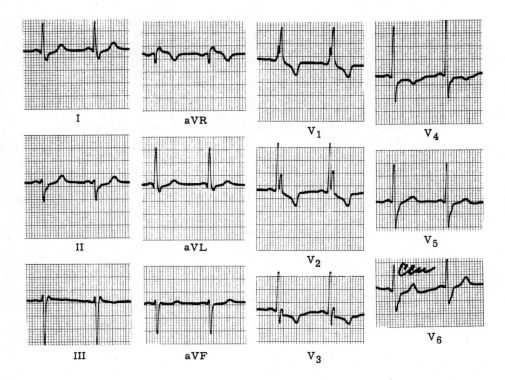

Figure 11–58. Bifascicular block. The ECG reveals a left anterior fascicular block and right bundle branch block. The patient had been admitted to a coronary care unit because of crescendo angina. (See Figs 11–59, 11–60, and 11–61.)

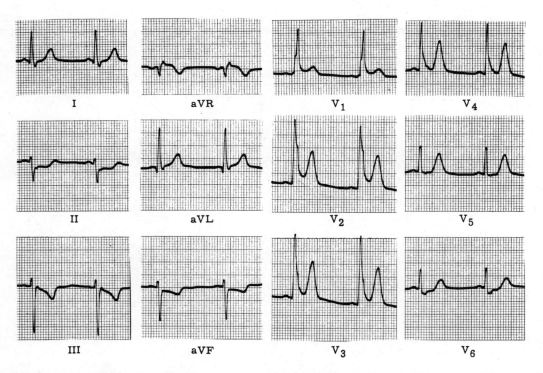

Figure 11–59. Acute infarction. This ECG was recorded 30 minutes after Fig 11–58. The patient was having severe chest pain. This record now reveals ST segment elevation in leads V_{1-3} with large (hyperacute) upright T waves in leads V_{1-5}. These changes are typical of acute anterior wall infarction.

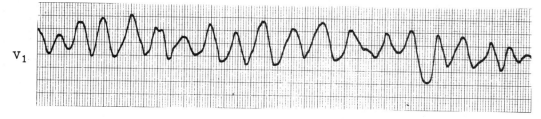

Figure 11–60. Ventricular fibrillation. This appeared 15 minutes after Fig 11–59. There had been no prior evidence of ventricular ectopy. It was immediately and successfully treated with DC shock.

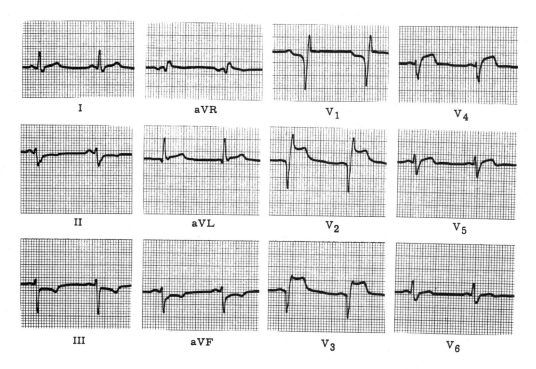

Figure 11–61. Acute infarction. This ECG was recorded 15 minutes after Fig 11–60. New deep Q waves are now evident in leads V_{1-3}. The ST segments remain elevated in leads V_{1-5}, but the hyperacute T waves are no longer present, illustrating the usual early and transient occurrence of the latter in acute myocardial infarction.

TRANSITORY ABNORMAL Q WAVES

Very uncommonly, abnormal Q waves may be seen that are consistent with myocardial infarction but disappear within hours. The Q waves are associated with clinical states of shock and disappear when the shock state has been successfully treated. It is believed that a stage of severe myocardial ischemia is reached in which the myocardium is "electrically dead" and is reflected in abnormal Q waves. However, with the restoration of myocardial blood flow, the myocardial ischemia is reversible and the Q waves disappear.

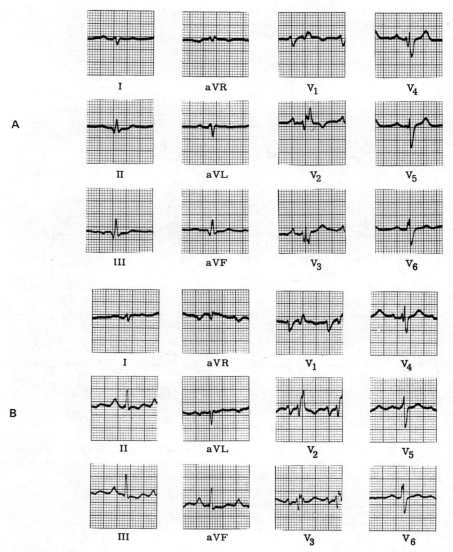

Figure 11–62. Transitory abnormal Q waves. *A:* The rhythm is sinus. The P–R interval = 0.24 s, indicating first degree heart block (see p 237). The notched P waves in frontal plane leads and the diphasic P with a wide negative deflection in V_1 are consistent with left atrial hypertrophy. The QRS interval = 0.15 s, and there is a wide S in I and wide, notched R' waves in V_{1-2}, indicating right bundle branch block. Wide Q waves are seen in II, III, and aVF and are consistent with inferior wall infarction. *B:* Taken 1 day after (A) (ECG 1 day before [A] was the same as [B]). The QRS interval has been reduced to 0.12 s, but the right bundle branch block persists. Normally small q waves are now seen in II, III, and aVF which do not indicate inferior wall infarction. *Clinical data:* The patient had mitral stenosis. At the time of tracing (A), he was in shock as a result of thromboembolism of the abdominal aorta. At the time of tracing (B), his blood pressure and peripheral perfusion had been temporarily improved. It is concluded that the Q waves seen in (A) resulted from severe myocardial ischemia which subsided at the time of record (B). *Autopsy findings:* Mitral stenosis with left atrial and right ventricular hypertrophy; extensive thrombosis of abdominal aorta; no myocardial infarction; no pulmonary embolization.

PSEUDOINFARCTION DUE TO INCORRECT LEAD PLACEMENT

Interchange of RA, LA, and LL electrodes results in marked changes in the frontal plane leads. Such will not alter the precordial leads, because the indifferent electrode is the sum of the potentials of RA + LA + LL, irrespective of the individual locations on the extremities. (See Figs 11–63 through 11–67.)

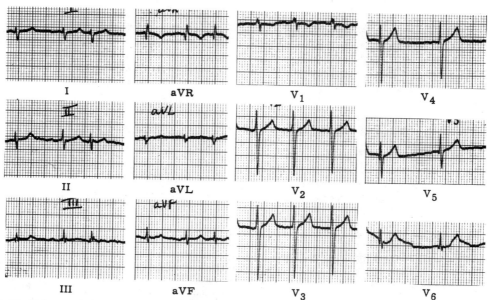

Figure 11–63. Right ventricular hypertrophy. The rhythm is atrial fibrillation. The frontal plane axis = +120 degrees. Even though the R:S ratio in V_1 is not over 1, the duration of the r wave in that lead is prolonged (0.05 s), indicating prominent anterior forces. All the above is consistent with right ventricular hypertrophy. *Clinical diagnosis:* Mitral stenosis in a 35-year-old woman. (See Fig 11–64.) .

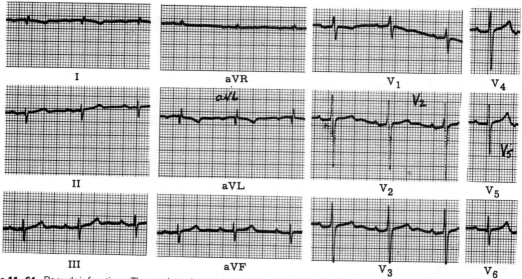

Figure 11–64. Pseudoinfarction. The patient (same as in Fig 11–63) had mitral valve replacement and an uneventful postoperative course. Two weeks after surgery, elective cardioversion was successfully accomplished. This ECG was taken 1 day later. Sinus rhythm is now present. A new Q wave with an inverted T wave is now evident in lead I. This was initially interpreted as indicating acute lateral myocardial infarction, probably secondary to coronary embolization following reversion to sinus rhythm. However, it is evident that the P wave is inverted in lead I and that leads II-III and aVR-aVL are reversed as a result of accidental interchange of the RA and LA electrodes (see p 80). This was confirmed by a repeat ECG taken correctly.

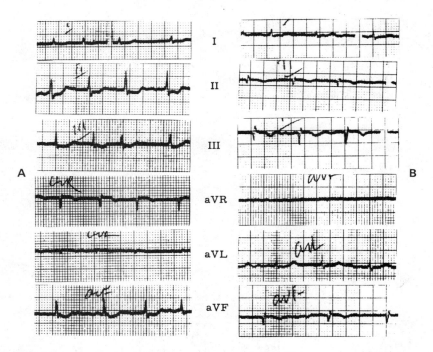

Figure 11–65. Pseudoinfarction. Only frontal plane leads are illustrated. Record A reveals atrial fibrillation. There are ST segment depressions consistent with digitalis effect. Record B is a repeat tracing several months later. No known clinical event had occurred. The ECG now reveals deep Q waves with T wave inversion in leads II, III, and aVF. This was initially interpreted as a new silent inferior myocardial infarction. However, leads aVR, aVL, and aVF of record A can be matched with aVF, aVR, and aVL, respectively, in record B. This error and its resultant effect on leads I, II, and III are illustrated in the following diagram.

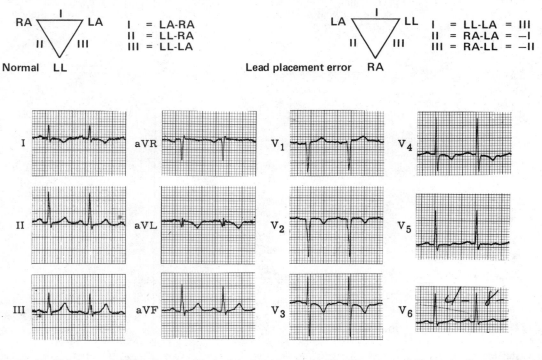

Figure 11–66. Old myocardial infarction. An elderly diabetic patient had suffered a myocardial infarction 3 years before this recording was made. The ECG reveals a QS complex in V_2 and T wave inversions in leads I, aVL, and V_{2-4}, all consistent with anterior wall infarction. (See Fig 11–67.)

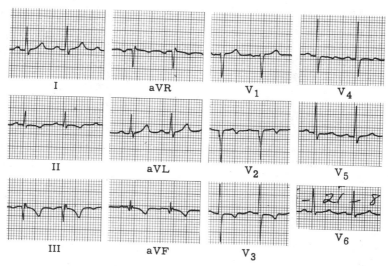

Figure 11–67. Pseudoinfarction. A repeat ECG was taken 3 weeks after the record in Fig 11–66 as a routine preoperative procedure. This now reveals new deep Q waves in III and aVF and new T wave inversion in II, III, and aVF. Although no clinical event had been recognized, the record was interpreted as a recent, silent inferior wall infarction, and surgery was canceled. More careful inspection indicates that leads aVL and aVF have been reversed. A repeat ECG confirmed the error. The resultant effect of this error is illustrated in the following diagram.

Normal

I = LA-RA
II = LL-RA
III = LL-LA

Lead placement error

I = LL-RA = II
II = LA-RA = I
III = LA-LL = −III

EFFECT OF FURTHER CORONARY INSUFFICIENCY
ON THE INFARCT PATTERN

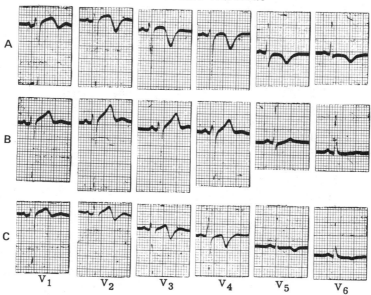

Figure 11–68. Coronary insufficiency superimposed upon infarction. (Only the precordial leads are illustrated.) *A:* The stable electrocardiographic pattern of a clinical myocardial infarct 2 months old. *B:* One day after initial tracing. The T waves are now upright (except in V₆) in precordial leads. The pattern looks more normal, but the inverted T waves of established infarction could not suddenly become upright in 1 day. This therefore indicates further coronary insufficiency (the patient was having chest pain at the time this record was taken). *C:* One day after (B). The T waves are again inverted in precordial leads, similar to (A).

PERIPHERAL LEFT VENTRICULAR CONDUCTION DEFECTS IN ASSOCIATION WITH MYOCARDIAL INFARCTION

Infarction of the myocardium can involve the anterior and posterior fascicles of the left bundle branch or the more distal Purkinje fibers in or about the area of infarction. Thus, myocardial infarction can be associated with (1) left anterior fascicular block, (2) left posterior fascicular block, or (3) peri-infarction block.

Anterior Infarction With Left Anterior Fascicular Block

The ECG will show evidence of anterior infarction, ie, abnormal Q waves in I, aVL, and precordial leads. Because of a block in the left anterior fascicle, the terminal forces of the QRS will be oriented to the left and superiorly, producing a mean frontal plane QRS axis > -30 degrees. The QRS interval is not abnormally lengthened, being under 0.12 s.

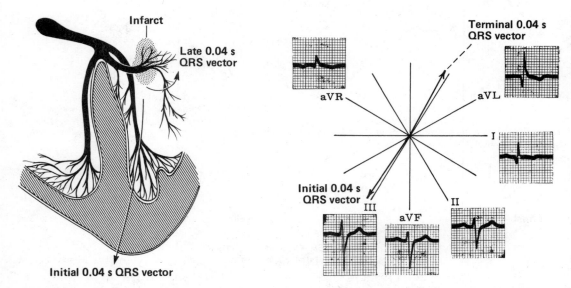

Figure 11–69. Anterior infarction with left anterior fascicular block illustrating orientation of initial and late QRS vectors in the frontal plane.

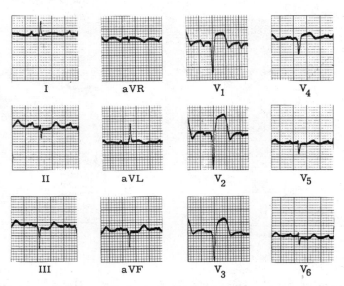

Figure 11–70. Anterior infarction with left anterior fascicular block. QS complexes with ST segment elevation and T wave inversion are present in V_{1-4}. This is evidence of acute anterior wall infarction. The mean frontal plane QRS axis = -45 degrees, indicative of a left anterior fascicular block.

Inferior (Posterior) Infarction With Left Posterior Fascicular Block

Inferior infarction will be evidenced by abnormal Q waves in aVF, posterior infarction by abnormally tall R waves in V_{1-2}. Because of a block in the left posterior fascicle, the terminal QRS forces will be oriented to the right (S in I), inferiorly (R in aVF), and posteriorly (S in V_{1-2}). The QRS interval is less than 0.12 s.

With multiple infarctions, various combinations of the above can occur.

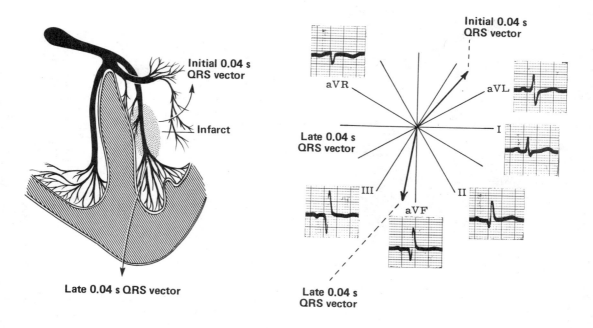

Figure 11–71. Inferior infarction with left posterior fascicular block illustrating orientation of initial and late QRS vectors in the frontal plane.

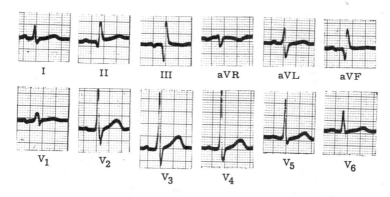

Figure 11–72. Inferior and posterior infarction with left posterior fascicular block. Deep and wide (0.04 s) Q waves are seen in leads II, III, and aVF, as evidence of inferior wall infarction. This indicates an initial 0.04 s QRS vector oriented superiorly. This same QRS vector produces the R wave in lead I, which indicates that this vector is also oriented to the left. This initial superior and left vector force is directed at a −50 degree axis in the frontal plane. The late 0.04 s QRS vector, producing the R waves in leads II, III, and aVF and the S wave in lead I, results in a late QRS vector directed at a +100 degree axis. The prominent R waves in V_{1-2} are the result of associated posterior wall infarction.

Myocardial Infarction With Opposite Fascicular Block

With multiple infarctions, various combinations of sites of infarction and left fascicular blocks can occur. A left anterior fascicular block can be seen in association with inferior (posterior) infarction or a left posterior fascicular block can occur in association with an anterior infarct. Such combinations indicate multiple lesions since a single lesion cannot explain the electrocardiographic findings.

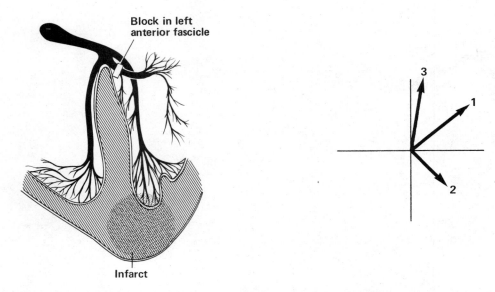

Figure 11–73. Inferior infarction with left anterior fascicular block illustrating orientation of initial, mid, and terminal QRS vectors in the frontal plane. *(1)* Initial 0.04 s QRS vector due to inferior wall infarct. *(2)* Midportion of QRS vector. *(3)* Terminal 0.04 s QRS vector due to left anterior fascicular block.

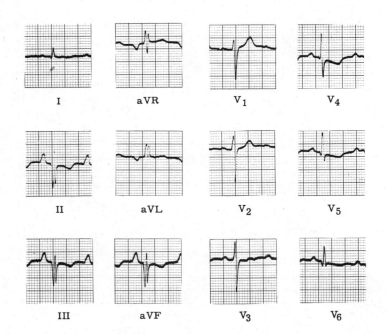

Figure 11–74. Inferior wall infarction with left anterior fascicular block. The initial 0.04 s QRS vector is oriented superiorly (Q waves in II, III, and aVF) and is evidence of inferior wall infarction. The midportion of the QRS is oriented inferiorly, producing the R waves in II, III, and aVF. The terminal 0.04 s QRS is again directed superiorly (S waves in II, III, and aVF). The mean frontal plane axis of this terminal force = −80 degrees and is indicative of a left anterior fascicular block. It is unlikely that one lesion could explain the latter and the inferior infarct. It is, therefore, indicative of 2 separate lesions.

Peri-infarction Block

Various definitions have been given for the term peri-infarction block. These include the following: (1) Peripheral left ventricular conduction defects that have been described in this text as infarction with left fascicular block; (2) an angle between the initial 0.04 s and terminal 0.04 s QRS vectors of greater than 110 degrees (not valid unless the tracing has abnormal Q waves, as evidence of the infarction); and (3) a QRS duration greater than 0.12 s in association with infarction. The author prefers this concept and definition: Conduction delay exists in and about the zone of in-

farction. Because conduction delay is longer in the intramural area than that resulting from block in the more proximal fascicles of the left bundle, the QRS will be prolonged over 0.12 s. The infarct will be evidenced by the abnormal initial 0.04 s QRS vector (ie, abnormal Q waves), and the terminal QRS vector is oriented opposite the site of infarction. Thus, the direction of initial and terminal forces will be the same as seen in infarction with left fascicular block, but the QRS interval will be prolonged because the block is more distal.

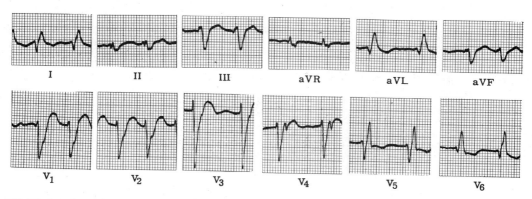

Figure 11–75. Anterior peri-infarction block. The rhythm is atrial fibrillation. The QRS interval = 0.16 s and resembles a left bundle branch block. However, there are deep, wide Q waves in I and aVL with minute r waves in V$_{5-6}$. This is evidence of anterior and lateral infarction. The terminal QRS vector is oriented to the left (R in I), and superiorly (S waves in II, III, and aVF) resulting in a mean QRS vector of −50 degrees. This is consistent with a left anterior fascicular block, but in view of the marked widening of the QRS interval it is indicative of more distal block in the area of infarction; hence the term peri-infarction block.

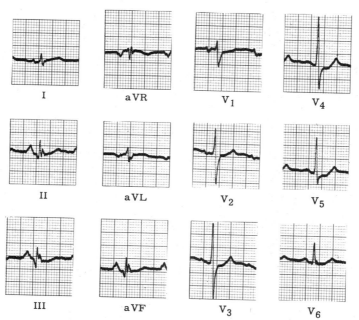

Figure 11–76. Inferior peri-infarction block. The QRS interval = 0.12 s. The Q waves in II, III, and aVF are indicative of inferior wall infarction. The terminal QRS forces are oriented inferiorly (notched R waves in II, III, and aVF) and slightly rightward (small s in I). This is consistent with a left posterior fascicular block, but in view of the QRS prolongation it is indicative of a more distal block in the area of infarction, ie, peri-infarction block.

Normal Cardiac Rhythm & the Atrial Arrhythmias

PHYSIOLOGY OF CARDIAC RHYTHM

In order to better understand disturbances of cardiac rhythm, a brief review of some of the physiologic properties of the heart is indicated. Some of these concepts have been discussed in Chapter 2.

Activation of heart muscle results from spontaneous discharge in a pacemaker and conduction of this impulse from cell to cell. Disturbances of cardiac rhythm are largely related to these basic processes—automaticity, conductivity, or both.

Automaticity

The basis for the automaticity of specialized cardiac cells is the spontaneous depolarization in phase 4 of the cell's action potential curve (see p 17). Normally, the sinus node acts as the primary pacemaker, but in certain situations secondary pacemakers assume automaticity. These are located in specialized conduction tissue in the atria, AV junctional areas, the common bundle, the bundle branches, and the peripheral Purkinje system.

The rate at which the sinus node (or secondary pacemakers) fires is dependent on the following: (1) the level of the threshold potential, (2) the slope of the diastolic depolarization in phase 4, and (3) the level of the membrane potential at the end of repolarization. If the threshold potential is reduced or the membrane potential is increased (or both) and the slope of diastolic depolarization is unchanged, the rate will slow since it will take longer for the potential to reach the threshold level. If the slope of diastolic depolarization is increased and both membrane and threshold potentials remain constant, the potential will reach the threshold level sooner and the rate will increase. Conversely, if the slope of phase 4 is reduced, the rate will slow. Important factors that influence automaticity are as follows:

A. Autonomic Nervous System: Vagal activity, by liberation of acetylcholine, decreases the slope of phase 4 and increases the diastolic membrane potential, thereby slowing the rate of discharge. This is most evident in the sinus node, producing sinus slowing. Increasing vagal activity results in further suppression of sinus activity; and, since the other areas of specialized conduction tissue are less affected, sec-

ondary pacemakers (escape phenomenon) can assume automaticity, producing ectopic atrial, AV junctional, or idioventricular rhythms. Large intravenous doses of acetylcholine can suppress all pacemaker activity, resulting in cardiac standstill. Sympathetic (beta-adrenergic) stimulation increases the slope of phase 4, resulting in an increase of the sinus rate or automatic discharge from secondary pacemakers (or both), resulting in ectopic atrial, AV junctional, or ventricular rhythms.

B. Temperature: Hypothermia decreases the slope of phase 4 and thereby slows the sinus rate. If significant sinus bradycardia occurs, there can be "escape" of secondary pacemakers in the atria or AV junctional areas (see p 291). A rise in temperature increases the slope of phase 4, producing sinus tachycardia.

C. Hypoxia and Hypercapnia: Both increase the slope of phase 4, thereby producing sinus tachycardia and ectopic discharge from secondary pacemaker sites. This explains the common clinical occurrence of arrhythmias in patients with pulmonary insufficiency.

D. Cardiac Dilatation: Myocardial stretch increases the slope of phase 4, similarly producing sinus tachycardia and ectopic discharge from secondary pacemakers. This is the reason for the common occurrence of sinus tachycardia and ectopic rhythms in patients with heart failure and their disappearance with therapy that reestablishes compensation and reduces cardiac dilatation.

E. Local Currents of Injury: Myocardial ischemia or necrosis in an area of myocardium can produce a current of injury (see p 140) that will increase the automaticity of neighboring specialized conduction tissue and initiate ectopic rhythms, as is commonly seen in patients with coronary artery disease.

F. Potassium Concentration: A reduction of extracellular potassium (hypokalemia) increases the slope of phase 4, thereby increasing automaticity and resulting in ectopic discharge. It also prolongs repolarization; and, if this occurs in a localized area of myocardium, an electrical gradient will result, increasing automaticity. Hypokalemia increases the membrane resting potential in ventricular muscle cells but not in Purkinje cells. A rise in extracellular potassium (hyperkalemia) has a differential sensitivity on various

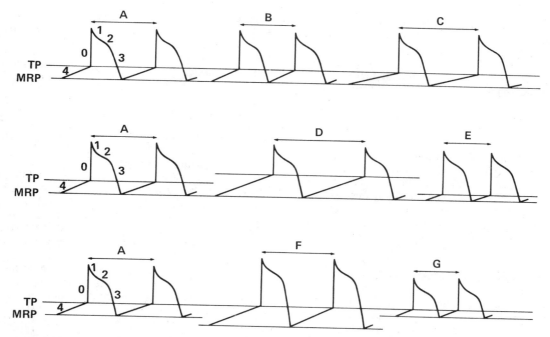

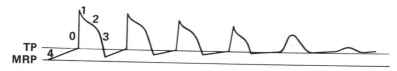

Figure 12–1. Diagrammatic illustrations of action potentials. (See p 18.) Effects of slope of phase 4, MRP, and TP on the rate of impulse formation. *A:* Basic rate of impulse formation is determined by slope of phase 4 and levels of MRP and TP. *B:* The slope of phase 4 is increased (as occurs with beta-adrenergic stimulation, hypoxia, hypercapnia, stretch, and hyperthermia). MRP and TP are the same as in (A). Less time is needed for the potential to reach threshold level, and the rate is therefore increased. *C:* The slope of phase 4 is decreased (as occurs with vagal stimulation, quinidine-like drugs, and hypothermia). MRP and TP are the same as in (A). More time is needed for the potential to reach threshold level, and the rate is therefore slowed. *D:* The threshold potential is reduced. MRP and the slope of phase 4 are the same as in (A). More time is required to reach threshold level, and the rate is therefore slowed. *E:* The threshold potential is increased. MRP and the slope of phase 4 are the same as in (A). This increases the rate. *F:* The MRP is increased. TP and the slope of phase 4 are the same as in (A). This decreases the rate and also increases the height of the action potential. *G:* The MRP is decreased. TP and the slope of phase 4 are the same as in (A). This increases the rate and decreases the height of the action potential.

Figure 12–2. Diagrammatic illustration of progressive (decremental) conduction in a series of Purkinje cells. Reduction in MRP results in progressive reduction in the height and rate of rise of the action potential, slowing conduction and leading to block.

cardiac cells. The Purkinje fibers and myocardial cells are most sensitive—the atrial muscle cells more so than the ventricular. The sinus node, atrial conducting tissues, AV node, and the bundle of His are least sensitive to hyperkalemia. In the sinus node, the slope of phase 4 is decreased; however, the distance between membrane resting potential and threshold potential is decreased, so that the net effect produces no change in the rate of sinus discharge. In Purkinje fibers, the slope of phase 4 is decreased and the distance between membrane resting potential and threshold potential increases, both of which result in a decrease in automaticity (and thereby slow conduction; see below).

G. Calcium Concentration: An increase in extracellular calcium (hypercalcemia) reduces threshold potential and thereby reduces the rate of automatic discharge. Hypocalcemia has the opposite effect. Hypercalcemia shortens the duration of the action potential by shortening phase 2; hypocalcemia lengthens phase 2 (see p 304). *prolong QT*

Conductivity

The rate of depolarization (phase 0 of action potential) and the amplitude of the action potential influence conductivity. A slowing of the rate of rise or of the amplitude of phase 0 decreases the speed of conduction and favors the production of block. A reduction in the magnitude of the membrane resting potential (phase 4) is a common cause for the above. A progressive decrease in the rate of rise and in the amplitude of phase 0 results in progressive impairment of conduction. This can occur in any portion of the conduction system or myocardium. It is termed decremental conduction. This is the explanation for the normal conduction delay in the AV node. Accentuation of this phenomenon produces increasing degrees of AV block.

Decremental conduction leads to progressive decrease in the speed of conduction and the eventual failure of conduction. This usually occurs in only one direction (unidirectional). This unidirectional block prevents conduction along a pathway in one direction but permits propagation in the opposite direction. It thereby permits reentry excitation and may explain the coupling of ectopic beats (bigeminy) or repetitive rapid rhythms (ectopic tachycardia).

Concealed conduction is the term used to explain the following electrophysiologic phenomenon. At times an impulse partially penetrates a portion of the conduction system (most commonly the AV node or AV junctional areas) but is not propagated, so that its effect is not evident at that time but is recognized by the

subsequent disturbance of the next conducted beat. *Examples:* (1) In atrial fibrillation, many impulses enter the AV node but are blocked within the AV node. Only a few impulses emerge from the AV node and result in ventricular excitation. (2) Interpolated ventricular premature beats (see p 254) can result in retrograde spread of the impulse into the AV nodal area. This can result in conduction delay for the next sinus beat which will be evident by a prolonged P–R interval. (3) Many complex arrhythmias are explained on the basis of such concealed conduction.

Hyperkalemia decreases the magnitude of the potential in phase 4. This results in a decrease in the rate of rise and in the amplitude of phase 0, resulting in a decrease in conduction velocity. This effect on conduction through the ventricular myocardium results in widening of the QRS; its maximal effect on atrial myocardium produces complete loss of excitation and the disappearance of the P wave (see p 299).

A decrease in conduction velocity with eventual block can occur when an impulse arrives at cells that have not reached complete repolarization from the previous beat and are thereby activated at a lower level of membrane potential. This is the mechanism for

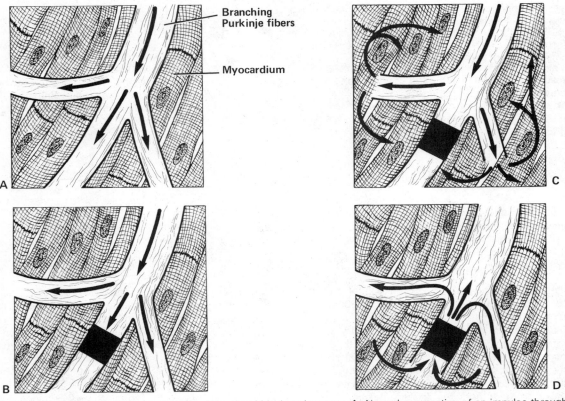

Figure 12–3. Diagrammatic illustration of unidirectional block and reentry. *A:* Normal propagation of an impulse through branching Purkinje fibers with activation of neighboring myocardium. *B:* The hatched area in one Purkinje fiber represents a zone of decremental conduction and unidirectional block. *C:* Propagation through the normally conducting fibers activates the myocardium. *D:* Since the block in the Purkinje fiber is unidirectional, the impulse that has spread through the normally conducting fibers can penetrate the affected fiber in a retrograde direction and reactivate the neighboring Purkinje fibers, producing a second myocardial response (reentry).

aberrancy of intraventricular conduction in association with supraventricular tachycardia (see Chapter 17).

It is probable that many arrhythmias result from alterations in both conductivity and automaticity. An increase in the slope of phase 4 leads to increased automaticity but may also reduce membrane potential, leading to slowed conduction, block, and reentry.

Electrophysiology of the AV Junction

The AV junctional area includes 3 distinct electrophysiologic zones: (1) an atrial-nodal (A-N) zone, consisting of distal atrial conducting fibers entering the AV node; (2) an internodal zone (N); and (3) a nodal-His zone (N-H), consisting of fibers leaving the AV node and entering the His bundle. Cells in the A-N and N-H zones have the property of diastolic depolarization and hence automaticity. Cells in the N region do not demonstrate diastolic depolarization and therefore are not capable of automatic discharge and impulse formation. They also have the property of slow conduction velocity, which explains the normal delay of impulse transmission in the AV node.

EFFECTS OF DRUGS ON CARDIAC RHYTHM

Digitalis

Digitalis has a dual effect on cardiac rhythm, one direct and the other indirect. Its direct effect is to slow conductivity through the atrial myocardium and to delay conduction through the AV node (N zone). Its indirect effect is strong vagal stimulation, which increases conductivity through the atrial myocardium and delays conduction through the AV node (N zone). The net effect of this dual action on the AV node is to slow the ventricular rate. The effect of digitalis on abnormal atrial rates is unique. At ectopic atrial rates of 160–200, digitalis can abolish the ectopic rhythm. At atrial rates of 300 or more, digitalis usually increases the atrial rate. Both of these latter effects are thought to be due to vagal stimulation.

Quinidine

Quinidine likewise has a dual action. Its direct effect is to slow conduction through the atrium, the AV node (A-N and N-H zones), the bundle of His, and the ventricular myocardium and to suppress myocardial irritability. This is accomplished by decreasing the slope of phase 4 (decreasing automaticity) and by a lowering of membrane potential which leads to a decrease in the rate of rise and height of the action potential (phase 0) and thereby slows conduction. It prolongs both the effective refractory period and repolarization, the former more than the latter, so that a response to stimulation occurs at a site of higher membrane potential. This effect occurs in both the atrial and ventricular myocardium and explains the effectiveness of quinidine in suppressing atrial and ventricular ectopic rhythms. Its indirect effect is that of weak vagal depression, which results in delayed conduction through the atrium and increased conduction through the AV node. The net effect on the atrium is to slow conduction, thus initially slowing and then abolishing an ectopic atrial rhythm. In atrial fibrillation, the usual effect of quinidine on the AV node is mainly vagolytic, resulting in improved AV conduction and a more rapid ventricular rate. With high doses of quinidine, the direct blocking action on the AV node may dominate, resulting in increasing degrees of AV block.

The physician must be aware of the interaction between digitalis and quinidine. When quinidine is given to an individual already receiving digoxin, the digoxin blood level is acutely increased as a result of multiple factors: displacement of digoxin binding sites by quinidine, reduction in renal clearance of digoxin, and alterations in the volume of distribution. This elevation in digoxin blood levels can lead to digitalis toxicity.

Procainamide (Pronestyl)

The effect of procainamide is similar to that of quinidine. However, procainamide is much more effective against the ventricular ectopic arrhythmias than those originating in the atria.

Table 12–1. Summary of effects of digitalis and quinidine.

	Quinidine	Digitalis
Vagal effect	Decreased	Increased
Absolute refractory period	No effect (or shortened)	Shortened
Conduction in atria	Delayed	1. Delayed (direct effect) 2. Accelerated (indirect effect)
Effect on AV node	1. Direct: delayed conduction 2. Indirect: accelerated conduction Net effect: slightly accelerated conduction	1. Direct: delayed conduction 2. Indirect: delayed conduction Net effect: markedly delayed conduction
Net effect on atrial rate*	Decreased	1. "Slow" rates (160–200): decreased 2. "Fast" rates (300+): accelerated
Net effect on ventricular rate*	May be accelerated owing to vagolytic effect on AV node	Decreased owing to marked effect on AV node

*In the presence of atrial tachycardia, flutter, or fibrillation.

Table 12–2. Comparative electrophysiologic properties of anti-arrhythmia drugs.

	Quinidine, Procainamide	Phenytoin, Lidocaine	Propranolol
Automaticity	Decreased	Decreased	Decreased
Duration of action potential	Increased	Decreased	Decreased
Effective refractory period	Increased	Decreased	Decreased
Conduction velocity	Decreased	No change or increased	Decreased
AV conduction time	No change, increased (direct), or decreased (indirect)	No change or decreased	No change or increased

Lidocaine (Xylocaine)

Lidocaine, like procainamide and quinidine, decreases automaticity by lowering the slope of phase 4 and therefore is effective in abolishing ectopic discharges, especially those of ventricular origin. In contrast to the latter drugs, it does not prolong the duration of the action potential, or it may even shorten the action potential and therefore, in the usual therapeutic doses, not produce conduction delay. It is also less hypotensive than the other 2 drugs, and its effect is of shorter duration.

Phenytoin (Dilantin)

This drug is of limited value in the control of ventricular arrhythmias except when they are the result of digitalis toxicity. It decreases automaticity by lowering the slope of phase 4. In contrast to quinidine-like drugs, it produces an increase in the rate of rise and height of the action potential (phase 0) even in the presence of a lowered membrane potential. This increases conduction velocity and thereby prevents reentry. It shortens repolarization and the effective refractory period of Purkinje fibers, the former more so than the latter, so that the earliest response to stimulation occurs at a site of higher membrane potential, thereby increasing conduction. By these mechanisms the drug depresses ventricular automaticity and abolishes reentry arrhythmias by increasing conduction velocity.

Propranolol (Inderal)

Propranolol is a beta-adrenergic blocking drug. It also has a quinidine-like action. It is effective in slowing the ventricular rate in atrial flutter and fibrillation by increasing the degree of AV block (A-N and N-H zones); it may be effective in converting atrial tachycardia to sinus rhythm; and it is of value in eliminating ventricular ectopic rhythms, especially those due to digitalis toxicity. It must be used with caution in the patient with heart failure since it depresses myocardial contractility and thereby can aggravate heart failure.

Disopyramide (Norpace)

This drug is similar to quinidine in its electrophysiologic action and clinical use. It causes less gastrointestinal disturbance than quinidine but has a greater negative inotropic action and a potent atropine-like effect.

Other Antiarrhythmia Drugs

Antiarrhythmia drugs are a subject of intensive research effort at present. Many drugs available in Europe are not yet approved for this indication in the USA, including tocainide, mexiletine, encainide, lorcainide, aprindine, and amiodarone. Verapamil (Calan, Osoptin) was recently approved and is being widely used.

NORMAL & ABNORMAL CARDIAC RHYTHMS

Diagram of Cardiac Conduction

Fig 12–4 illustrates the electrocardiographic tracings of normal and abnormal conduction.

SINUS RHYTHMS

Regular Sinus Rhythm

This is the normal rhythm of the heart. The average rate is 60–100 beats/min.

Sinus Tachycardia

A regular sinus rhythm with a rate in excess of 100. Sinus tachycardia does not usually exceed 160 beats/min in the adult.

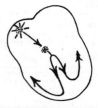

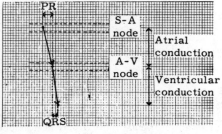

Figure 12–4. Diagram of cardiac conduction. (The normal delay in the AV node is not illustrated.)

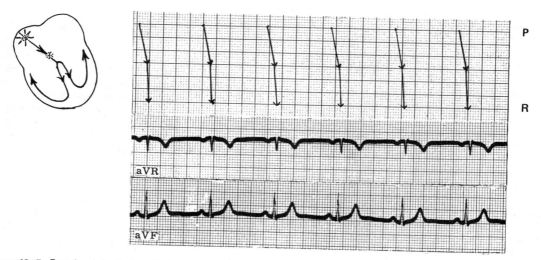

Figure 12–5. Regular sinus rhythm. R –R = 0.96 s. Rate = 63. The P is normally inverted in aVR and normally upright in aVF.

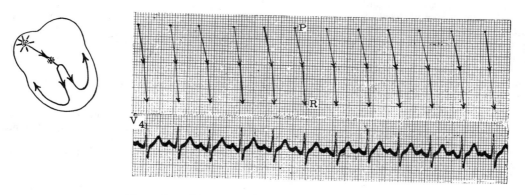

Figure 12–6. Sinus tachycardia. R –R = 0.48 s. Rate = 125.

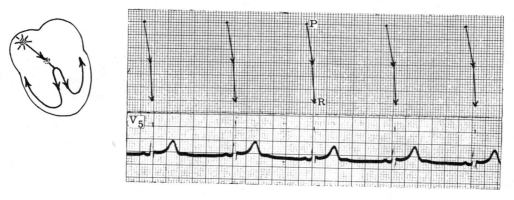

Figure 12–7. Sinus bradycardia. R –R = 1.2 s. Rate = 50.

100. Sinus tachycardia does not usually exceed 160 beats/min in the adult.

Sinus Bradycardia

A regular sinus rhythm with a rate under 60/min.

Sinus Arrhythmia

The impulse arises normally in the SA node. The arrhythmia is manifested by alternating periods of slower and more rapid heart rates. The variations are usually related to respiration, the rate increasing with inspiration and decreasing with expiration. This condition is more common in children than adults and is frequently associated with sinus bradycardia.

Clinical Significance

Sinus tachycardia, sinus bradycardia, and sinus arrhythmia do not in themselves indicate any organic heart disease.

Sinoatrial (SA) Block

In this situation, the sinus node discharges regularly, but, as a result of exit block, all do not result in atrial depolarization. There can be partial or complete SA block. Since the sinus node discharge is not evident in the ECG, this arrhythmia is recognized by group beating of sinus-conducted beats followed by pauses without P waves.

Partial SA block (Wenckebach type): The Wenckebach phenomenon (see p 239) describes a conduction disturbance in which conduction is delayed for increasingly prolonged intervals from beat to beat until it is completely blocked for one beat, whereupon the cycle is repeated. The greatest increase in the progressive conduction delay is in the second complex of the cycle. The ECG will record sinus rhythm with a constant PR interval. There will be progressive shortening of the R–R intervals until a beat is dropped. In 2:1 SA block, sinus bradycardia will be evident and the diagnosis can only be made if sinus rhythm at twice the rate is seen in other parts of the record.

Complete SA block: For variable periods of time, consecutive sinus node discharges do not result in atrial depolarization. This results in atrial standstill, which is often followed by an escape rhythm, usually from an AV junctional pacemaker. It is impossible to differentiate between complete SA exit block (implying continued sinus node discharges with no atrial capture) and failure of impulse formation in the SA node.

Clinical Significance

SA exit block is commonly the result of increased vagal tone. It can occur in normal individuals, can be produced by carotid sinus or eyeball pressure (eg, eye surgery) or other vagal reflexes, or can be the result of drug toxicity (digitalis, quinidine) or organic heart disease involving the SA nodal area secondary to inflammation or ischemia. It is one manifestation of the "sick sinus syndrome."

ABNORMAL ATRIAL RHYTHMS

ATRIAL PREMATURE BEATS

An atrial premature beat (premature contraction or premature depolarization) results from a secondary stimulus arising in an ectopic focus anywhere in either atrium. An atrial excitation (P') takes place prematurely. Usually it will initiate a ventricular complex

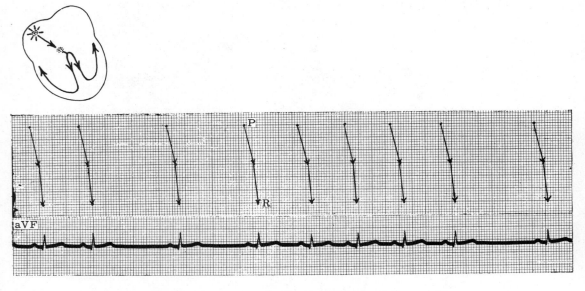

Figure 12–8. Sinus arrhythmia. Slowing of the rate during expiration.

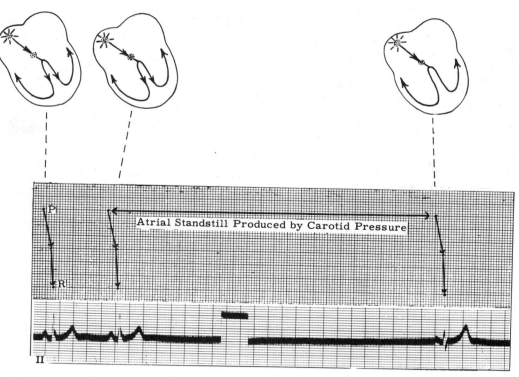

Figure 12–9. Atrial standstill (lead II). The patient was a 25-year-old "vagotonic" individual. The rhythm at the start of the record is regular sinus with a rate of 63. Following right carotid sinus pressure, complete asystole is produced for 4.6 s. The first beat following asystole is sinus-conducted but shows aberrant intraventricular conduction. (See Chapter 17.)

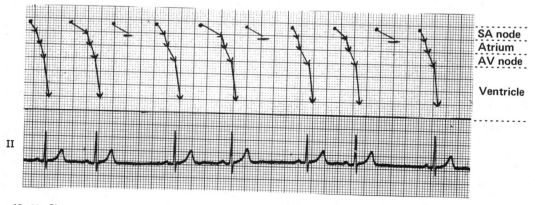

Figure 12–10. Sinus node exit block (3:2 Wenckebach type). Repetitively, 2 sinus-conducted beats are followed by a pause. All P waves are of the same form, the P–R interval is constant, and no blocked atrial premature beats are evident. In this instance, the sinus node is firing regularly (but cannot be seen in the ECG). There is a progressive SA block with the result that every third SA discharge is not conducted.

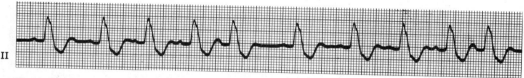

Figure 12–11. Sinus node Wenckebach block. Cycles of 5 sinus-conducted beats are seen followed by a pause. The P–R interval is constant. The R–R interval between the first 2 beats of the cycle is longest because the greatest increment of conduction delay occurs with the second beat. A left bundle branch block is also present.

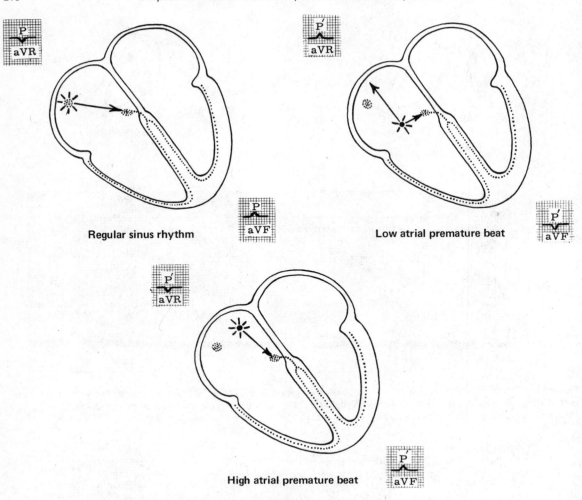

Figure 12–12. Regular sinus rhythm and ectopic atrial rhythms.

with a normal or basic* QRS configuration. Since the normal spread of excitation is from the upper end to the lower end of the atrium, the P wave is normally inverted in aVR and high esophageal leads and upright in aVF and low esophageal leads. An atrial ectopic stimulus arising in the upper end of the atrium will result in P′ waves having this same normal direction. An impulse arising in the lower end of the atrium will stimulate the atrium in a foot-to-head direction, producing upright P′ waves in aVR and high esophageal leads, and inverted P′ waves in aVF and low esophageal leads. The P′–R interval may be shorter or longer than the basic P–R interval. In most instances, there is not a full compensatory pause (see p 254) in association with this arrhythmia. That is, the R–R

*The term "basic" is used to describe the configuration of the QRS complex associated with the regular sinus-conducted beats. Thus, in a bundle branch block, the basic QRS complex will be wide and slurred and an atrial premature beat will likewise produce a QRS complex of the bundle branch type.

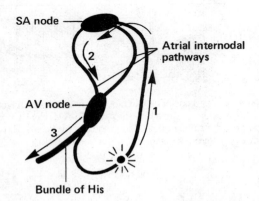

Figure 12–13. Diagrammatic illustration of low atrial ectopic beat, producing a normally directed P wave. *(1)* Rapid retrograde passage of impulse up an internodal pathway. *(2)* Resultant depolarization of the atria in a normal direction. *(3)* Normal anterograde spread of impulse to AV node and bundle of His.

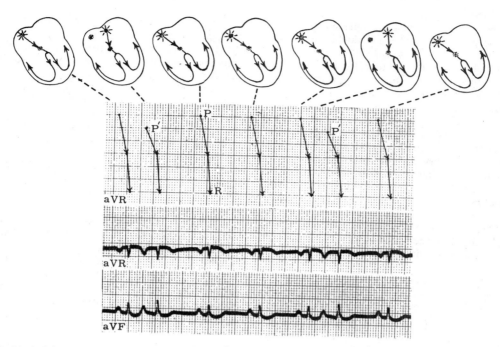

Figure 12–14. Atrial premature beats: High atrial ectopic focus. The rhythm is predominantly regular sinus. The rate is 75. The P–P interval is 0.8 s. The P′ wave occurs 0.64 s after the preceding P, ie, it occurs prematurely. The P′–R interval is longer than the normal P–R interval. P′ is inverted in aVR and upright in aVF, indicating a high atrial ectopic focus. The normal configuration of the QRS complex of the premature beat indicates that conduction through the AV node and ventricles is normal.

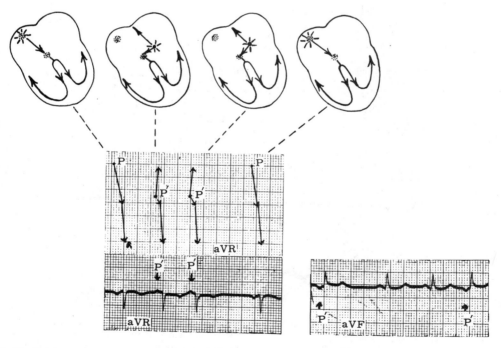

Figure 12–15. Atrial premature beats: Low atrial ectopic focus. The predominant rhythm is regular sinus. The rate = 81. The P–P interval = 0.74 s. The P′ waves occur prematurely. The P′ is upright in aVR and inverted in aVF. This is the reverse of the normal P wave and indicates a low atrial ectopic focus. The QRS complexes are normal.

interval between the normal beats preceding and following the premature beat is not double the normal R–R interval.

The polarity (ie, direction) of the P vector is not always predictive of the site of origin of an atrial ectopic beat. It has been shown experimentally that production of an atrial ectopic beat by electrical stimulation in certain low atrial areas can produce a P wave of normal direction which is therefore upright in aVF. The P–R interval is usually shortened. This is explained by the theory that the stimulus arises in, or close to, one of the internodal pathways. The impulse rapidly spreads upward (retrograde) in this tract to the high atrial area or sinus node; atrial depolarization then results in a normal (anterograde) direction, producing an upright P wave in aVF. The AV node, bundle of His, and ventricle are activated by the ectopic stimulus in a normal anterograde direction.

Blocked Atrial Premature Contractions

If the P′ wave occurs very soon after a normal beat, the AV node and the ventricle will still be refrac-

tory and will not respond. This is known as a blocked atrial premature beat.

Premature atrial foci arising in the middle of the atrium will produce flat or diphasic P′ waves in aVR and aVF.

Aberrant intraventricular conduction may be associated with atrial premature beats. This will be discussed in Chapter 17.

At times, the P′ waves may not be apparent in any given lead. Therefore, the pause following this may be mistaken for SA exit block. Usually, another lead will more clearly demonstrate the ectopic P wave (Fig 12–17).

Clinical Significance

Atrial premature beats frequently occur in normal individuals. At times, they may occur secondary to stimulation from emotional disturbances, tobacco, tea, or coffee. Digitalis uncommonly produces this arrhythmia. Almost any form of organic heart disease may be responsible, and in such instances this arrhythmia may be the precursor of paroxysmal atrial

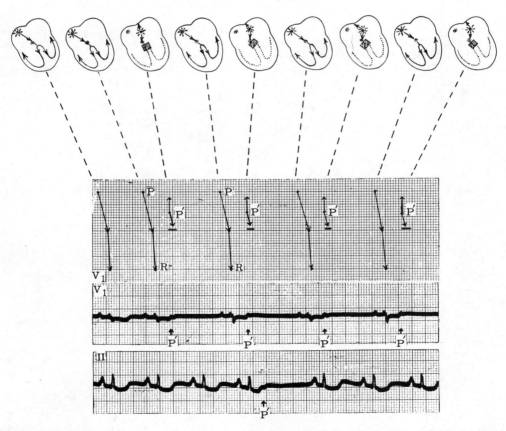

Figure 12–16. Blocked atrial premature contractions: V₁. The first 2 beats are sinus-conducted. The P–P interval = 0.68 s. An atrial complex (P′) follows the second QRS complex. The P–P′ interval = 0.36 s. This atrial complex is occurring prematurely. Since it follows so closely after the QRS, the AV node and ventricle are still refractory and do not respond. A full compensatory pause does not follow. The cycle is repeated for the next 3 sinus-conducted beats, producing an atrial bigeminal rhythm, ie, one regular sinus-conducted beat followed by one blocked atrial premature beat. In lead II, one blocked premature atrial contraction is seen.

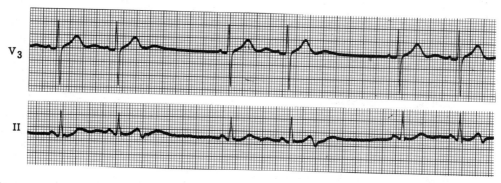

Figure 12–17. Blocked atrial premature beats. Two sinus-conducted beats are followed by a long pause. In lead V$_3$, this simulates SA block; in lead II, the blocked atrial premature beats are clearly evident.

tachycardia and atrial fibrillation. As a general rule, a diagnosis of organic heart disease must not be made solely on the electrocardiographic finding of atrial premature contractions.

WANDERING PACEMAKER

In this disturbance of cardiac rhythm, some of the impulses originate in the SA node whereas others originate from various foci in the atrium and even in the AV junction. As a result, there will be a variation in rhythm, a changing configuration of the P' wave and a changing P'–R interval. Normally inverted P or P' waves in aVR and upright P or P' waves in aVF will result from impulses arising in the SA node and the upper portion of the atrium; upright P' waves in aVR and inverted P' waves in aVF will result from impulses arising in the lower portion of the atrium or AV junction.

Clinical Significance

This arrhythmia may occur in normal individuals. It can result from increased vagal tone. Digitalis may be the etiologic factor. Various forms of organic heart disease, notably acute rheumatic fever, can also produce this arrhythmia.

PAROXYSMAL ATRIAL TACHYCARDIA

Paroxysmal atrial tachycardia is characterized by a regular atrial rhythm at a rate of 160–220. In most instances there is 1:1 AV conduction. Less commonly, atrial tachycardia is associated with AV block of varying degree, usually 2:1.

Etiology & Incidence

Paroxysmal atrial tachycardia most commonly occurs in normal individuals who show no clinical evidence of heart disease. It may occur in relation to

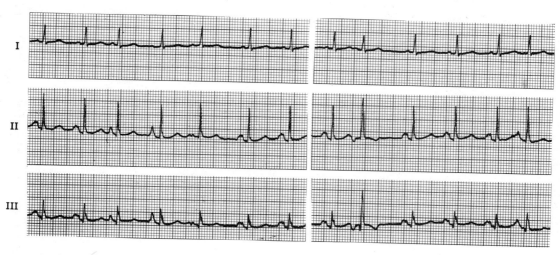

Figure 12–18. Wandering pacemaker. Each QRS complex is preceded by an atrial wave. However, the configuration of the P wave frequently changes in height and direction, and the P–R interval varies. This indicates that the pacemaker is shifting from the sinus node to varying portions of the atrium.

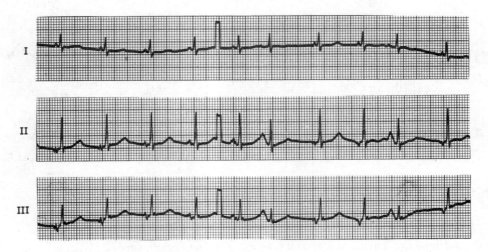

Figure 12–19. Wandering atrial pacemaker. The rhythm is irregular. Each QRS complex is preceded by a P wave, but there is a marked variation in the morphology of the P waves. Some are tall and upright (of sinus origin) in leads II and III; others are inverted or diphasic in these leads and have shorter P–R intervals. The above is indicative of varying atrial pacemakers (from sinus node to AV junctional sites). It is possible that some of the P waves represent fusion between 2 atrial foci. *Clinical diagnosis:* Severe chronic obstructive lung disease.

emotional trauma. Rheumatic mitral valvular disease, pulmonary embolization, cardiac surgery, thyrotoxicosis, and coronary artery disease are less common etiologic factors. It is the common arrhythmia associated with the WPW syndrome (see p 272). Atrial tachycardia with AV block is a common manifestation of digitalis toxicity (see pp 292–295).

Mechanism

Two mechanisms can be invoked to explain the occurrence of atrial tachycardia: **(1) Ectopic mechanism:** An ectopic focus located in either atrium discharges at the above-mentioned rate. Each atrial stimulus activates the ventricle, resulting in a regular ventricular rhythm. There are rare exceptions to the typical regularity of atrial tachycardia. These are (a) multiple atrial foci instead of a single focus, producing an atrial tachycardia of the wandering pacemaker type (occasionally seen in patients with cor pulmonale); and (b) introduction of premature beats from other foci, interrupting the regularity of the rhythm. **(2) Reentry mechanism:** Evidence based on multiple intracardiac recordings indicates that a reentry mechanism is a more common—if not the major—explanation for atrial tachycardia. The tachycardia is initiated by one atrial premature beat with a prolonged P–R interval. The ventricle is activated in a normal fashion through the AV node, bundle of His, bundle branches, and Purkinje fibers. In addition, the stimulus is able to reenter the bundle of His in a retrograde direction (possibly spreading through fibers that had not been depolarized by the initial anterograde stimulus) and activate nonrefractory sites in the bundle of His, AV junctional regions, or the atria, and is then propagated in a normal anterograde direction to result in a second ventricular capture. Perpetuation along this reentry pathway results in atrial tachycardia. It is also possible that the pathway may exist within the atria only. Reentry atrial tachycardia due to an accessory pathway in the preexcitation syndromes will be discussed in Chapter 16.

Electrocardiographic Pattern

Paroxysmal atrial tachycardia resembles a continuous run of atrial premature beats. With the rare exceptions of the above-mentioned conditions, each P' wave will be followed by a ventricular complex. As is true also of atrial premature beats (see p 216), the direction of the P' waves in leads aVR, aVF, and esophageal leads will indicate the site of origin (high or low) of the atrial ectopic focus (with the exception as stated on p 216).

The QRS complexes and T waves usually are of normal (or basic) configuration. However, with prolonged tachycardia, the ST segment may become depressed and the T waves inverted in left ventricular epicardial leads as a result of ischemia. Aberrancy of intraventricular conduction can occur with atrial tachycardia (see p 283) and thereby simulate ventricular tachycardia.

In this arrhythmia, the impulse spreads through atrial muscle more slowly than a normal sinus beat or an atrial premature beat. Thus, the P'–R interval is often prolonged. The P' wave may therefore be buried in the preceding ventricular (QRS) complex, simulating an AV junctional tachycardia (see p 250).

Following reversion of an episode of paroxysmal atrial tachycardia to sinus rhythm, the ECG may show transient deep T wave inversions in many leads, whereas such inversions were not present before or during the tachycardia. These posttachycardia changes in ventricular repolarization are not evidence of new

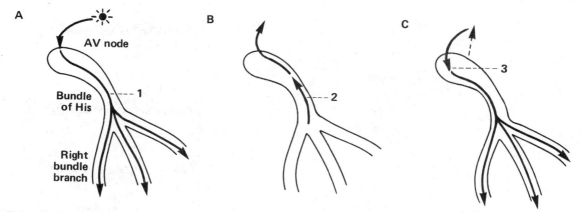

Figure 12–20. Diagrammatic illustration of the reentry mechanism. *A:* An atrial ectopic beat activates the ventricle *(1)* in a normal fashion. *B:* The same activation wave reenters the bundle of His and spreads through the AV node to the atrium *(2)*. *C:* The retrograde atrial activation reenters atrial pathways and is conducted in a normal anterograde direction through the AV node, bundle of His, and intraventricular conducting pathways to again depolarize the ventricle *(3)*. This second activation wave reenters the bundle of His (as in [B]), perpetuating the reentry cycle. It is possible that this reentry pathway can exist within AV junctional sites or within the bundle of His.

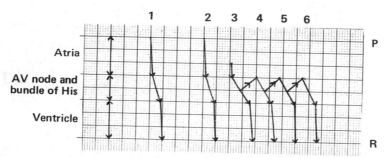

Figure 12–21. Normal and atrial ectopic beats. *1 and 2:* Normal sinus beats. *3:* Atrial ectopic beat with prolonged P–R interval. *4, 5, and 6:* Reentry mechanism which produces atrial tachycardia.

myocardial disease, however, since this phenomenon occurs in clinically normal individuals.

Differential Diagnosis

A. Sinus Tachycardia: A paroxysmal atrial tachycardia arising from an initial ectopic focus high in the atrium and therefore producing normally directed P′ waves may be indistinguishable from a sinus tachycardia at rates of approximately 140–160 in one single ECG. A constant R–R interval will favor a diagnosis of paroxysmal atrial tachycardia. The response to carotid sinus pressure may solve this problem. In paroxysmal atrial tachycardia, this maneuver may abruptly terminate the attack. In sinus tachycardia there may be some gradual and slight sinus slowing. If there is no response to carotid sinus pressure, one must then compare the pattern of the P (or P′) waves of the tachycardia to the pattern present during slower regular sinus rhythm. If there is a difference in configuration of the atrial complexes in the 2 tracings, a diagnosis of paroxysmal atrial tachycardia is justified. The above refers to an electrocardiographic differential diagnosis and does not include the points

of clinical difference between these 2 rhythms.

B. Junctional and Ventricular Tachycardia: These will be discussed under their respective headings.

Clinical Significance

The tachycardia may last for a few seconds, minutes, hours, or days. Persistence of this arrhythmia in an individual with a diseased myocardium can precipitate congestive heart failure and coronary insufficiency. Even in a normal individual, the persistence of the tachycardia for days can produce heart failure. It is therefore urgent that this arrhythmia be diagnosed and treated promptly.

Prognosis

The prognosis of paroxysmal atrial tachycardia depends on the status of the heart irrespective of the tachycardia. If properly treated and if there is no known underlying cause, this arrhythmia will in no way reduce the patient's life expectancy. Such patients are prone to have recurrences unless controlled by digitalis or quinidine (or both) in maintenance doses.

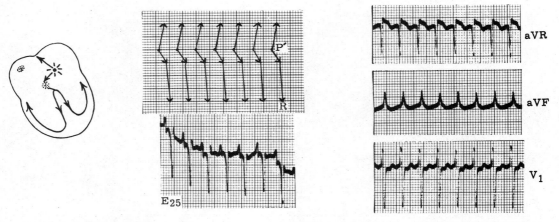

Figure 12–22. Paroxysmal atrial tachycardia. The ventricular rhythm is regular at a rate of 215. The QRS complexes are normal. No definite evidence of atrial activity can be seen in leads aVR, aVF, and V_1. Lead E_{25} shows an upright P′ preceding each QRS complex, indicating a low atrial ectopic focus.

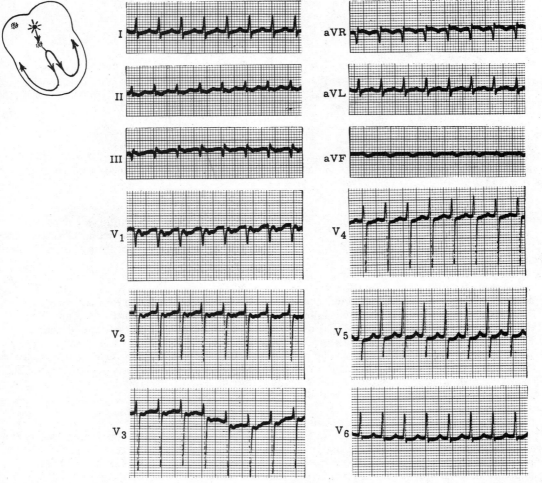

Figure 12–23. Paroxysmal atrial tachycardia. A regular ventricular rhythm is seen with a ventricular rate of 188. The QRS complexes are not widened. P′ waves are evident in V_{1-2}. The minor ST depressions seen in precordial leads could be the result of prominent T_a waves or could represent myocardial ischemia secondary to the tachycardia.

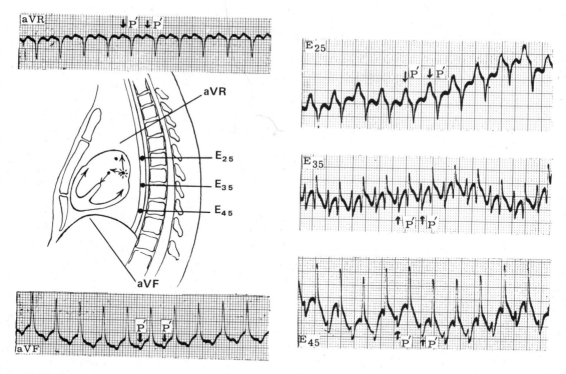

Figure 12–24. Paroxysmal atrial tachycardia. The atrial and ventricular rates are 170. The P' waves (indicated by arrows) are upright in aVR, inverted in aVF and E₄₅, diphasic in E₃₅, and upright in E₂₅, indicating an ectopic focus low in the atrium (or AV junction).

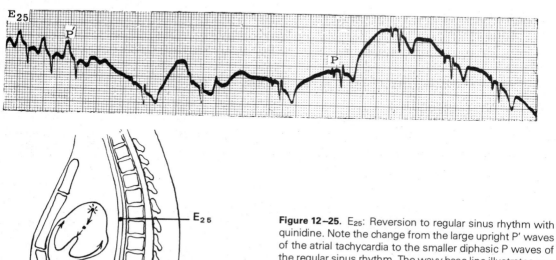

Figure 12–25. E₂₅: Reversion to regular sinus rhythm with quinidine. Note the change from the large upright P' waves of the atrial tachycardia to the smaller diphasic P waves of the regular sinus rhythm. The wavy base line illustrates one of the technical difficulties encountered in taking esophageal leads.

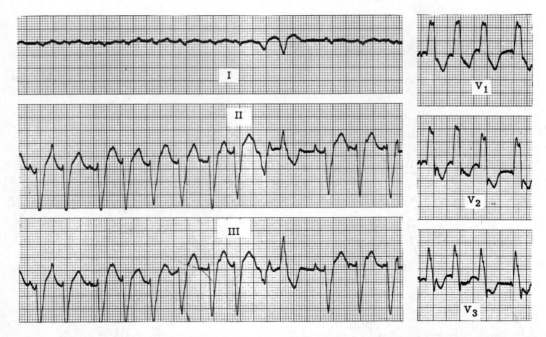

Figure 12–26. Chaotic atrial tachycardia. The ventricular rate is 130 and totally irregular. Each QRS is preceded by a P wave. The P waves are of variable configuration and direction. The P–P, P–R, and R–R intervals are not constant. There is an intraventricular conduction defect indicative of right bundle branch block and left anterior fascicular block. The ninth and tenth QRS complexes in I, II, and III show further aberrancy. *Clinical and autopsy diagnosis:* 80-year-old man with severe chronic obstructive lung disease and coronary artery disease.

These patients must be assured that their paroxysms are not indicative of heart disease and that the prognosis is excellent.

CHAOTIC ATRIAL RHYTHM

A chaotic atrial rhythm is one in which there are 3 or more different types of P waves that activate the ventricles. In addition to the variation in P wave morphology, the P–P, P–R, and R–R intervals are not constant. There is usually 1:1 AV conduction, but occasional P waves that fall in the refractory period of the previous beat are blocked. Aberrancy of intraventricular conduction may occur with single or multiple beats. This arrhythmia simulates a wandering atrial pacemaker rhythm and multiple atrial ectopic beats, but it is differentiated by the inability to select a dominant P wave.

Clinically, this arrhythmia is seen in elderly individuals who have chronic obstructive lung disease and coronary artery disease. The ventricular rate is often rapid, and when the rate exceeds 120, the rhythm is called chaotic (or multifocal) atrial tachycardia. Digitalis is relatively ineffective in slowing the ventricular rate. Antiarrhythmia drugs are of limited value. Digitalis toxicity is a rare cause of this arrhythmia.

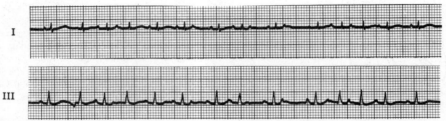

Figure 12–27. Multifocal atrial tachycardia. The ventricular rate is 140; the ventricular rhythm is irregular. Each QRS is preceded by a P wave. The P waves vary in configuration and direction. The P–R interval varies from beat to beat. Some of the P waves do not activate the ventricle (blocked atrial beats). This tracing represents an atrial tachycardia resulting from multiple atrial foci (ie, wandering pacemaker). *Clinical diagnosis:* Severe chronic lung disease with hypoxia and hypercapnia. The patient was not receiving digitalis.

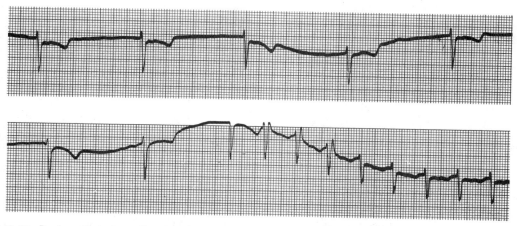

Figure 12–28. Bradycardia-tachycardia syndrome. Continuous recording of lead V₁. In the upper strip, a regular ventricular rhythm is evident at a rate of 38. The QRS complexes are narrow and are followed by retrograde P waves, indicating an AV junctional rhythm. In the lower strip, there are upright P waves which represent independent sinus activity. The bradycardia abruptly changes to a supraventricular tachycardia, rate = 125.

BRADYCARDIA–TACHYCARDIA SYNDROME

Marked sinus bradycardia or slow AV junctional rhythms may occur as a result of diseases that involve the SA node or the atria and may significantly lower cardiac output and produce symptoms of dizziness and syncope. Unless the bradycardia is the result of some reversible factor, such as drug toxicity, pacing is indicated. This disorder is often referred to as the sick-sinus syndrome.

In addition to periods of bradycardia, the patient may also experience episodes of supraventricular tachycardia. This is called the bradycardia-tachycardia syndrome. Medical therapy for the tachycardia could seriously worsen the bradycardia phase of the syndrome. Therefore, pacing is indicated to prevent serious bradycardia and permit medical therapy of the tachycardia.

ATRIAL FLUTTER

Atrial flutter is manifested by a regular atrial rate, usually 220–350 (the author has observed one case with an atrial rate of 430), with varying degrees of AV block, usually 2:1 or 4:1. The ventricular rhythm is most often regular, being one-half to one-fourth the atrial rate. Occasionally, as a result of a constantly changing AV block, the ventricular rhythm is irregular.

Etiology & Incidence

Atrial flutter may occur in normal individuals. However, there is usually underlying organic disease, notably coronary artery disease, rheumatic mitral valvular disease, pulmonary embolization, cardiac surgery, or associated hyperthyroidism. It commonly occurs during the course of quinidine therapy for atrial fibrillation. It is seen much less commonly in association with trauma to the heart, metastatic malignancy involving the heart, and the various myocarditides.

Mechanism

Since the work of Sir Thomas Lewis, it had been accepted that atrial flutter results from a "circus" movement in the atrium. The work of Scherf and Prinzmetal had shown that atrial flutter results from a single ectopic atrial focus. Thus, except for the difference in AV conduction, atrial tachycardia and atrial flutter differ only in frequency of atrial rates. Sir Thomas Lewis' still valid observations of the influence of the atrial rate upon AV conduction testify further to the identity of the basic mechanism of the 2 conditions. With atrial rates of 160–220 (atrial tachycardia), vagal stimulation produces asystole followed by reversion to regular sinus rhythm; with rates of 220–300, varying degrees of AV block result without a change in the atrial rate; with rates of 340 or more, atrial fibrillation results. This explains the reversion of paroxysmal atrial tachycardia to regular sinus rhythm with carotid sinus pressure (vagal influence), the abrupt but temporary slowing of the ventricular rhythm in atrial flutter with carotid sinus pressure (vagal influence), and the conversion of atrial flutter to atrial fibrillation with digitalis (vagal influence).

The above "ectopic" unitarian concept was never universally accepted. As in the case of atrial tachycardia, intracardiac recordings favor the presence of a reentry mechanism. The reentry pathway could lie within the atria, thereby confirming Lewis' original work. Thus, it is possible to explain both atrial tachycardia and atrial flutter on the basis of a "uni-

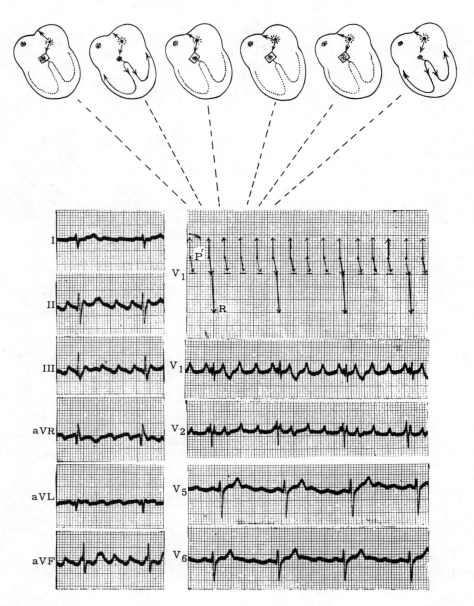

Figure 12–29. Atrial flutter. The atria are beating regularly at a rate of 240. The P' waves have a "saw-toothed" appearance in II, III, and aVF. The ventricles are beating regularly at a rate of 60. Every fourth atrial stimulus penetrates the AV node and results in ventricular stimulation. Thus, this a 4:1 atrial flutter. In addition, the pattern is that of an incomplete right bundle branch block (rsR' in V₁; QRS = 0.08 s). *Clinical diagnosis:* Mitral stenosis.

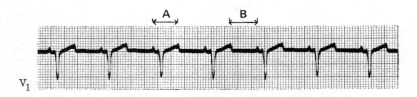

Figure 12–30. Atrial flutter with inconstant atrial rate. A 2:1 atrial flutter is present. The ventricular rhythm is regular at a rate of 75. The P'–P' interval in which a QRS complex intervenes (A) is 0.38 s. The P'–P' interval with no intervening QRS complex (B) is 0.41 s. This difference in rate is thought to result from a reflex mechanism induced by the ventricular contraction.

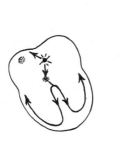

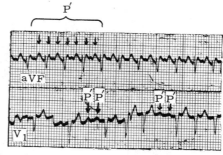

Figure 12–31. Atrial flutter (with 2:1 AV block). Lead aVF: The ventricular rhythm is regular; the rate = 215. At first glance, only one atrial contraction is seen for each QRS complex. However, upon closer inspection, another P' wave may be present immediately following the QRS complex. Lead V₁: With carotid pressure the degree of AV block is temporarily increased and an atrial rate of 430 is present. This proves that the pattern in aVF is an atrial flutter with 2:1 AV block.

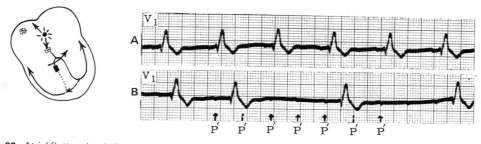

Figure 12–32. Atrial flutter simulating regular sinus rhythm. *A:* The ventricular rate is 72; the pattern is that of a right bundle branch block. Only one atrial wave is seen preceding each QRS complex, which suggests regular sinus rhythm. Other leads offered no further information. *B:* Taken during carotid sinus pressure. This produces further AV block and clearly demonstrates a flutter with an atrial rate of 144. This proves that the rhythm in (A) is a 2:1 atrial flutter (or tachycardia).

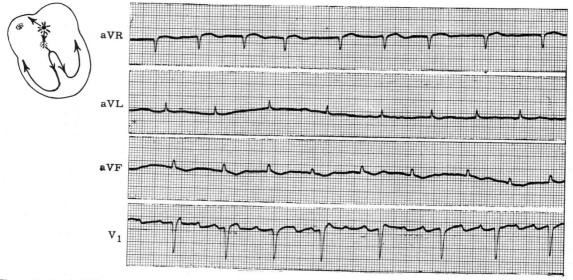

Figure 12–33. Atrial flutter simulating atrial fibrillation. Leads aVR, aVL, and aVF reveal an irregular ventricular rhythm with no evidence of regular atrial activity. Other leads, except V₁, showed a similar pattern. This would be termed atrial fibrillation. Lead V₁ shows a regular atrial rhythm at a rate of 210. The ventricular rhythm is irregular. This is an atrial flutter with irregular ventricular response.

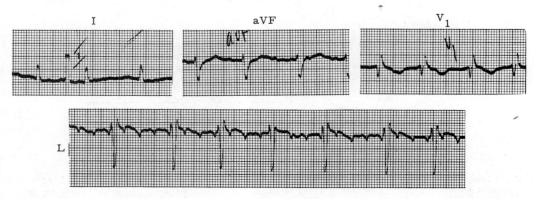

Figure 12–34. Value of Lewis lead. Leads I, aVF, and V₁ indicate some atrial activity which cannot be defined with certainty. A Lewis lead (L, see p 4) clearly indicates an atrial flutter with irregular ventricular response.

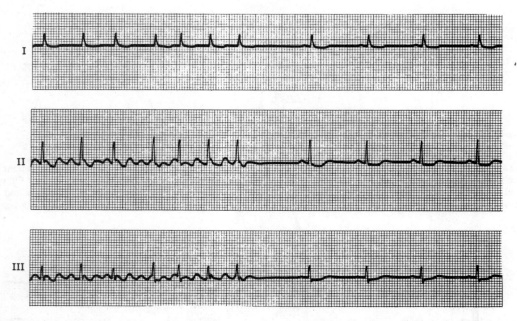

Figure 12–35. Atrial flutter. The initial portion of the record indicates atrial flutter (or flutter-fibrillation) with spontaneous reversion to sinus rhythm.

tarian reentry'' concept rather than invoking a ''unitarian ectopic'' mechanism or differing mechanisms.

Electrocardiographic Pattern

With atrial rates of less than 200, the P' waves of atrial flutter will be identical with those of atrial tachycardia. As the atrial rate increases, a more prominent T_a wave will appear. The direction of the T_a wave is opposite to that of the P'. As the atrial rate continues to increase (over 300), the amplitude of the T_a wave will be equal to that of the P' wave, producing a ''saw-toothed'' appearance. The direction of the P' wave will indicate the site of origin of the ectopic atrial focus. An alternative explanation for the appearance of the rapid atrial depolarizations is that it is a result of a reentry phenomenon within the atria. The QRS com-

plexes are of normal (or basic) configuration if no other cardiac abnormalities exist. This resulting electrocardiographic pattern is consistent with either a reentry or single ectopic mechanism.

Differential Diagnosis of Atrial Flutter

A. Paroxysmal Atrial Tachycardia: Basically, there is no difference between atrial tachycardia and atrial flutter except for the atrial rate and the difference in the site of reentry. Therefore, both of these rhythms can be defined as atrial tachycardia of a given atrial rate with a certain degree of AV block, ie, 1:1, 2:1, 4:1, etc. At times, such a rhythm with a 2:1 block may be mistaken for an atrial tachycardia with 1:1 conduction or even regular sinus rhythm because one of the P' waves is buried in the QRS complex. In such an in-

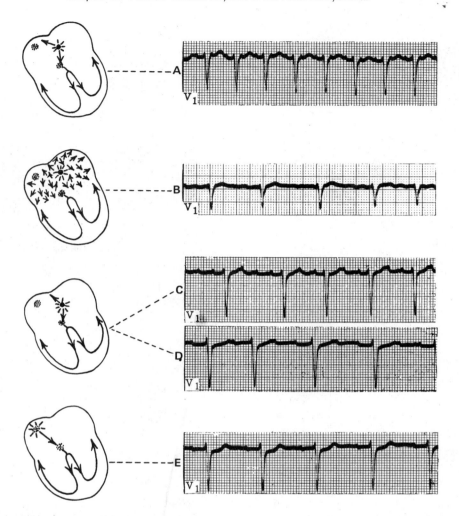

Figure 12–36. Atrial flutter: Response to digitalis and quinidine. **A:** Before therapy: Atrial flutter with 2:1 AV block. The atrial rate is 272; the ventricular rate is 136. **B:** After digitalization: The rhythm is now atrial fibrillation; the ventricular rate has been slowed to 80. **C:** During initial quinidine therapy: Quinidine has changed the atrial fibrillation to atrial flutter. The atrial rate is 272 (as in [A]), but owing to the blocking action of digitalis on the AV node there is 3:1 and 4:1 AV block, resulting in a ventricular rate of 85. **D:** During continued quinidine therapy: Atrial flutter persists, but the atrial rate has been reduced to 200. There is 2:1 and 3:1 AV block, resulting in a ventricular rate of 75. **E:** Further quinidine therapy: The rhythm has reverted to regular sinus.

stance, carotid sinus pressure will be helpful in making the differentiation by increasing the degree of AV block.

B. Atrial Fibrillation: With rapid atrial rates, many leads of the ECG will not clearly show the regularly recurring P′ waves. If the ventricular response is irregular, this will simulate atrial fibrillation. Lead V₁, which most commonly best records the atrial impulses, will usually show the regular P′ waves even though no other lead of the 12-lead ECG will. Carotid sinus pressure, by increasing the degree of AV block, is also of aid.

Clinical Significance

Atrial flutter may be paroxysmal or chronic. The

urgency of therapy will depend upon the ventricular rate, as in paroxysmal atrial tachycardia.

Prognosis

The prognosis of atrial flutter will depend on the nature of the underlying heart disease. If no heart disease is present, the prognosis is the same as that of paroxysmal atrial tachycardia.

ATRIAL FIBRILLATION

Atrial fibrillation is a totally irregular atrial rhythm manifested by an irregular ventricular rhythm

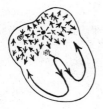

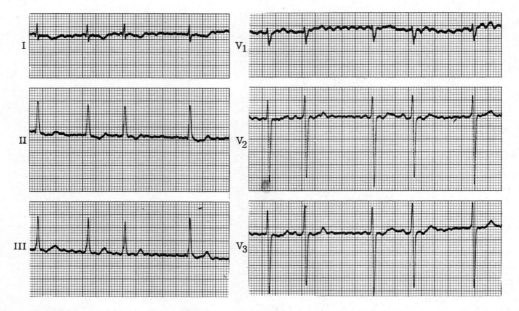

Figure 12–37. Atrial fibrillation. Atrial activity is manifested by rapid, small, irregular waves. The ventricular rhythm is completely irregular.

occurring at rates of less than 50 to more than 200.

Etiology & Incidence

Atrial fibrillation is most commonly seen in association with coronary artery disease, rheumatic mitral valvular disease, and hyperthyroidism. It may also occur in perfectly normal persons, either in paroxysmal or chronic, persistent form. Less common etiologic factors include those listed under atrial flutter (see p 225).

Mechanism

The human atrium can respond regularly to a stimulus only up to a certain rate. This is usually in the range of 350–400/min. At faster rates than this, the atrium can no longer respond completely to each stimulus. A chaotic disturbance with asynchronous contractions of the atria results.

The ventricular rhythm is totally irregular because the majority of the atrial impulses reaching the AV node are blocked because of refractoriness of the AV node. Only occasional impulses will meet nonre-

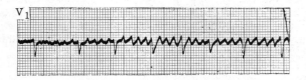

Figure 12–38. Atrial flutter-fibrillation. On the right-hand portion of the strip, regularly recurring atrial complexes are seen that simulate flutter waves. These occur at a rate of 500/min. This is too rapid for true flutter. The atrial complexes on the left-hand portion of the strip are typical of atrial fibrillation. It is simplest to call the above atrial fibrillation. It could also be called "flutter-fibrillation," "coarse fibrillation," or "impure flutter."

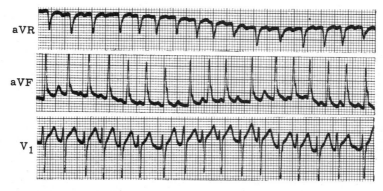

Figure 12–39. Rapid atrial fibrillation simulating tachycardia. A rapid ventricular rhythm is present at a rate of 200. At first glance, this has the appearance of paroxysmal atrial tachycardia. However, upon more careful inspection, it is seen that the ventricular rhythm is not regular, indicating a rapid atrial fibrillation.

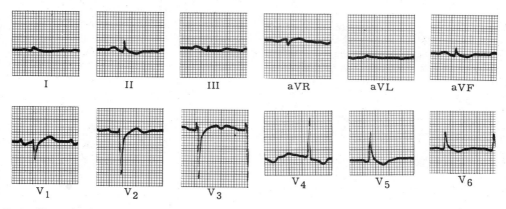

Figure 12–40. The patient has hemodynamically significant mitral stenosis. Because of past episodes of atrial fibrillation, the patient is receiving digitalis and quinidine. The ECG reveals sinus rhythm; the P waves are consistent with left atrial hypertrophy; ST segment depression, T wave inversion, and prolongation of ventricular repolarization (prominent U waves) are indicative of digitalis and quinidine effect.

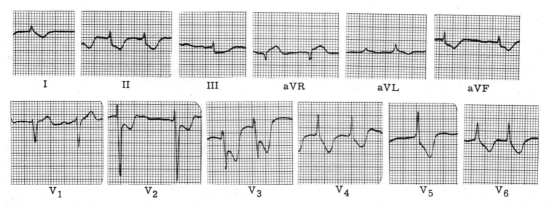

Figure 12–41. This tracing was taken within 15 minutes after recurrence of atrial fibrillation. The ventricular rate averages 110. There is marked ST depression—up to 5 mm in V_3. This is indicative of severe myocardial ischemia. At this time, the patient was in shock. Reversion to sinus rhythm was immediately accomplished with DC shock. Within minutes, the ECG reverted to that seen in Fig 12–40, and all clinical signs of shock disappeared. Follow-up clinical studies revealed no other cause for this episode (eg, pulmonary embolus). These tracings illustrate the profound electrocardiographic changes of ischemia that result from a marked fall in cardiac output secondary to the onset of atrial fibrillation in association with tight mitral stenosis.

fractory sites and be conducted distally to activate the ventricles. This is an example of "concealed" conduction.

Electrocardiographic Pattern

The atrial impulses are recorded as small waves that are totally irregular and vary in size and shape from beat to beat. These are called F waves. They are usually most prominent in V_1 in the routine ECG. The ventricular rhythm is irregular. The QRS complexes and T waves are usually of normal or basic configuration (see p 216, note). With rapid sustained atrial fibrillation, ST segment and T wave changes can occur as the result of secondary myocardial ischemia. As in the other atrial arrhythmias, aberrancy of intraventricular conduction may exist (see p 281).

Differential Diagnosis

A. Atrial Flutter: This has already been discussed (see p 225). At times, the rhythm may alternate between flutter and fibrillation in a single tracing. There are borderline cases in which a precise differentiation cannot be made. In such instances, the terms "flutter-fibrillation," "coarse fibrillation," or "impure flutter" may be used. However, it is better to reserve the term "flutter" for those records with perfectly regular atrial depolarizations, and fibrillation for all those that are irregular. The presence of coarse fibrillatory waves favors an etiologic diagnosis of rheumatic mitral valve disease or thyrotoxicosis. Fine fibrillatory waves are more commonly associated with arteriosclerotic or hypertensive cardiovascular disease.

B. Atrial Tachycardia: A rapid atrial fibrillation with a ventricular rate of 200 may simulate an atrial tachycardia. However, on careful measurement of many R–R intervals, the former rhythm will show variation, whereas the latter will be perfectly regular. Carotid sinus pressure may terminate a tachycardia but will produce only some ventricular slowing in atrial fibrillation.

Clinical Significance

Atrial fibrillation is a much less efficient cardiac mechanism than regular sinus rhythm because it reduces cardiac output. It also leads to the formation of atrial thrombi, with the danger of pulmonary and systemic arterial embolism. Even in the normal person, atrial fibrillation persisting for years can lead to cardiac dilatation and hypertrophy. For these reasons, an attempt to revert this arrhythmia to regular sinus rhythm is indicated in most cases.

Artifactual Atrial Arrhythmias

Skeletal muscle contractions, as seen in patients with various neurologic diseases (eg, Parkinson's disease), are often detected by the ECG. At times, these occur at a rate and regularity which simulate atrial arrhythmias. A monitored lead is more apt to pick up this artifact.

Prognosis

The prognosis of atrial fibrillation depends on the nature of any underlying disease. If the ventricular rate can be kept in a normal range, the prognosis from the atrial fibrillation is by no means poor. However, one can never be certain of this, since such a patient may dislodge a mural thrombus from either atrium and develop serious or even fatal pulmonary or systemic embolism.

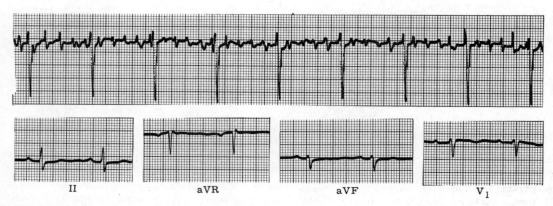

II   aVR   aVF V_1

Figure 12–42. The top strip is a monitored (modified CL_1) lead from a patient in an intensive care unit. The ventricular rhythm is regular; rate = 65. Also regular "atrial" activity is seen at a rate of approximately 300. This tracing could be interpreted as atrial flutter. The bottom strip illustrates leads II, aVR, aVF, and V_1, recorded simultaneously with the above-mentioned lead. The rhythm is clearly normal sinus. The apparent "atrial flutter" in the monitored lead was due to skeletal muscle contractions in a patient with Parkinson's disease.

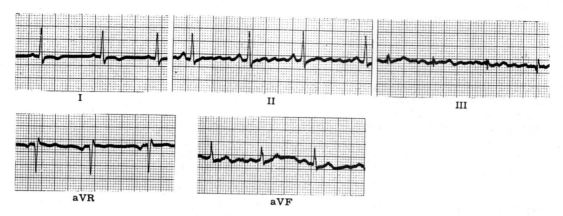

Figure 12–43. Lead III and, to a lesser degree, leads II and aVF show an undulating base line suggesting atrial fibrillation. However, leads I, aVR, and aVL indicate regular sinus rhythm. This ECG was recorded on a patient whose left leg was in a cast. Skeletal muscle contractions of the left leg (which are common to leads II, III, and aVF) explain the artifact in these leads.

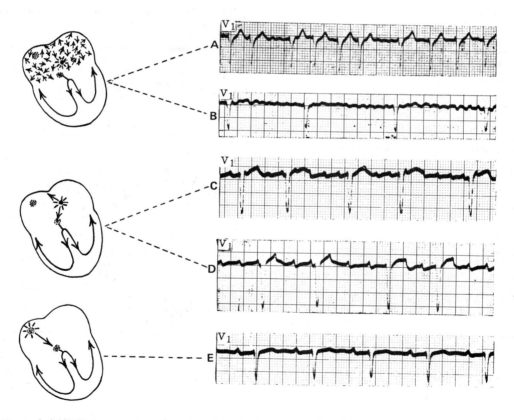

Figure 12–44. Atrial fibrillation: Treatment with digitalis and quinidine. *A:* Before therapy: Atrial fibrillation; ventricular rate = 120. *B:* After digitalization: Atrial fibrillation; ventricular rate = 50. *C:* During initial quinidine therapy: Atrial flutter; atrial rate = 300; there is a varying AV block (3:1 to 5:1), resulting in a ventricular rate of 75. *D:* During continued quinidine therapy: Atrial flutter persists, but the atrial rate has been reduced to 210; there is a varying AV block, resulting in a ventricular rate of 65. *E:* Further quinidine therapy: Regular sinus rhythm; rate = 68.

SUMMARY OF THE ATRIAL ARRHYTHMIAS

An ectopic focus in the atrium with reentry is responsible for the development of atrial premature contractions, atrial tachycardia, atrial flutter, and atrial fibrillation. The rate at which this reentry pathway operates and the site of reentry will determine the type of the atrial arrhythmia.

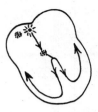

Figure 12–45. Initial ectopic focus in the atrium (upper end).

Table 12–3. Summary of the atrial arrhythmias, illustrated by portions of the continuous esophageal (E_{35}) ECG of a patient who manifested all the rhythms illustrated within a single 5-minute period.

Rate of Discharge of Atrial Ectopic Focus	Arrhythmia
Occasional discharge at a rate slower than the basic sinus rhythm Atrial premature contractions (at arrows)	E_{35}
About 160 to about 220 (with reentry) Atrial tachycardia (with 1:1 conduction)	E_{35}
About 220 to about 350 (with reentry) Atrial flutter	E_{35}
Over 350 Atrial fibrillation	E_{35}

ATRIOVENTRICULAR BLOCK

Atrioventricular block is a disturbance in conduction between the normal sinus impulse and the eventual ventricular response. It may be complete or incomplete.

Classification
    A. Incomplete:
        1. First degree.
        2. Second degree.
          a. Mobitz type II.
          b. Mobitz type I (Wenckebach block).
    B. Complete (third degree).

Etiology & Incidence
First degree AV block may occur in the absence of any evidence of organic heart disease. Practically every known acute infectious disease may cause this abnormality. It is quite common in acute rheumatic fever. Digitalis and quinidine may produce a first degree AV block. Coronary artery disease and certain congenital heart lesions may be etiologic factors.

Second and third degree AV blocks are usually on an organic basis. Digitalis toxicity, infectious diseases (especially diphtheria), coronary artery disease, and myocardial infarction resulting from occlusion of the right coronary artery (the major blood supply to the AV node) are common causes of the abnormal rhythm.

Mechanism
AV block results from either a functional or pathologic defect in the atria, AV node, bundle of His, or bundle branches with resulting delay in conduction of the impulse. Functional block can occur as the result of increased vagal stimulation. The AV block produced by digitalis toxicity is in part due to vagal stimulation.

The degree of delay in AV conduction will determine the type of AV block: (1) If all atrial impulses are conducted to the ventricles but the conductivity is delayed (ie, P–R > 0.2 s), a first degree AV block results. (2) If some of the atrial impulses are conducted to the ventricles and others are not, second degree AV block results. (3) If all atrial impulses are blocked, a second cardiac pacemaker, either in an AV junctional site, in the bundle of His, bundle branches, or in the ventricle, stimulates the ventricles; complete (third degree) AV block is the result.

Site of AV Block
The normal P–R interval is that period that includes atrial depolarization and passage through the AV node with its physiologic delay, bundle of His, bundle branches, and Purkinje fibers. With bundle of His recordings, simultaneous ECGs are usually recorded from one or more body surface leads, a high atrial and a low atrial location. The P–R interval can then be subdivided into 3 segments: (1) the time from the beginning of the P wave as recorded in a body surface lead or high atrial electrode to the beginning of atrial depolarization as seen in a low atrial recording (A), P–A time representing intra-atrial conduction; (2) the time from the beginning of low atrial depolarization to the bundle of His spike (A–H); and (3) the time from the bundle of His spike to the beginning of ventricular depolarization (H–V). With normal P–R intervals, the P–A interval is 20–30 ms. This measurement is usually of little clinical significance. The average normal A–H interval is 70–120 ms and the H–V interval 40–55 ms. These measurements are of major clinical significance. In the presence of first degree AV block (prolonged P–R interval), the block may either be (1) above the His bundle (therefore in the AV node), giving a prolonged A–H interval and normal H–V interval; (2) below the His bundle (therefore in the intraventricular conduction system), giving a normal A–H interval and a prolonged H–V interval; or (3) a combination of both with prolonged A–H and H–V intervals. (See Fig 13–1.) Even in the presence of a normal P–R interval, either the A–H or the H–V interval may be prolonged.

His bundle recordings, although not available as a routine clinical tool, have resulted in clarification of the mechanisms and sites of block in first, second, and third degree heart block.

Differential Diagnosis
The diagnosis of first degree AV block is rarely made clinically. Second degree AV block may clinically be mistaken for any other arrhythmia with an irregular ventricular rhythm. A complete AV block with a ventricular rate of ±50 may be mistaken for a

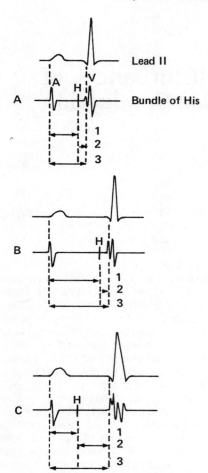

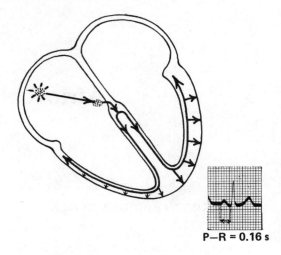

Figure 13–2. Normal AV conduction. No abnormal delay in spread of impulse from the SA node through the AV node and bundle of His. This produces a normal P–R interval.

Figure 13–1. Diagrammatic illustrations of bundle of His recordings. *A:* Normal AV conduction: (1) = A–H interval, approximately 120 ms. (2) = H–V interval, approximately 50 ms. (3) = P–R interval, 170 ms. *B:* First degree AV block: (1) A–H interval prolonged. (2) H–V interval normal. (3) Total P–R interval prolonged. The block is therefore proximal to the His bundle in the AV node. *C:* First degree AV block: (1) A–H interval normal. (2) H–V interval prolonged. (3) Total P–R interval prolonged. The block is therefore distal to the His bundle in the intraventricular conduction system. The QRS interval is prolonged; this is often associated with AV block distal to the bundle of His.

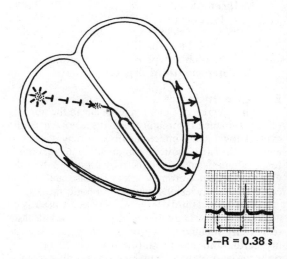

Figure 13–3. First degree AV block. Delay in conduction through the AV node or bundle of His (or through atria). This produces a lengthening of the P–R interval.

sinus bradycardia. Therefore, an ECG is essential for the correct diagnosis.

Clinical Significance & Prognosis

The clinical significance and the prognosis of AV block depend on the cause. That due to vagal stimulation is of no clinical significance in itself. Heart block due to digitalis toxicity, if properly treated, does not alter the prognosis of the individual patient. The sudden change from a regular sinus rhythm to a complete heart block is one cause for the clinical entity known as the Stokes-Adams syndrome.

First degree heart block occurring in association with many acute infectious diseases (except in rheumatic fever) is of little clinical significance in itself. The finding of a first or second degree AV block in acute rheumatic fever is an indication of rheumatic myocarditis. The AV block usually disappears as the disease becomes inactive, but occasionally this disturbance in conduction persists long after all other signs of rheumatic activity have disappeared. Heart block in diphtheria indicates a severe myocarditis. However, with recovery from the disease, there is no evidence of resulting chronic myocarditis.

The significance and prognosis of heart block in association with coronary artery disease will depend upon the severity and location (see below) of the latter disease.

The Stokes-Adams syndrome associated with complete AV block carries a serious prognosis. Death may occur as a result of ventricular standstill or ventricular fibrillation.

ELECTROCARDIOGRAPHIC PATTERNS

First Degree Block

In this condition there is a disturbance in conduction between the SA and the AV nodes or a delay in conduction through the AV node, bundle of His, or intraventricular conduction system. This results in prolongation of the P–R interval above the upper limit of normal (0.2 s). With slow heart rates the interval may be prolonged to 0.6 s. Rare instances of P–R intervals of 0.7–0.8 s have been reported. The rhythm remains regular. No dropped beats occur.

Second Degree Block (Mobitz Type II)

Periodically, the ventricle fails to respond to the atrial stimulation. This may occur at any interval. For example, only 5 ventricular complexes may follow 6 atrial complexes, the sixth P wave not being followed by a QRS complex. The seventh to eleventh subsequent atrial contractions will again initiate ventricular responses, but the twelfth will not. The above

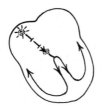

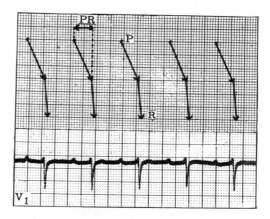

Figure 13–4. First degree AV block. The P–R interval is prolonged to 0.28 s.

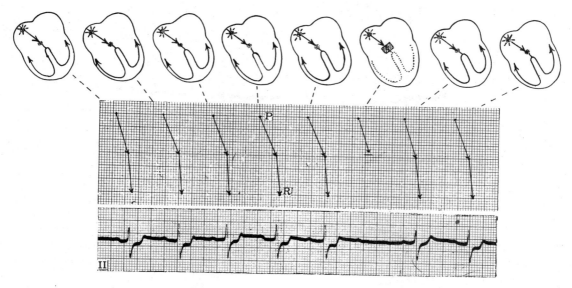

Figure 13–5. Second degree AV block of Wenckebach type. The P–P interval is constant, but the P–R interval progressively lengthens. After 5 sinus-conducted beats, the sixth atrial impulse is blocked, indicating a 6:5 AV block.

example would be termed a 6:5 AV block. The P–P and P–R intervals are constant throughout. This rhythm is not uncommonly associated with first degree AV block. This type of second degree block (also known as Mobitz type II), when associated with acute myocardial infarction (more commonly anterior wall infarction), has a much more serious prognosis than does a second degree block of the Wenckebach type (Fig 13–5). The site of block, as shown by bundle of His recordings (Fig 13–10), is distal to the His bundle. Pathologically, significant irreversible disease is usually present in the branches of the intraventricular conduction system, and this is manifested by electrocardiographic evidence of intraventricular conduction defects.

Second Degree Constant Block (See Fig 13–6.)

The above term is used to define a constant 2:1 AV block. As such it is impossible to differentiate between a Mobitz I and Mobitz II, since no 2 consecutive P–R intervals are recorded. If there is an associated intraventricular conduction defect, a Mobitz II block is more likely. A His bundle recording is necessary to establish an exact differential.

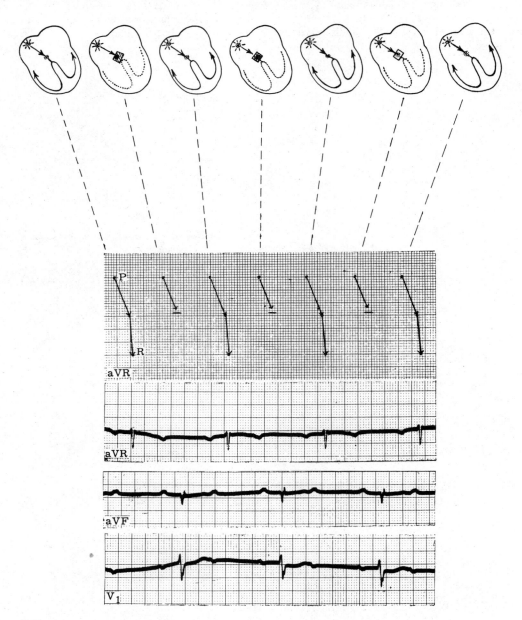

Figure 13–6. 2:1 AV block. The atrial rhythm is regular at a rate of 82. Every second atrial beat produces ventricular stimulation.

Second Degree Wenckebach Type of Block (Mobitz Type I)

A single ventricular beat is dropped in a cyclic fashion. With the first atrial impulse of the cycle there is usually a normal P–R interval. With each succeeding beat the P–R interval becomes progressively longer, until after several (usually 3–6) beats an atrial depolarization fails to initiate a ventricular response. A

long diastolic pause results, and the cycle is then resumed. The increment in P–R lengthening is greatest with the second beat of the cycle. This results in a longer R–R interval between the first and second beats than with subsequent beats of the cycle. The number of beats in each cycle is not necessarily constant. Its occurrence in association with acute myocardial infarction (more commonly inferior wall infarction due

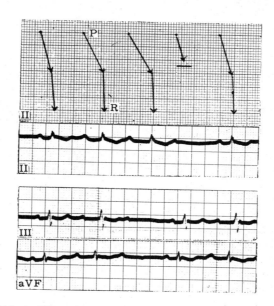

Figure 13–7. Second degree AV block of Wenckebach type. The atrial rhythm is regular. In lead II, the first P–R interval = 0.18 s, the second = 0.28 s, and the third = 0.36 s. The fourth atrial beat fails to activate the ventricle. In leads III and aVF, the cycle consists of only 2 sinus-conducted beats followed by the dropped ventricular beat.

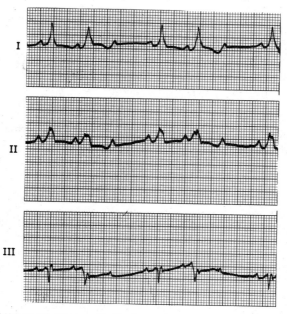

Figure 13–8. Second degree AV block (Mobitz type II). The P–P interval is constant, and the P–R interval of the conducted beats is constant. Every third atrial impulse is blocked, resulting in 3:2 AV conduction. The constant P–R interval and the additional left bundle branch block indicate that the site of block is distal to the His bundle and involves the left bundle branch.

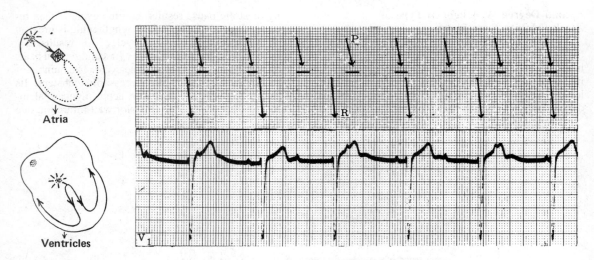

Figure 13–9. Diagram of complete heart block. The atria are activated by impulses arising normally in the SA node. In this example, the atrial rate = 72. The atrial impulses do not activate the ventricles. A second cardiac pacemaker is located near the AV node and stimulates the ventricles. The ventricular rate = 54. The atrial and ventricular rhythms are independent of each other.

to right coronary artery disease) usually represents reversible ischemia in the AV node and is much less serious than the Mobitz II type of block. Bundle of His recordings (see below) prove that the site of block is proximal to the His bundle and therefore within the AV node.

Complete (Third Degree) Block (See Fig 13–9.)

In this condition the atria and ventricles beat entirely independently of one another. The atrial rhythm is usually regular, and the atrial rate is that of average regular sinus rhythm. However, the atrial rhythm may at times be an atrial tachycardia or atrial fibrillation. The ventricular rhythm is usually quite regular but of much slower rate (20–60). The ventricle may respond to a pacemaker in an AV junctional site, producing QRS complexes that appear normal; or may respond to a pacemaker in either ventricle, producing QRS complexes that have the appearance of ventricular premature beats. The latter is termed idioventricular rhythm. Bundle of His recordings (see below) will localize the site of block. The presence of His bundle spikes preceding each QRS complex will indicate an AV junctional pacemaker which activates the ventricles. The absence of His bundle spikes will indicate a pacemaker distal to the bundle of His, either in a branch of the intraventricular bundle system or in the ventricle.

Heart Block (Second & Third Degree) in Association With Myocardial Infarction

The prognosis of heart block in association with acute myocardial infarction is well correlated with the location of the infarct. Inferior and posterior infarction (right coronary artery disease) results in ischemia, which is usually reversible, of the AV node. Anterior infarction (left anterior descending coronary artery

disease) produces greater and usually permanent damage to the bundle branches, is often associated with electrocardiographic evidence of bundle branch block, and carries a much more serious prognosis.

Bundle of His Recordings in Second & Third Degree Block

Bundle of His recordings, when available in special cardiac laboratories, localize the site of block, ie, above or below the bundle of His. (See Fig 13–10.)

(1) Mobitz type I (Wenckebach) second degree heart block: Characteristically, the block is proximal to the bundle of His in the AV node, and no bundle of His spike is recorded following the P wave which does not activate the ventricle. The lengthened P–R intervals relate to progressively longer A–H intervals and normal H–V intervals.

(2) Mobitz type II: Typically, the block is distal to the bundle of His in a part of the trifascicular divisions of the intraventricular conduction system. A bundle of His spike will be recorded following each P wave, including the P waves that do not activate the ventricle. The H–V interval of the conducted beats is prolonged.

(3) Second degree constant block, eg, 2:1 AV block: In this form of heart block it is impossible to determine whether the block is in the AV node (type I) or distal to the bundle of His (type II) without bundle of His recordings. The presence of a His bundle spike following the nonconducted P wave indicates type II, and absence of the His spike following the nonconducted P wave indicates type I block.

(4) Complete heart block: As in (3), above, exact location of the site of block requires bundle of His recordings. Absence of His spikes indicates a pacemaker distal to the bundle of His, either in the

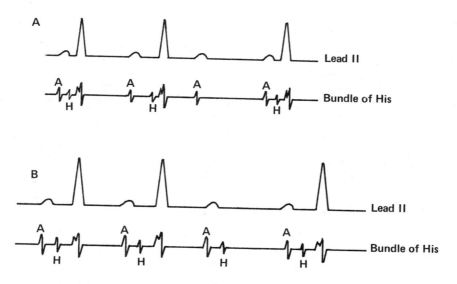

Figure 13–10. Diagrammatic illustrations of bundle of His recordings in second degree AV block. *A:* Mobitz type I (Wenckebach) block: The first complex has a normal P–R interval with normal A–H and H–V intervals. The second complex has a prolonged P–R interval due to lengthening of the A–H interval. The third P wave is not conducted and is not followed by a bundle of His spike. This indicates that the site of block is proximal to the His bundle, in the AV node. *B:* Mobitz type II block: The first 2 beats are sinus-conducted with a prolonged P–R interval due to lengthening of the H–V interval. The third P wave is not conducted and is followed by a His spike. This indicates that the block is distal to the His bundle. The P–R interval is constant for the conducted beats, and the QRS interval is prolonged.

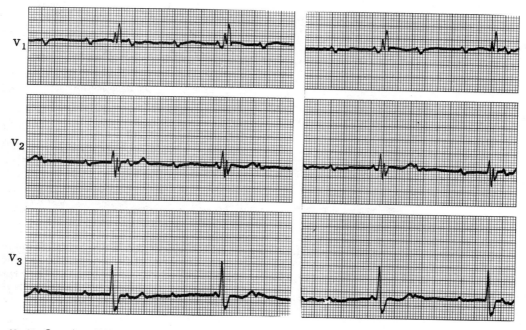

Figure 13–11. Complete AV block with an intraventricular conduction defect. Two strips (not continuous) of leads V_{1-3} are illustrated. The atrial rhythm is regular at a rate of 88. The ventricular rhythm is regular at a rate of 37 but is completely independent of the atrial rhythm. The QRS complexes are wide and simulate a right bundle branch block. This could indicate an idioventricular pacemaker in the left ventricle. However, a junctional pacemaker with an associated right bundle branch block cannot be excluded, although the slow ventricular rate would favor the former. A bundle of His recording would be necessary for definitive differential diagnosis. Absence of His bundle spikes would indicate an idioventricular focus. Presence of His spikes preceding each QRS with a constant H–V interval would indicate a junctional pacemaker.

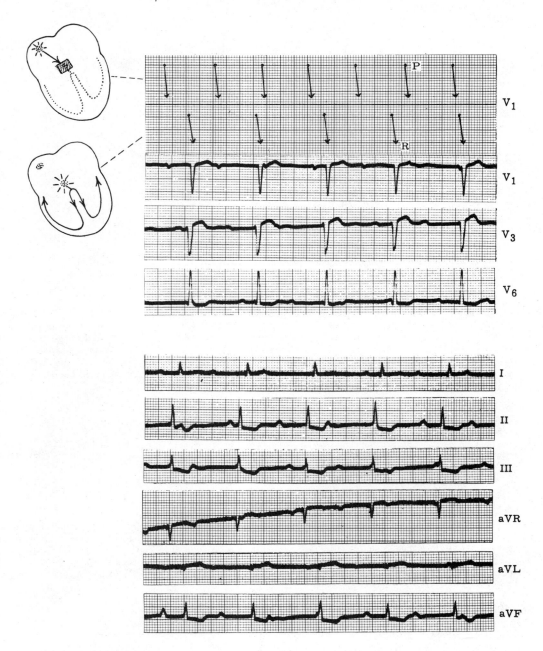

Figure 13–12. Complete AV block. The atrial rhythm is regular at a rate of 82. The ventricular rhythm is regular at a rate of 60. There is no relationship between the 2 rhythms, the atria responding to the sinus node and the ventricles responding to a second independent pacemaker. Since the QRS complexes are of normal duration, this latter pacemaker is in the AV junction or bundle of His. The apparent widening of some of the QRS complexes (fifth QRS in lead III and third QRS in lead aVF) is the result of fortuitous superimposition of the P wave and the QRS complex.

bundle branches or Purkinje fibers. Presence of His spikes indicates a pacemaker in or above the bundle of His. Since these are not routinely available, a good general rule can be applied for (3) and (4). If the QRS is normal, the block is most likely proximal to the His bundle in the AV node. If the QRS interval is prolonged (over 0.12 s), the block is most likely distal to the His bundle, ie, in the bundle branches.

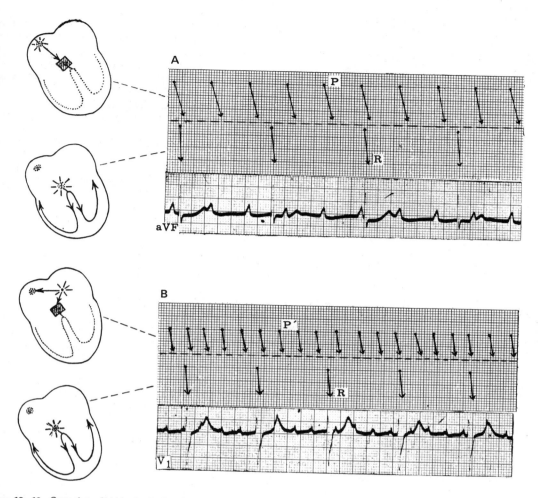

Figure 13–13. Complete AV block. *A:* A regular sinus atrial rhythm at a rate of 107 exists with an independent ventricular rhythm at a rate of 43. *B:* The atrial rate is now rapid at a rate of 230. This indicates atrial tachycardia. The ventricular rhythm is regular at a rate of 55. This is still a complete heart block and not 4:1 AV conduction since there is no constant relationship between the QRS complex and the preceding atrial wave. (Note that the atrial rhythm is not perfectly regular. This is a rare exception to the general rule that the atrial rhythm of atrial tachycardia is regular.) It is believed that the ventricular contractions "reflexly" alter the P'–P' interval (see p 227).

ATRIOVENTRICULAR JUNCTIONAL RHYTHMS

Intracellular potentials recorded from the main body of the AV node show absence of diastolic depolarization (phase 4). It is therefore concluded that automaticity does not exist in this area and that cells in the AV node cannot act as pacemakers or originate ectopic discharge. The zone in which atrial fibers enter the AV node (A-N zone) and the zone in which the AV node extends into the bundle of His (N-H zone) are zones of automaticity and can act as pacemakers or be the site of ectopic discharge. Hence, the older terminology of AV nodal rhythms has been replaced by AV junctional rhythms (A-N or N-H).

Junctional Beats

In this condition an ectopic focus arises in junctional sites (A-N or N-H zones). The impulse then spreads upward into the atrium and downward into the ventricle. This usually produces an upright P′ in aVR and high esophageal leads and an inverted P′ in aVF and low esophageal leads. The QRS–T complexes are of normal (or basic) configuration.

Junctional beats may be either premature, ie, occurring earlier than the next anticipated sinus beat, or escape beats. The latter occur when the sinus rate slows or when increased automaticity of the junctional site develops (eg, digitalis toxicity).

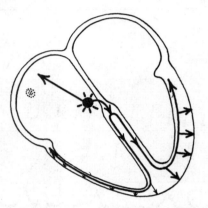

Figure 13–14. Cardiac impulse arising in AV junctional zones.

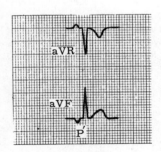

High AV junctional focus (A-N). Note upright P′ in aVR and inverted P′ in aVF preceding the QRS complex.

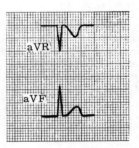

AV junctional focus. P′ buried in QRS complex. The impulse is arising in either the A-N or N-H zones and activating the atria and ventricles simultaneously.

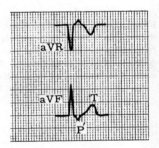

Low AV junctional focus (N-H). Note upright P′ in aVR and inverted P′ in aVF following the QRS complex.

Figure 13–15. Electrocardiographic patterns of impulses arising in various junctional sites.

High AV Junctional Beats

The ectopic focus is believed to arise in the A-N zone. The atrium is activated in a retrograde fashion prior to activation of the ventricle. This produces a normal or short P'–R interval. Such a beat is indistin-guishable from an atrial ectopic beat arising from a low atrial focus and therefore is best referred to as a supraventricular or AV junctional beat. It may be either a premature or an escape beat.

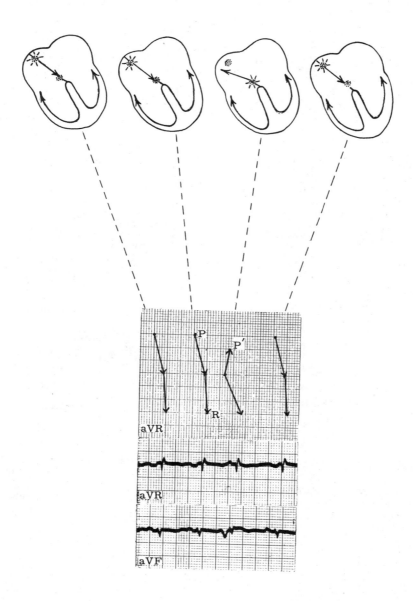

Figure 13–16. High AV junctional premature beats. The first, second, and fourth beats are sinus-conducted; the P–R interval = 0.14 s. The third beat has an upright P' in aVR and an inverted P' in aVF, indicating retrograde atrial conduction. The P'–R interval = 0.08 s. The QRS–T complexes are normal. It is postulated that the impulse arises in the A-N zone and produces retrograde atrial stimulation prior to ventricular stimulation. An identical pattern could result from an ectopic focus low in the atrium. A more inclusive term would be "supraventricular or AV junctional premature beats."

AV Junctional Beats

The P' wave is buried in the QRS complex and may not be visible. It may be either a premature or an escape beat.

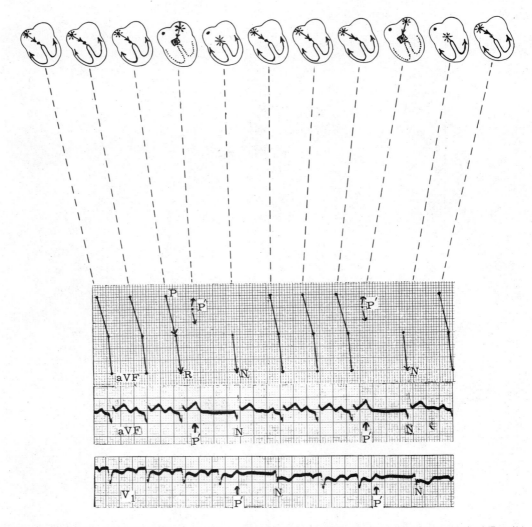

Figure 13–17. AV junctional beats. Blocked premature atrial contractions (P') are indicated by the arrows in aVF and V_1. Each is followed by a ventricular complex (N) which is similar to those of the regular sinus beats. However, no evidence of atrial activity can be seen preceding or following the ventricular complex. These beats are AV junctional escape beats with impulse formation in either the A-N or N-H zones with resulting ventricular activation. In addition, lead aVF reveals a deep, wide Q wave indicative of inferior wall infarction.

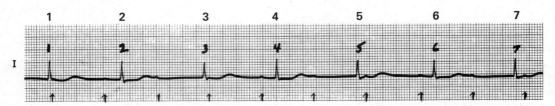

Figure 13–18. AV block with junctional escape beats. Regular atrial activity is evident by P waves (arrows) with a constant P–P interval. Complexes 2, 4, and 6 are sinus-conducted beats. Complexes 1, 3, 5, and 7 are junctional escape beats due to second degree AV block. The R–R intervals between 2–3, 4–5, and 6–7 are longer than between 1–2, 3–4, and 5–6.

Low AV Junctional Beats

The P' wave follows the QRS complex. The atria are stimulated in a retrograde fashion but are activated after ventricular excitation. The site of impulse formation is probably in the N-H zone. As stated above, it may be either a premature or an escape beat.

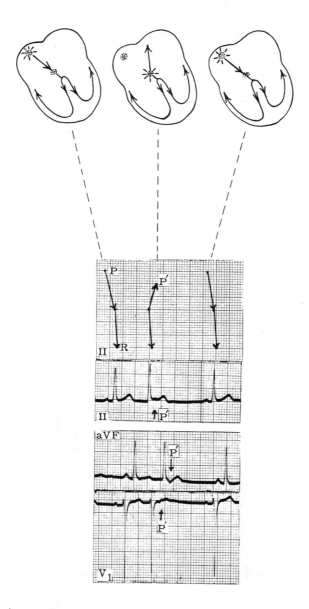

Figure 13–19. Low AV junctional premature beats. One premature beat is seen in each lead. The QRS complex is normal and is not preceded by an atrial wave, indicating that it is arising from an ectopic stimulus in the N–H zone. Each such QRS complex is followed by a P' wave (indicated by arrow). This is inverted in aVF, indicating retrograde atrial conduction.

The above classification of high and low AV junctional beats is an oversimplification. It must be appreciated that the time relation between the P' wave and the QRS not only depends on the site of origin (A-N or N-H zones) but also on the relative speed of conduction retrogradely into the atria and distally to the ventricles. Even though the P' precedes the QRS and favors an A-N zone focus, it is possible that the ectopic discharge occurs in the N-H zone, and retrograde conduction into the atria is more rapid than anterograde conduction to the ventricles.

Clinical Significance

Junctional premature beats have the same clinical significance as atrial premature beats. Escape beats are protective in that they represent secondary pacemaker takeover when the primary pacemaker (sinus node) slows or fails.

Reciprocal Beats

The P' wave may follow the QRS complex by a fairly long interval. If the AV node, bundle of His, and bundle branches are no longer refractory, the atrial stimulation resulting from the AV junctional stimulus may in turn reactivate the ventricle and produce another QRS–T complex of normal (or basic) configuration. This is known as a reciprocal (or echo) beat.

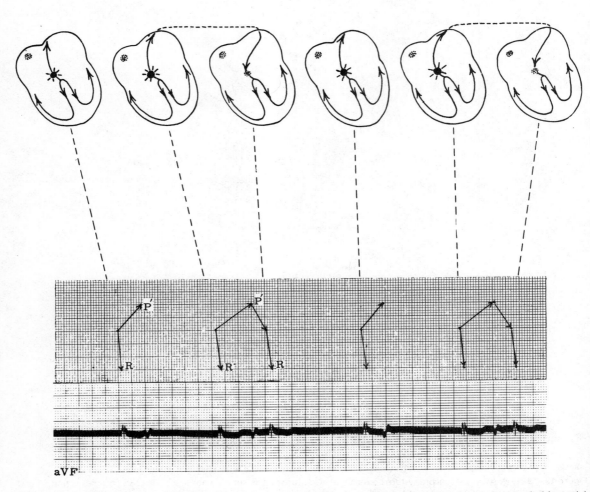

Figure 13–20. AV junctional rhythm with reciprocal beats. The first 2 ventricular complexes are not preceded by atrial activity. Both are followed by P' waves produced by retrograde atrial conduction. The second atrial beat follows the ventricular beat by a sufficiently long period of time to allow the ventricle to respond again to this retrograde atrial impulse. The cycle is then repeated.

AV Junctional Rhythm

The AV junctional sites act as the cardiac pacemaker. Each complete complex has the same appearance as a junctional premature beat. The rhythm is regular, and the rate may vary from 40–80. Similar to the types of junctional premature beats, an AV junctional rhythm may arise from a high (A-N) or low (N-H) junctional focus. That arising from a high junctional focus has been termed "coronary sinus" rhythm.

Clinical Significance

Junctional rhythm may be transient or permanent. Transient junctional rhythm may be seen in normal people. It may be produced by carotid sinus pressure (protective escape phenomenon) or may result from digitalis (increased automaticity of junctional site) or quinidine administration. Transient or permanent junctional rhythm results from a variety of organic heart diseases, eg, rheumatic fever, other acute infectious myocarditides, and coronary artery disease.

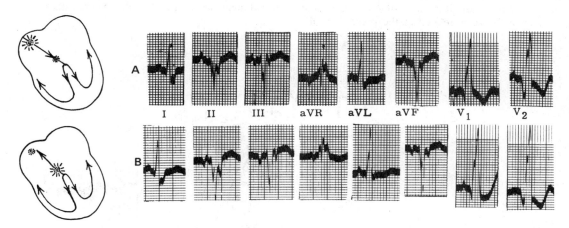

Figure 13–21. AV junctional rhythm (coronary sinus rhythm). *A:* The rhythm is regular sinus, as evidenced by the upright P waves in II, III, and aVF and the inverted P in aVR. In addition, the pattern is that of a right bundle branch block (wide, notched R in V_{1-2}; QRS = 0.15 s), left anterior fascicular block (axis of the initial 0.05 s QRS in the frontal plane = −70 degrees) with anterior wall infarction (deep, wide Q in V_{1-2}). *B:* The P′ waves are now inverted in II, III, and aVF and upright in aVR. This is indicative of a high AV junctional rhythm.

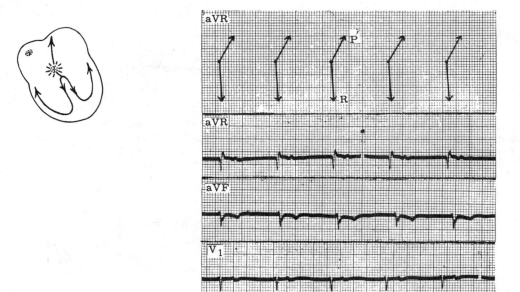

Figure 13–22. AV junctional rhythm. A regular ventricular rhythm is present at a rate of 70. No atrial activity precedes the QRS complexes. An atrial wave intermingled with the T wave is seen following each QRS complex. The P′ is upright and the T is inverted in aVR; the P′ and T are inverted in aVF, indicating retrograde atrial conduction.

ATRIOVENTRICULAR JUNCTIONAL TACHYCARDIA

In AV junctional tachycardia the A-H or N-H zone acts as the primary cardiac pacemaker. The rate can vary from 120–200. The ventricular rhythm is regular. The P' waves may precede, be buried in, or follow the QRS complexes, depending on the site of origin. The electrocardiographic pattern of each entire complex is identical with that of a junctional premature beat. With a rapid rate it is impossible to tell whether any given P' wave is related to the preceding QRS complex or to the following complex. Actually one cannot differentiate the electrocardiographic pattern produced by junctional tachycardia from that produced by an atrial tachycardia arising in a low atrial ectopic focus. Therefore, the more inclusive term, supraventricular tachycardia, is applicable.

Clinical Significance

The clinical significance is the same as for atrial tachycardia (see p 222). Slower junctional rhythms at rates of 100–120 (also known as nonparoxysmal junctional tachycardia) are often the result of digitalis toxicity.

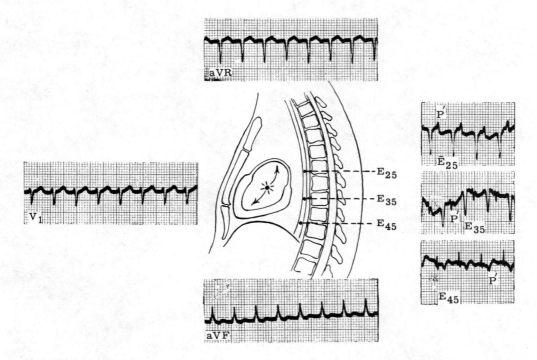

Leads aVR, aVF, and V₁ reveal a tachycardia with a ventricular rate of 182. No atrial activity can be identified. In esophageal leads the atrial waves are readily visible. At E₄₅ the P' is inverted, and at E₂₅ the P' is upright. This is the reverse of the normal direction, indicating an ectopic focus in the A-N or N-H zone or lower portion of the atrium.

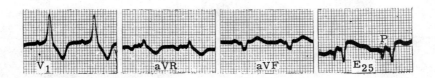

After conversion with intravenous digitalis. The P wave is now normally inverted at E₂₅. The basic pattern is that of a Wolff-Parkinson-White syndrome. (See p 276.)

Figure 13–23. Supraventricular (AV junctional or low atrial) paroxysmal tachycardia.

The Ventricular Arrhythmias | 14

VENTRICULAR PREMATURE BEATS

Ventricular premature beats (depolarizations or contractions) are those that arise from an ectopic focus in any portion of the ventricular myocardium.

Etiology & Incidence

Ventricular premature beats are commonly seen in association with any form of organic heart disease, especially coronary artery disease and any of the myocarditides. They are often the result of drug intoxication, digitalis being the most common offender and quinidine a less common cause. They may occur in normal individuals, but much less commonly than supraventricular premature beats.

Mechanism

Ventricular premature beats result from an irritable focus in any portion of the ventricular myocardium. The impulse arising from this ectopic focus will activate the ventricles. Since this impulse usually does not activate the atria and depolarize the SA node, the regular sinoatrial rhythm is not disturbed. The regular sinus impulse following the premature beat will usually not activate the ventricle since the latter is still refractory from the premature contraction. The ventricle will respond to the next normal sinus impulse. Therefore, the interval between the 2 sinus beats preceding and following the premature beat will be exactly twice the regular sinus rate. This is known as a compensatory pause (Fig 14–5). The premature ventricular depolarization may result in partial depolarization of the AV node. The following sinus beat, which depolarizes the ventricle, meets further delay in the AV node (because of this concealed conduction), resulting in a prolongation of the P–R interval.

Differential Diagnosis

Clinically, ventricular premature beats may be mistaken for atrial premature beats. The presence of numerous ventricular premature beats may lead to a mistaken clinical diagnosis of atrial fibrillation. Electrocardiographically, there is little difficulty in diagnosis. Accelerated conduction beats (Fig 16–12) and atrial premature beats with aberrant conduction (see p 280) may be mistaken for ventricular premature depolarizations.

Clinical Significance

Digitalis is a common cause of ventricular premature depolarizations and characteristically produces ventricular bigeminy. On the other hand, one may see frequent ventricular premature beats (or even bigeminy) in a patient with congestive heart failure who has not received digitalis. These may then disappear following digitalization. One can see how important an accurate history is in such a circumstance, since the ventricular premature beats as a manifestation of heart failure could indicate a need for digitalis or could indicate digitalis intoxication.

Ventricular ectopic beats occurring in association with acute myocardial infarction require immediate therapy since they may be the precursors of such serious or even fatal arrhythmias as ventricular tachycardia or ventricular fibrillation.

The following classification of ventricular premature depolarizations (as proposed by Lown) is commonly used as a clinical guide to indicate the severity of the ventricular ectopy:

Class 0: No ectopy.
Class 1: Less than 30/h.

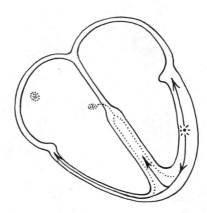

Figure 14–1. Ectopic focus in ventricle producing ventricular premature beat.

Class 2: More than 30/h.
Class 3: Multiformed complexes.
Class 4A: Couplets.
Class 4B: Runs of 3 or more (ventricular tachy-
          cardia).
Class 5: R on T phenomenon.

Prognosis

The nature of the underlying heart disease rather than the presence of the ventricular premature beats as such will determine the prognosis. The presence of numerous and multiformed ventricular premature beats in the presence of serious heart disease (eg, acute

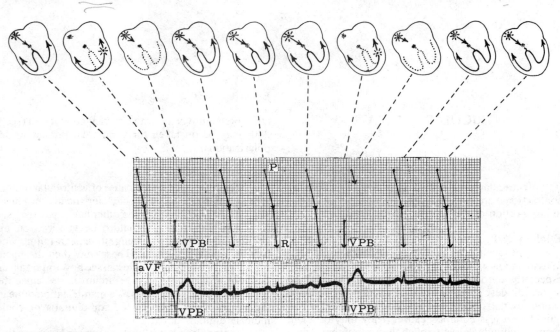

Figure 14–2. Unifocal ventricular premature beats. Two ventricular premature beats (VPB) are seen in association with a regular sinus rhythm. Both are the same configuration and direction, indicating a single focus.

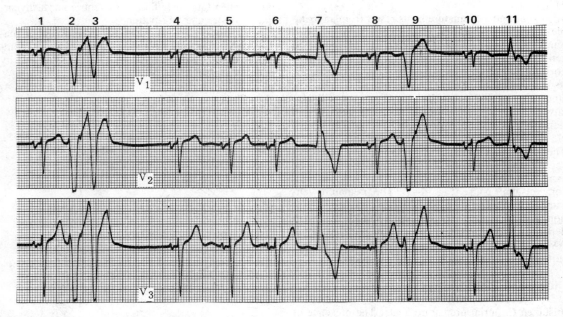

Figure 14–3. Multifocal (multiformed) ventricular premature beats. Complexes 1, 4, 5, 6, 8, and 10 are sinus-conducted beats. Complexes 2, 3, and 9 are ventricular premature beats that are oriented posteriorly (deep S waves in V_{1-3}) and indicate a right ventricular ectopic focus. Complexes 7 and 11 are ventricular premature beats that are oriented anteriorly (tall R waves in V_{1-3}) and indicate a left ventricular ectopic focus.

myocardial infarction) worsens the prognosis. In the absence of organic heart disease, ventricular premature beats usually have no significance and do not affect the prognosis.

ELECTROCARDIOGRAPHIC PATTERNS

The QRS complex is prolonged over 0.1 s and has a bizarre appearance, being notched and slurred. The ST segment and the T wave are usually displaced in the direction opposite to the main deflection of the QRS complex.

Ventricular premature beats arising from a single ectopic focus have the same configuration in any one lead. Those arising from different ectopic foci show differing patterns in any one lead. However, special electrophysiologic studies have shown that repetitive discharge from a single focus, because of altered pathways of conduction, can result in different forms of the QRS complex. Therefore, the term multiformed is commonly used in place of multifocal.

Depending upon when the ventricular premature beat occurs, the independent normal atrial beats may precede, be hidden in, or follow the QRS. A retrograde P' may follow the QRS. The occurrence of a normal P wave preceding the QRS complex of the premature ventricular beat is purely fortuitous. It may be impossible to distinguish such a beat from a preexcitation beat (Fig 16–12).

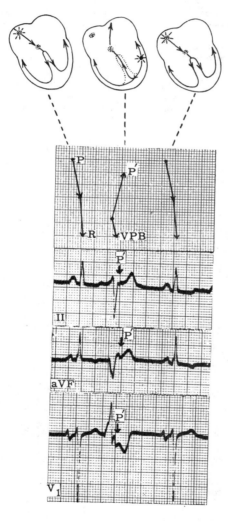

Figure 14–4. Ventricular premature contractions. In the illustrated leads a wide slurred QRS complex is seen between 2 regular sinus beats. These are not preceded by an atrial complex and hence are premature ventricular contractions. P' waves are seen following each of these. The direction of the P' wave (inverted in II and aVF) is opposite that of the normal P, indicating a reverse direction of atrial stimulation. These are retrograde atrial contractions resulting from the premature ventricular beat.

Since the normal sinus rhythm is usually not disturbed, a full compensatory pause follows the ventricular premature beat.

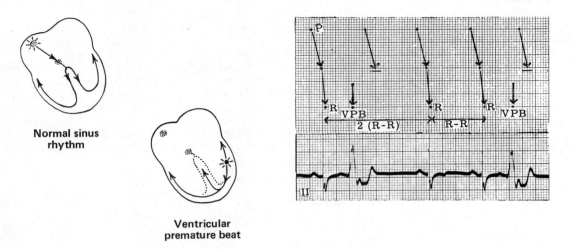

Figure 14–5. Ventricular premature beats; compensatory pause. Ventricular premature beats are seen following the first and third sinus beats. The R–R interval for the sinus rhythm (measured between the second and third sinus beats) = 0.8 s. The R–R interval between the first and third sinus beats = 1.6 s. Hence, a full compensatory pause exists.

If the sinus rhythm is slow, a ventricular premature beat can occur between 2 normal sinus beats without altering the R–R interval. This is known as an interpolated beat.

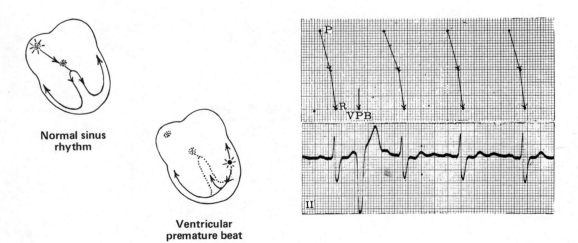

Figure 14–6. Interpolated ventricular premature beat. A ventricular premature beat is seen between the first and second sinus beats. A compensatory pause does not follow the premature contraction. The slight variation in the R–R interval is due to sinus arrhythmia. The QRS interval of the sinus beats = 0.15 s, indicating an intraventricular conduction defect. The P–R interval of the third and fourth sinus-conducted beats = 0.18 s. The P–R interval of the second sinus beat (the one following the ventricular premature beat) is 0.22 s. This prolongation is due to conduction delay in the AV nodal area resulting from retrograde penetration into the AV nodal area from the premature beat. This is an example of concealed conduction.

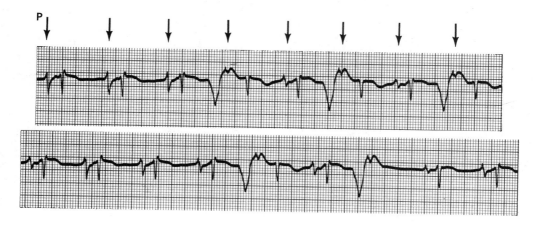

Figure 14–7. Ventricular premature beats; right atrial ECG. The above is a continuous recording from a catheter electrode in the right atrium. The rhythm is regular sinus (arrows indicate P waves) with ventricular ectopic beats. The first 4 ectopic beats are followed by a sinus P wave that activates the ventricle after a P–R interval of 0.3 s (the basic P–R interval is 0.2 s). This prolongation of the P–R interval is due to partial depolarization of the bundle of His or AV node by retrograde activation from the ectopic beat, thereby impairing conduction for the next sinus beat. This is an example of concealed conduction. The fifth ventricular ectopic beat is followed by a sinus P wave that does not activate the ventricle because the bundle of His or AV node is completely refractory. The following P wave activates the ventricle after a basic P–R interval of 0.2 s and produces a compensatory pause.

Ventricular premature beats may occur in association with any other arrhythmia.

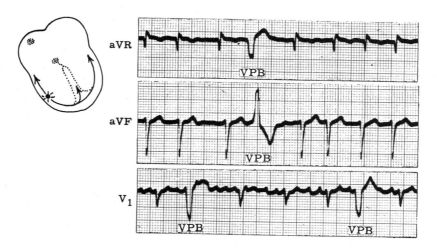

Figure 14–8. Ventricular premature contractions in association with atrial fibrillation.

Ventricular Premature Contractions During the Vulnerable Period

Since the Q–T interval approximates the refractory period of the heart cycle, a ventricular premature contraction usually occurs after the T wave of the preceding beat. However, on occasion, a ventricular ectopic beat will begin at the peak or downstroke of the preceding T wave. This portion of the T wave coincides with the vulnerable or supernormal excitability period described for intracellular potentials (see p 17). Such an ectopic beat is prone to initiate repetitive discharge, ie, ventricular tachycardia and fibrillation, and therefore has a much more serious clinical significance. This is known as the R on T phenomenon.

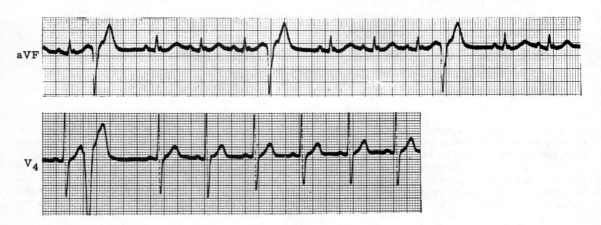

aVF

V_4

Figure 14–9. Ventricular premature contractions during the vulnerable period. Above are 2 electrocardiographic strips from 2 patients. Ventricular ectopic beats are seen occurring before completion of the T wave of the preceding beat.

Differentiation of Site of Ectopic Beat

One can distinguish between ventricular premature beats arising in either the left or right ventricle. If the major QRS deflection is upright in right precordial leads (V_1) and downward in left precordial leads (V_{5-6}), the ectopic focus is in the left ventricle. The reverse is true for right ventricular premature beats.

Thus, a left ventricular ectopic beat will mimic the QRS pattern of a right bundle branch block and a right ventricular ectopic beat will simulate the QRS pattern of a left bundle branch block. This is well illustrated by electrical pacing of either the right or left ventricle (see p 311).

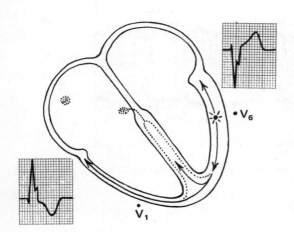

Figure 14–10. Ectopic focus in left ventricle. The main spread of the impulse is away from the electrode at V_6, resulting in a downward QRS deflection; it is toward the electrode at V_1, resulting in an upright QRS deflection.

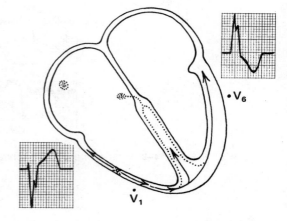

Figure 14–11. Ectopic focus in right ventricle. The main spread of the impulse is away from the electrode at V_1, resulting in a downward QRS deflection; it is toward the electrode at V_6, resulting in an upright QRS deflection.

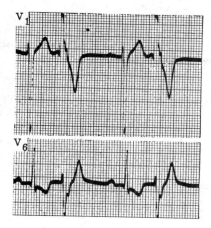

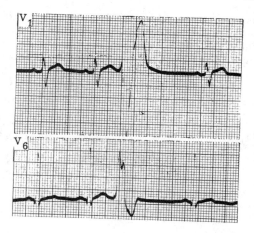

Figure 14–12. Ventricular premature beats of left ventricular origin. The main deflection of the ventricular premature beats is upright in V₁ and downward in V₆, indicating an ectopic focus in the left ventricle.

Figure 14–13. Ventricular premature beats of right ventricular origin. The main deflection of the ventricular premature beats is downward in V₁ and upright in V₆, indicating an ectopic focus in the right ventricle.

Ventricular Bigeminy

The rhythm alternates between a regular sinus beat (or any basic arrhythmia) and a ventricular premature beat. There is usually a constant interval between the sinus beat and the ventricular premature beat, ie, fixed coupling, indicating that the sinus beat controls the discharge of the ventricular ectopic focus by a reentry mechanism within the ventricular myocardium (see p 210).

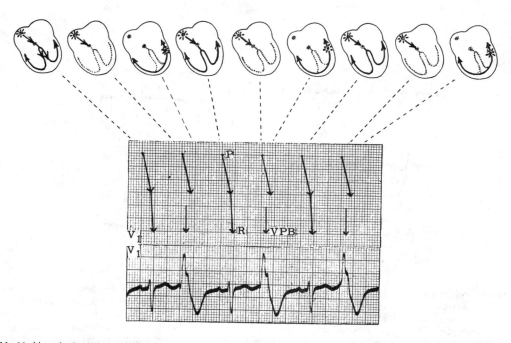

Figure 14–14. Ventricular bigeminy. The rhythm is a regular sinus beat followed by a ventricular premature beat, a pause, and then repetition of this sequence. The time interval between the sinus beat and the ventricular premature beat is perfectly constant (fixed coupling). The P waves of the sinus rhythm fortuitously precede the first 2 ectopic beats. The P wave is buried in the QRS complex of the third ectopic beat.

Premature Contractions of Myocardial Infarction

In the presence of myocardial infarction, a ventricular premature beat may show some of the typical features of an infarct pattern, ie, a QR. As mentioned above (see p 195), one cannot usually diagnose an infarct in the presence of a left bundle branch block. However, a ventricular beat in such a circumstance may show the infarct pattern.

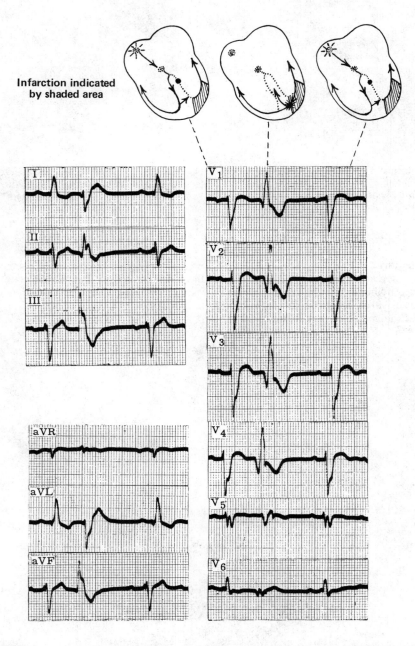

Figure 14–15. Ventricular premature contractions as an indication of myocardial infarction. The first and third complexes in each lead are sinus-conducted beats. The pattern is indicative of a left bundle branch block. An electrocardiographic diagnosis of infarction cannot be made in the presence of this pattern. The second complex in each lead is a premature ventricular contraction. The major QRS deflection is upright in V_1 and downward in V_6, indicating a left ventricular focus. Deep Q waves are part of the complex of these beats and are characteristic of an infarct pattern. Although an electrocardiographic diagnosis of infarction based on the appearance of premature ventricular contractions is not conclusive, it is strongly suggestive. *Clinical diagnosis:* Arteriosclerotic heart disease; history of myocardial infarction 1 year previously.

Postextrasystolic T Wave Change

Occasionally, the T wave of the basic complex following a premature ventricular contraction will have a different configuration than the basic T wave of the other sinus-conducted beats. For example, the basic T wave will be upright and the T wave of the complex following the premature beat will be inverted. Although initially thought to represent myocardial disease, more recent studies have shown that this finding has no specific clinical significance.

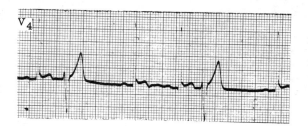

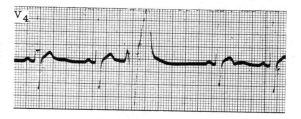

Figure 14–16. Change in the T wave following a ventricular premature beat. The T waves of the complex preceding the premature beat are upright. Those following are diphasic to inverted. The strips illustrated are from 2 different patients. Both were clinically diagnosed as idiopathic myocarditis.

VENTRICULAR TACHYCARDIA

Ventricular tachycardia is a rapid heart action, with a rate usually varying from 140–220 beats/min. The rhythm is usually slightly irregular.

Etiology & Incidence

Ventricular tachycardia is most commonly associated with recent myocardial infarction. It may occur in association with hypertensive and arteriosclerotic heart disease. Digitalis toxicity or quinidine toxicity may induce ventricular tachycardia. It is rarely seen in individuals with no clinical evidence of organic heart disease. In the latter instance, it has been reported to occur in association with the Wolff-Parkinson-White syndrome (see p 272).

Mechanism

Ventricular tachycardia results from a rapidly discharging focus (usually single) in the ventricular myocardium. It is likely that ventricular tachycardia is initiated by a single ventricular ectopic beat and that perpetuation of repetitive ventricular discharge, ie, ventricular tachycardia, is the result of a reentry mechanism within the ventricular myocardium.

Clinical Significance

Ventricular tachycardia is practically always indicative of serious organic heart disease or serious drug (digitalis or quinidine) intoxication.

Prognosis

Ventricular tachycardia is a very serious arrhythmia. Unless successfully terminated, the mortality rate will be very high. Prognosis depends also upon the nature of the underlying heart disease.

ELECTROCARDIOGRAPHIC PATTERNS

The rhythm is a rapid succession of ventricular premature beats, each complex having the exact appearance of a ventricular premature beat. With a rapid rate, it may be impossible to separate the QRS complexes from the ST segments and T waves, and the tracing has the appearance of a series of wide, large undulations. The ventricular rhythm is usually slightly irregular.

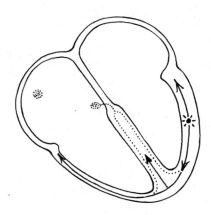

Figure 14–17. Propagation of impulse from left ventricular focus.

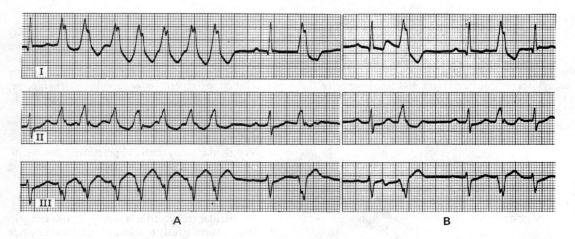

Figure 14—18. Ventricular tachycardia and ventricular premature beats. *A:* Following one sinus beat, there are 7 consecutive ventricular premature beats, indicating ventricular tachycardia. The ventricular rate is 150, and the rhythm is irregular. *B:* The above is followed by sinus rhythm with ventricular bigeminy. The configuration of the ventricular ectopic beats is identical to that of the tachycardia. This indicates that both are arising from the same ventricular focus.

The normal sinus rhythm usually continues independently of the ventricular tachycardia. The P waves may not be seen with any regularity in the standard 12-lead ECG, but esophageal leads will clearly record the sinus beats. Retrograde P′ waves may occur just as in an isolated ventricular premature beat or a junctional premature beat.

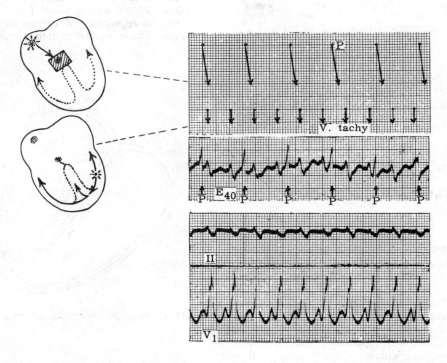

Figure 14—19. Ventricular tachycardia. Leads II and V₁ reveal a tachycardia with a ventricular rate of 173. There is suggestive evidence of atrial activity, but one could not be positive of this. The QRS complexes are wide and slurred. Esophageal lead E₄₀ clearly identifies the atrial contractions (indicated by arrows). They occur regularly at a rate of 95 and are totally independent. This, therefore, is a ventricular tachycardia. The ventricles respond to an ectopic left ventricular focus discharging at a rate of 173. The atria respond to the normal sinus pacemaker at a rate of 95.

Ventricular tachycardia may occur independently in the presence of any atrial arrhythmia. However, it is usually impossible to diagnose the atrial arrhythmia at this time without the use of esophageal or intracardiac leads.

Bidirectional ventricular tachycardia is the term applied to a form of ventricular tachycardia in which the QRS complexes in any one lead alternate in opposite directions; ie, the QRS complex of one ventricular beat is upright and that of the following is downward.

It had been assumed that tachycardia originating in the left ventricle would result in QRS complexes simulating right bundle branch block and that tachycardia originating in the right ventricle would mimic left bundle branch block. However, specialized endocardial and epicardial catheter mapping procedures have shown that the above need not be correct. Such studies have indicated that all ventricular tachycardias with right bundle branch block morphology do originate in the left ventricle, but most with left bundle branch block morphology arise in the left septal or paraseptal regions, especially in association with a left ventricular aneurysm. Some tachycardias with left bundle branch block morphology do arise in the right ventricle and such are associated with less serious heart disease.

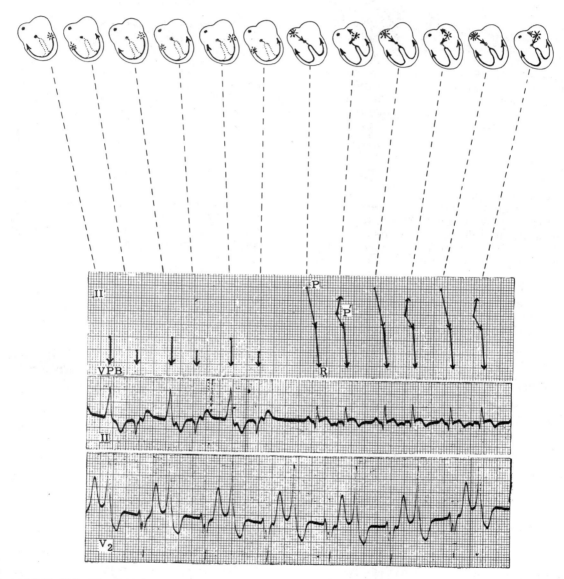

Figure 14–20. Bidirectional ventricular tachycardia. The first portion of II and all of V₂ show a series of ventricular premature contractions occurring in a bidirectional fashion. The ventricular rate is 128. The bidirectional ventricular tachycardia did not result from digitalis in this case. The second half of the lead II strip reveals a regular sinus rhythm alternating with atrial premature contractions. The Q and inverted T in II is evidence of inferior wall infarction.

Ventricular Ectopic Discharge Due to Central Venous Pressure Catheter

Any foreign body within the ventricle can initiate ventricular ectopic discharge. With the common use of central venous pressure monitoring, the catheter may inadvertently advance into the right ventricle and produce ventricular ectopic beats or ventricular tachycardia. Anti-arrhythmia drug therapy, such as intravenous lidocaine, is usually ineffective in abolishing the arrhythmia. It is essential that the physician be alert to this possibility in such a patient, since the simple maneuver of pulling the catheter out of the right ventricular chamber immediately corrects this potentially serious arrhythmia.

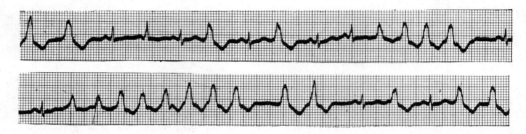

Figure 14–21. The above is a continuous recording of lead II in a postoperative patient with a central venous catheter in place. Frequent ventricular ectopic beats and runs of ventricular tachycardia are evident. Initially, the cause of this arrhythmia was not known to the physician, and intravenous lidocaine therapy was ineffective. X-ray observation indicated that the catheter was within the right ventricular cavity. When the catheter was pulled back into the superior vena cava, the arrhythmia promptly disappeared.

Differential Diagnosis

A. Atrial Fibrillation (or Supraventricular Tachycardia) With Bundle Branch Block: Such a pattern may be indistinguishable from a ventricular tachycardia. If the ectopic focus is arising in the upper portion of the atrium and the P′ waves are clearly recorded (as in esophageal leads), the P′ waves will indicate a normal direction of atrial stimulation (inverted in aVR and high esophageal leads; upright in aVF and low esophageal leads) and therefore identify the rhythm as atrial in origin.

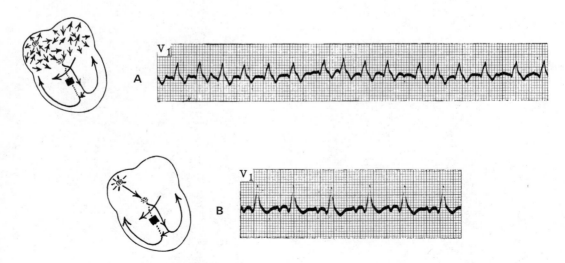

Figure 14–22. Rapid atrial fibrillation with a right bundle branch block simulating ventricular tachycardia. *A:* An irregular rhythm is seen with a ventricular rate of 170. The QRS complexes are wide and notched. This could represent a ventricular tachycardia, but the degree of irregularity would be unusual. *B:* The rhythm is now regular sinus. The QRS complexes remain wide and are similar to those seen in (A). (The wide Q and absent initial r indicate the presence of anterior wall infarction in association with right bundle branch block.)

However, if the supraventricular tachycardia is the result of an ectopic focus in the lower portion of the atrium (or AV junctional area), the P' waves will indicate the reverse direction of atrial stimulation and are indistinguishable from retrograde P' waves resulting from ventricular tachycardia. One will therefore have to rely on other criteria for the differential diagnosis.

(1) Supraventricular tachycardia is practically always perfectly regular, ie, the R–R interval is constant. Ventricular tachycardia is usually slightly irregular, ie, the R–R interval is not absolutely constant.

(2) Carotid stimulation may terminate an episode of supraventricular tachycardia but will have no effect on a ventricular tachycardia.

(3) Differentiation may be impossible until the tachycardia stops and the subsequent QRS complexes can be observed.

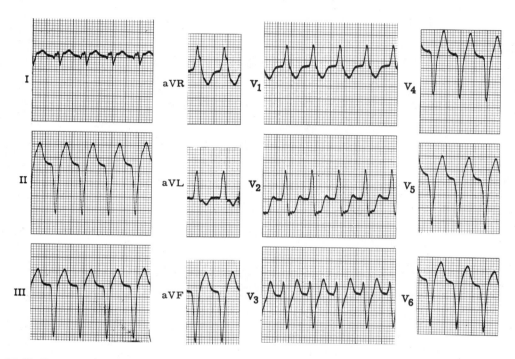

Figure 14–23. Paroxysmal ventricular versus supraventricular tachycardia. The ventricular rate = 150 and regular; QRS = 0.14 s. The QRS vector is oriented to the right (S waves in I and V₆), superiorly (QS complexes in aVF), and anteriorly (R wave in V₁). Suggestive P waves are seen in V₁₋₂ immediately following the QRS. (See Figs 14–24 and 14–25.)

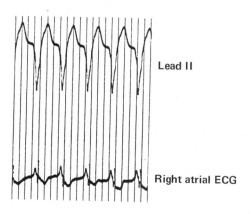

Lead II

Right atrial ECG

Figure 14–24. Paroxysmal ventricular versus supraventricular tachycardia (same patient as in Fig 14–23). Right atrial ECG with simultaneous lead II. A definite P wave is seen following each QRS. However, it is impossible to know whether this P wave activates the ventricle with a P–R = 0.26 s, indicating supraventricular tachycardia, or the P wave represents retrograde atrial depolarization from ventricular tachycardia.

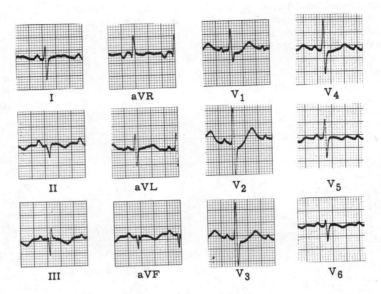

Figure 14–25. Paroxysmal ventricular versus supraventricular tachycardia (same patient as in Figs 14–23 and 14–24). After DC conversion. The rhythm is now regular sinus. The Q waves with inverted T waves in aVF indicate inferior infarction, and the tall R waves in V_{1-2} indicate posterior wall infarction.

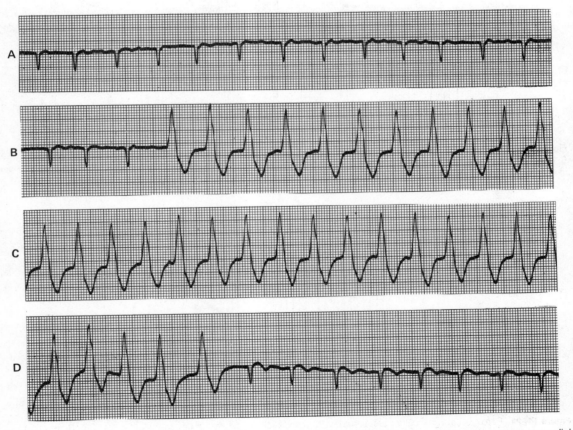

Figure 14–26. Accelerated idioventricular rhythm. Continuous recording of lead V_1 in a patient with acute myocardial infarction. *A:* Atrial fibrillation with irregular ventricular response, rate = 100. *B–C:* Appearance of idioventricular rhythm which initially has a rate of 100 and then increases to 120. *D:* Spontaneous reversion.

B. Supraventricular Tachycardia or Atrial Fibrillation With Aberrant Intraventricular Conduction or Accelerated Conduction: Such a pattern will simulate supraventricular tachycardia or fibrillation with bundle branch block and ventricular tachycardia (see p 282).

ACCELERATED IDIOVENTRICULAR RHYTHM

In contrast to the slow (30–40/min) idioventricular rhythm seen in association with complete heart block (see p 240) and rapid (140–220/min) ventricular tachycardia (see p 259), an intermediate type of idioventricular rhythm occurs at rates of 60–120. As in the former 2 arrhythmias, the QRS complexes are wide and slurred, regular or slightly irregular, and entirely independent of any atrial activity.

Accelerated idioventricular rhythm is most commonly seen in association with acute myocardial infarction. It is usually transient and may not require any therapy if the clinical status is stable. It is a much more benign arrhythmia than the slow idioventricular rhythm of complete heart block and rapid ventricular tachycardia. Although therapy may not be indicated initially, constant observation of the patient is necessary to detect clinical deterioration or worsening arrhythmias which will require treatment.

It may be impossible to differentiate an accelerated idioventricular rhythm from an AV junctional rhythm with aberrancy of intraventricular conduction without a His bundle recording. The QRS complexes

of idioventricular rhythm will not be preceded by His bundle spikes.

VENTRICULAR FIBRILLATION

Ventricular fibrillation is a rapid, irregular cardiac rhythm. The diagnosis must be made electrocardiographically since the peripheral pulses are not palpable and the heartbeat is inaudible.

Etiology & Incidence

The same conditions that give rise to ventricular tachycardia can result in ventricular fibrillation. The most common cause is acute myocardial infarction and is an explanation for many of the sudden deaths in this disease. It can occur as the terminal manifestation of any organic heart disease. Digitalis or quinidine toxicity can produce this rhythm. It occurs during surgical procedures performed under general anesthesia, in which case hypoxia is the common precipitating factor. Electric shock may produce ventricular fibrillation. Hypothermia, either naturally occurring or induced as an adjunct to surgery (unless a bypass circulation is used), commonly produces ventricular fibrillation when the body temperature falls below 28 °C.

Mechanism

Ventricular fibrillation results from a rapid discharge of impulses from single or multiple foci in the ventricles. The ventricles are unable to respond completely and effectively to each stimulus.

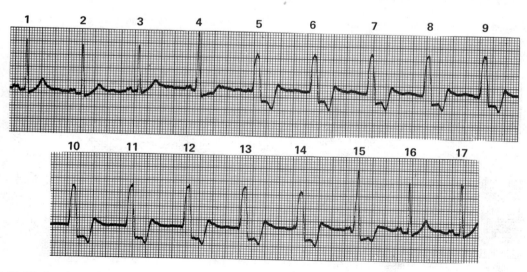

Figure 14–27. Accelerated idioventricular rhythm. Continuous recording of lead II. Complexes 1, 2, 3, 16, and 17 are sinus-conducted beats which precede and follow the arrhythmia. Beats 5 through 14 have wide QRS complexes, are not preceded by P waves, and are regular at a rate of 75. Complexes 4 and 15 are preceded by sinus P waves but with the P–R interval shorter and the QRS interval longer than the sinus-conducted beats. These are fusion beats, ie, ventricular depolarization in part results from sinus conduction and in part from the idioventricular focus.

Electrocardiographic Pattern

Since the ventricular contractions are erratic, the ECG shows bizarre ventricular patterns of varying size and configuration. The rate is rapid and irregular. The atria may continue to respond to sinus node stimulation, but P waves are not visible without the aid of esophageal leads.

Differential Diagnosis

Since there is no palpable or auscultatory evidence of cardiac action, ventricular fibrillation cannot be clinically differentiated from ventricular standstill. It is essential to differentiate these 2 conditions electrocardiographically, since the treatment will differ. Ventricular standstill may respond to isoproterenol, atropine, or electrical pacing whereas ventricular fibrillation requires immediate electrical defibrillation.

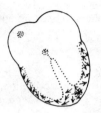

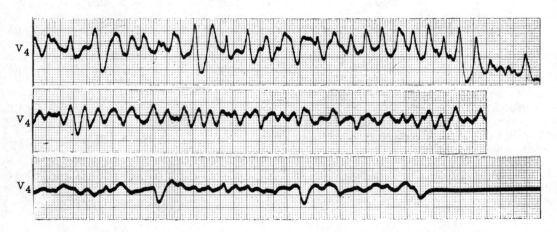

Figure 14–28. Ventricular fibrillation. Portions of a continuous strip of lead V₄ taken on a patient dying of a myocardial infarct. The ventricular complexes are rapid, irregular, and bizarre. This is typical of ventricular fibrillation. The tracing terminates with asystole.

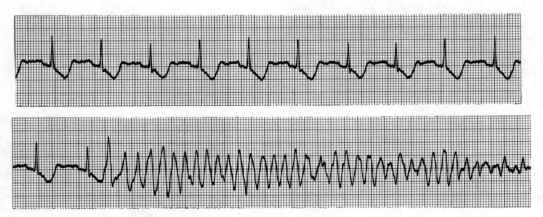

Figure 14–29. Ventricular fibrillation. Continuous monitor lead (similar to V₅) in a patient with acute myocardial infarction. The rhythm in the upper strip is regular sinus with a rate of 80. There is ST depression and T wave inversion indicative of ischemia. Following the second sinus beat in the lower strip, a ventricular ectopic beat occurs within the T wave of the previous beat, ie, in the vulnerable period. This initiates ventricular fibrillation. The patient was immediately and successfully defibrillated with DC shock and then had an uneventful convalescence.

Clinical Significance

Ventricular fibrillation is the most serious arrhythmia that occurs. Since it is often preceded by ventricular premature beats and ventricular tachycardia, the latter rhythms in the presence of serious organic heart disease (eg, acute myocardial infarction) must be treated promptly. Treatment of patients in coronary care units has reduced the mortality rate from acute myocardial infarction largely by the immediate recognition and treatment of the ventricular arrhythmias.

Ventricular fibrillation may occur in transient paroxysms and be the cause of the Stokes-Adams syndrome.

Prognosis

The prognosis is exceedingly poor in the presence of ventricular fibrillation. Since recovery is rare if this arrhythmia has continued for 5 minutes, immediate electrocardiographic diagnosis and prompt therapy is necessary for recovery.

The prognosis is better when this arrhythmia occurs in the operating room or in intensive care units where immediate resuscitation measures, including electrical defibrillation, can be instituted. With experienced professional personnel and equipment on open hospital wards and training of paramedical and lay personnel in treatment of cardiac arrest, many such patients are now being salvaged.

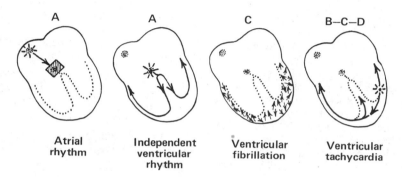

Atrial rhythm — Independent ventricular rhythm — Ventricular fibrillation — Ventricular tachycardia

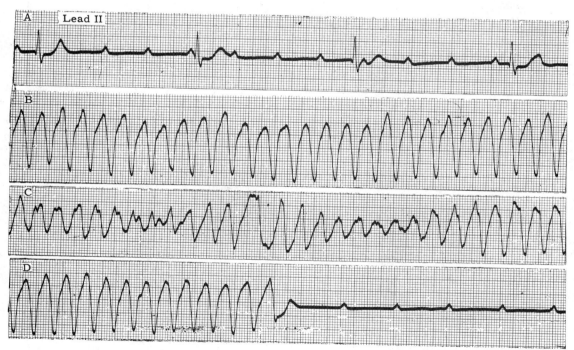

Figure 14–30. Stokes-Adams syndrome. Complete heart block with ventricular tachycardia, ventricular fibrillation, and ventricular asystole. *A:* Complete heart block: The atrial rate is 92, the ventricular rate 25. *B:* Ventricular tachycardia: The ventricular rate is 200. The QRS complexes are wide, undulating waves. *C:* Ventricular fibrillation interspersed with ventricular tachycardia: The QRS complexes are more bizarre during the period of ventricular fibrillation and vary in size and configuration from beat to beat. *D:* Ventricular tachycardia terminating in ventricular asystole: Atrial activity is now seen. The patient died shortly thereafter. This tracing illustrates the arrhythmias associated with the Stokes-Adams syndrome. This record was taken in 1949, before the availability of electrical pacing.

15 | The Pararrhythmias

A pararrhythmia is an abnormal rhythm in which 2 pacemakers discharge independently of each other; each at differing times can activate the ventricles. One center is usually in the SA node. By definition, a pararrhythmia need not disturb the conduction of the normal sinus impulse. Complete AV block, a common example of 2 independent rhythms, is therefore not a pararrhythmia since it "blocks" conduction of the sinus impulse through the AV node.

Such a mechanism, consisting of 2 independent pacemakers activating the heart at different times, could not exist unless the more rapid rhythm were somehow prevented from assuming complete control of the heart. The protective mechanism that prevents this from happening is known as a "protective block" or "entrance block."

There are 2 types of pararrhythmias: (1) parasystole and (2) AV dissociation, complete or incomplete.

PARASYSTOLE

A parasystolic rhythm is a pararrhythmia in which one pacemaker is in the SA node and the second is in an ectopic site.

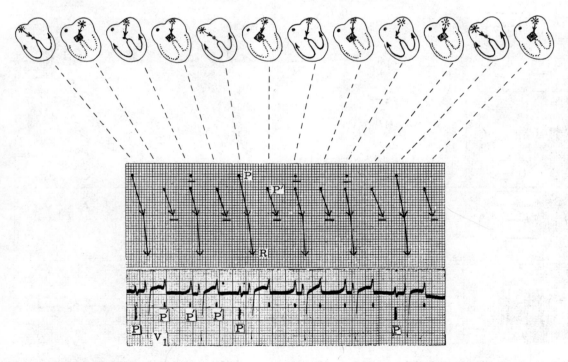

Figure 15–1. Atrial parasystole. Two types of atrial complexes are seen. The normal P waves occur at intervals of 1.56 s and 2.34 s. These are both multiples of 0.78 s, indicating a normal sinus rhythm at a rate of 77/min. Each P wave is not visible at the 0.78-s interval because the ectopic atrial (parasystolic) pacemaker is discharging more rapidly. This latter focus produces the P' waves. These occur at a rate of 150/min. The ventricle responds only to every second P' wave (atrial tachycardia with 2:1 AV block). The P and P' waves are both competing for the ventricular response; since the rate of the P' waves is more rapid, it dominates the ventricular response. This is an uncommon example of parasystole because (1) the ectopic focus is in the atrium and (2) the atrial ectopic focus rate is more rapid than the SA pacemaker rate.

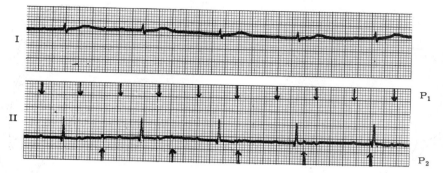

Figure 15–2. Atrial parasystole. The ventricular rhythm is regular at a rate of 53. Two independent and regular P waves are present. P_1 identifies regular P waves occurring at a rate of 106 (2 times the ventricular rate). This P wave precedes each QRS complex by a constant interval of 0.32 s. This is 2:1 AV block. In addition, there are P waves (P_2) which occur regularly at a rate of 60/min. These latter P waves do not activate the ventricle.

Incidence & Significance

Parasystole is an uncommon form of arrhythmia. It is most commonly seen in association with organic heart disease of varying etiology. An iatrogenic type of parasystole can occur in patients with an implanted asynchronous pacemaker (Fig 19–3). Patients with heart transplants demonstrate an atrial parasystole resulting from SA node impulse formation and atrial activation from the donor heart and the recipient's residual SA node and atria. However, the P wave that results from depolarization of the recipient's own residual atria never results in ventricular capture.

Mechanism & Electrocardiographic Patterns

The most common type of parasystole is one in which the slower ectopic center (more often in the ventricle than the atrium) competes with the more rapid SA center for control of the heart. The ventricles will be activated by one or the other pacemaker, depending upon the refractoriness of the AV node and ventricles at any particular moment. The slower ectopic center will produce an electrocardiographic complex having the appearance of an ectopic beat. The electrocardiographic criteria of parasystole are (1) that there is no constant time relationship between the sinus beat and the ectopic beat (in contrast to fixed coupling; see p 257); (2) that the time interval between ectopic beats (ie, parasystolic contractions) will be constant or will be an exact multiple of a common denominator (the least common denominator will represent the actual rate of discharge of the ectopic focus); and (3) that fusion beats representing depolarization from both sites are commonly seen.

A less common form of parasystole is one in which the rate of impulse formation of the ectopic focus is more rapid than that of the normal SA pacemaker. In an attempt to explain why the more rapid ectopic pacemaker does not assume complete

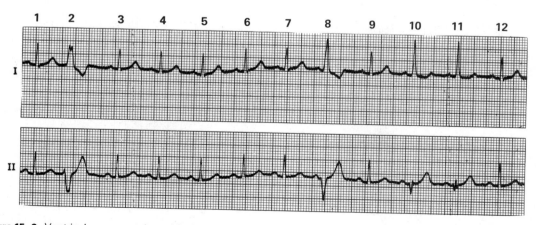

Figure 15–3. Ventricular parasystole and fusion. Beats 1, 3, 4, 5, 6, 7, 9, and 12 are sinus-conducted. Beat 2 is a typical ventricular ectopic beat. Beats 8, 10, and 11 are preceded by sinus P waves but show variable QRS morphology. These are fusion beats. The ventricles are depolarized in part from the ventricular ectopic focus and in part from normal sinus conduction. The interval between the ectopic beat and the preceding sinus beat is not constant. The intervals between 1 and 2 = 0.48 s, 7 and 8 = 0.54 s, and 9 and 10 = 0.64 s. The interectopic intervals between 2 and 8 = 3.90 s, between 8 and 10 = 1.30 s, and between 10 and 11 = 0.65 s. These intervals are all multiples of 0.65 s, indicating a parasystolic rate of 92/min.

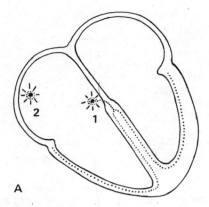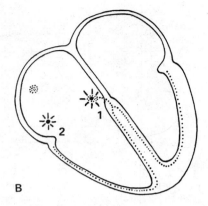

Figure 15–4. AV dissociation. *A:* (1) Pacemaker in AV junction. (2) Second pacemaker in SA node. *B:* (1) Pacemaker in AV junction. (2) Second pacemaker in lower end of atrium. Either pacemaker (1 or 2) may activate the ventricles.

control of the heart and produce an entirely ectopic rhythm or ectopic tachycardia, it has been postulated that some of the impulses originating in the ectopic center are blocked and that this allows the normal SA center to activate the heart at that given moment. This is known as "exit block."

ATRIOVENTRICULAR DISSOCIATION

AV dissociation is a pararrhythmia in which the dominant pacemaker is in the AV junction (or ventricle) and controls ventricular activation and another pacemaker (SA node or atrial) controls the atria. It may be complete or incomplete. It must not be confused with complete heart block. The latter implies complete inability of a supraventricular focus to activate the ventricle, owing to total AV block. Such need not occur with AV dissociation. Therefore, all instances of complete heart block are associated with AV dissociation, but all instances of AV dissociation are not related to complete heart block (see Mechanism, below).

Incidence & Significance

This uncommon arrhythmia most often occurs as a result of coronary artery disease, rheumatic carditis, other myocarditides, and digitalis or quinidine poisoning.

Mechanism

Two pacemakers exist, one an AV junctional or idioventricular site and the other in the atrium, usually in the SA node. The AV junctional pacemaker is the dominant one, either because of (1) suppression of the sinus pacemaker and escape of the junctional pacemaker or (2) increased automaticity of the junctional pacemaker. The atrial mechanism may be sinus or any

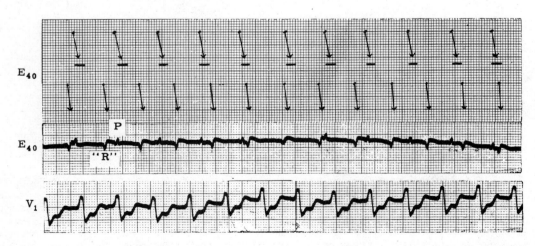

Figure 15–5. Complete AV dissociation. The ventricular rhythm is regular at a rate of 113. An independent atrial rhythm is present at a rate of 94. There is no relationship between the 2 rhythms. Since the ventricular rhythm is regular and of AV junctional origin, it is evident that no atrial impulse has activated the ventricle. The arrhythmia can readily be diagnosed in E_{40} but could not be resolved by V_1 alone.

atrial arrhythmia. In complete AV dissociation the atrial focus never activates the ventricle because the AV node is constantly refractory from the dominant junctional pacemaker. Incomplete AV dissociation occurs when the sinus (or ectopic atrial) focus arrives at the AV node when the latter is nonrefractory and therefore can be conducted to activate the ventricle. In the presence of independent sinus rhythm, the junctional pacemaker is more rapid. In contrast to complete heart block with independent sinus rhythm, the latter is more rapid but can never activate the ventricle.

Electrocardiographic Pattern

The basic rhythm is AV junctional or idioventricular (eg, accelerated idioventricular rhythm). An independent slower atrial rhythm is present. On occasion, the ventricle responds to the atrial stimulus, thereby interfering with the regularity of the AV junctional rhythm. This explains the older terminology of interference dissociation instead of the preferable term of incomplete AV dissociation.

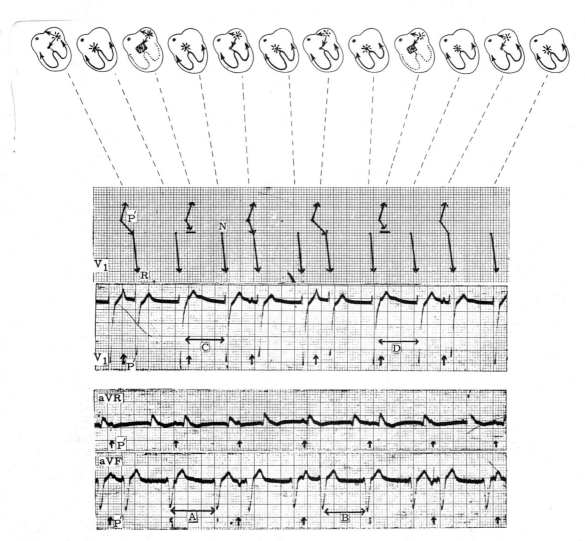

Figure 15–6. Incomplete AV dissociation (interference dissociation). Two rhythms are evident on study of this record. (1) A regular atrial rhythm (indicated by arrows) is present at a rate of 60. The P' waves are upright in aVR and inverted in aVF, indicating an ectopic focus low in the atrium. These atrial stimuli initiate some of the ventricular complexes seen. P'–R varies from 0.1–0.28 s. (2) In addition, QRS complexes are seen that are of the same configuration as those resulting from the above atrial stimuli. They are not preceded by P' waves and therefore are of AV junctional origin. The AV junctional rate can be determined when 2 junctional beats are seen in sequence. These are marked at (A), (C), and (D). The R–R interval is 0.7 s, resulting in a basic AV junctional rate of 85. (B) has the same R–R interval, but this is fortuitous since the first ventricular beat results from the atrial stimulus. In this illustration, there is an AV junctional rhythm at a basic rate of 85. However, the ectopic atrial focus interferes with this rhythm by also stimulating the ventricles. This produces an irregular ventricular rhythm. *Clinical diagnosis:* Arteriosclerotic heart disease.

16 | Preexcitation Syndromes

The preexcitation syndromes include the following clinical and electrocardiographic features: (1) Wolff-Parkinson-White (WPW) syndrome, which by definition requires the electrocardiographic pattern plus supraventricular arrhythmias; (2) Lown-Ganong-Levine (LGL) syndrome; and (3) recurrent supraventricular tachyarrhythmias in the absence of the typical electrocardiographic findings of preexcitation during sinus rhythm.

Etiology & Incidence

The incidence of WPW syndrome is approximately 1–3 per 1000 in the population. It is a congenital anomaly that usually is not associated with other evidence of organic heart disease. It has been associated with certain congenital lesions such as Ebstein's anomaly and prolapsed mitral valve syndrome. Development of the syndrome secondary to acquired heart disease has never been documented.

Mechanism

Since the original description of WPW syndrome in 1930, many theories have been offered in an attempt to explain how it comes about. In recent years, specialized electrophysiologic techniques and surgery have proved that in most cases the syndrome is the result of accessory pathways that bypass the AV node. These include the following:

(1) Lateral or paraseptal connections between the atrial myocardium and a portion of the ventricular myocardium. There may be more than one such accessory pathway in any given individual. This is the typical finding in WPW syndrome.

(2) Mahaim fibers are accessory connections between the distal AV node or His bundle and a portion of the ventricular myocardium. This will permit normal conduction through the AV node; thus, one electrocardiographic feature of WPW syndrome (the short P–R interval) will not be present.

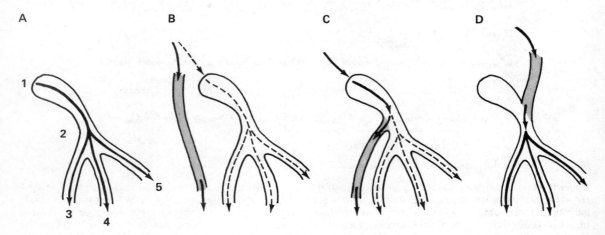

Figure 16–1. Diagrammatic illustrations of accessory pathways. *A:* Diagram of normal conduction from atrium to (1) AV node, (2) bundle of His, (3) right bundle branch, (4) left anterior fascicle, and (5) left posterior fascicle. *B:* Diagram of lateral accessory pathway. This bypasses the AV node and enters a site in the ventricular myocardium (typical WPW). *C:* Diagram of Mahaim fibers connecting the distal AV node or His bundle with a portion of the ventricular myocardium. *D:* Diagram of accessory pathway connecting the atrium with the distal AV node or His bundle (LGL).

(3) Accessory pathways connect the atrial myocardium and the His bundle. These bypass the AV node but permit normal intraventricular conduction. It is possible that preferential conduction through the normal posterior internodal tract (see p 36) could be the pathway involved. The resulting electrocardiographic pattern with its pertinent clinical relevance is LGL syndrome.

(4) Accelerated conduction: It has been postulated that rapid conduction occurs through a portion of the AV node and that this results in premature excitation of a portion of the ventricular myocardium. This concept has not been well documented.

Electrocardiographic Patterns

In typical WPW syndrome, the impulse arises normally in the SA node. Because there is little or no conduction delay in the accessory pathway (in contrast to normal AV nodal conduction delay; see p 24), the

atrial impulse rapidly traverses the accessory pathway and results in premature depolarization (preexcitation) of that portion of the ventricular myocardium into which this connection enters. Part or all of the remainder of ventricular depolarization may result from this excitation. More commonly, normal conduction through the AV node and the His-Purkinje system follows. The entire ventricular complex is therefore a fusion beat in which ventricular depolarization results from the accessory and normal pathways. The amount of fusion, ie, the extent of ventricular myocardium depolarized by each of the pathways, may vary from time to time. The above results in (1) a short P–R interval, less than 0.12 s; (2) slurring of the initial portion of the QRS complex (the delta wave); and, frequently, (3) associated ST segment and T wave changes deflected in a direction opposite to that of the QRS complex.

Two types of preexcitation patterns have been

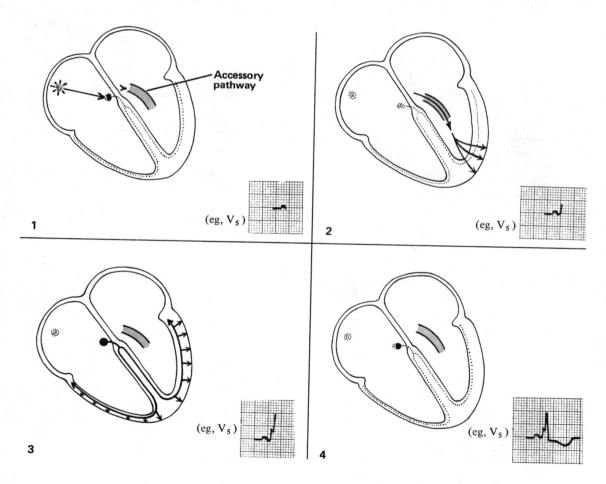

Figure 16–2. Diagram of preexcitation. (1) The impulse arises normally in the SA node and traverses a normal pathway to the AV node and to the accessory pathway. (2) Rapid conduction through the accessory pathway bypasses the AV node and results in premature activation of a portion of the ventricular myocardium. (3) The AV node, which has been activated in a normal fashion and has delayed transmission of the impulse, now activates the intraventricular conducting system in a normal manner, completing ventricular depolarization. (4) Depolarization and repolarization are complete.

described in the past. In type A there are tall R waves in V_{1-2}; in type B there are tall R waves in left precordial leads and negative QRS complexes in V_{1-2}. However, there are many variations of the above. When indicated, specialized electrophysiologic studies are essential to determine the location of such pathways in order to evaluate medical or surgical therapy.

The delta wave may be oriented superiorly and thereby produce Q waves in II, III, and aVF. This will simulate inferior wall infarction. In the presence of an ECG that demonstrates WPW syndrome, an electrocardiographic diagnosis of infarction is never justified on the basis of such Q waves. Such misinterpretation has resulted in unwarranted cardiac invalidism.

The usual preexcitation beat has a normal P–J interval, ie, the interval from the beginning of the P wave to the end of the QRS complex is the same in any one individual for a preexcitation beat and a normally conducted sinus beat. Thus, the common pattern is a short P–R interval, a wide and slurred QRS complex, and a normal P–J interval.

Variations of the above pattern may occur, as follows:

(1) Short P–R interval with wide QRS and shortened P–J interval: It is postulated that the premature ventricular stimulation excited the remainder of the ventricular myocardium before the latter could be activated through a normal pathway. This shortens the P–J interval. However, one cannot know whether this P–J interval is short or normal unless normally conducted sinus beats are seen in the same tracing or in serial tracings.

(2) Short P–R interval with normal QRS–T complexes and a short P–J interval: It is believed that the fibers that bypass the AV node enter and activate the bundle of His prematurely, and ventricular activation occurs normally. This (except for the short P–R interval) is indistinguishable from a normally conducted sinus rhythm. If the P–R interval is about 0.12 s, it cannot be so distinguished unless normally conducted sinus beats are seen with longer P–R intervals.

Clinical Significance

The electrocardiographic pattern of preexcitation syndrome has no clinical significance itself. However, individuals who have this pattern (WPW or LGL) are prone to have paroxysmal attacks of an atrial arrhythmia. This is usually paroxysmal atrial tachycardia (ie, 1:1 conduction) and, less commonly, atrial flutter or atrial fibrillation (see p 250). The mechanism of the tachycardia is explainable by a reentry mechanism in one of 2 directions: (1) The tachycardia is initiated by an atrial ectopic beat with a longer P–R interval or a ventricular ectopic beat. The latter is then conducted in a retrograde manner through the anomalous pathway back to the atrium, leading to its reactivation and, in turn, activation of the AV node and ventricles. Perpetuation of this leads to the common type of atrial tachycardia with normal QRS complexes. (2) Less commonly, the atrial impulse is conducted through the anomalous pathway with resultant ventricular activation and retrograde conduction back to the atria via the AV node. Perpetuation of this mechanism produces atrial tachycardia with wide QRS complexes, mimicking ventricular tachycardia.

Patients with atrial flutter or fibrillation are at high risk. The accessory pathway does not have the

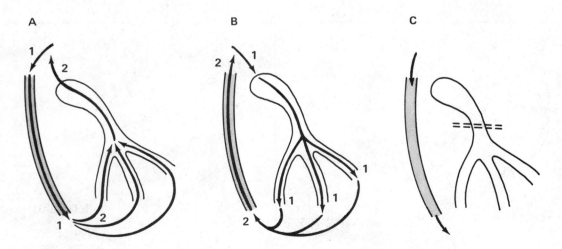

Figure 16–3. Diagrams of mechanism of tachycardias. *A:* Antegrade conduction via the accessory pathway (1) and retrograde conduction through the bundle of His and AV node (2). The QRS complexes will show the preexcitation pattern. *B:* Antegrade conduction via the normal pathway (1) and retrograde conduction through the accessory pathway (2). The QRS complexes will be normal. *C:* In the presence of atrial fibrillation or flutter, the accessory pathway can conduct the rapid atrial impulses with resultant rapid ventricular rates. The QRS complexes will show the preexcitation pattern. A similar situation occurs when the bundle of His has been surgically sectioned.

property of conduction delay comparable to the normal AV node. Thus, impulses at the rate of 250–300 can be conducted antegrade through the accessory pathway and can result in extremely rapid ventricular rates. The latter can induce congestive heart failure or deteriorate into ventricular fibrillation. This is the usual mechanism of death in patients with this syndrome. It is essential that such patients have specialized electrophysiologic studies, not only to identify and localize the accessory pathways but also to evaluate the response of induced atrial arrhythmias to various drugs. In general, digitalis is contraindicated in patients with atrial fibrillation or flutter. Among currently available drugs in the USA, quinidine and propranolol are the most effective drugs for this purpose. Verapamil and ajmaline (neither available in the USA) are promising.

There is a group of patients with recurrent supraventricular tachycardia due to an accessory pathway whose ECGs during sinus rhythm show no evidence of preexcitation. Electrophysiologic studies have documented this. Antegrade conduction is via the normal pathway. The accessory pathway conducts in a retrograde direction and is only functional during the tachycardia.

Prognosis

The preexcitation syndromes—as an isolated electrocardiographic finding and in the absence of tachyarrhythmias—do not alter life expectancy. However, recurrent atrial tachycardias that are unresponsive to conventional drug therapy can be incapacitating. Rapid ventricular rates secondary to atrial fibrillation or flutter can result in serious hemodynamic consequences and deterioration into ventricular fibrillation. This is fatal unless it is recognized and treated immediately with DC shock. Therefore, all such patients should have the benefit of specialized studies that can identify and localize the accessory pathways and permit proper surgical or medical therapy.

Surgical interruption of the accessory pathways has resulted in the elimination of the electrocardiographic pattern of preexcitation and the associated arrhythmias. When surgery is indicated and has been unsuccessful in identifying or sectioning the accessory pathway, surgical division of the bundle of His combined with ventricular pacing has been successfully accomplished. However, in this situation, if the accessory pathway is still functional, supraventricular tachycardias with antegrade conduction through the accessory pathway may continue. The ECG will show a continuous preexcitation pattern and mimic ventricular tachycardia.

Mahaim Pathways

If the accessory pathway originates in the distal portion of the AV node or His bundle, the normal conduction delay will occur in the AV node and the P–R interval will not be shortened. Ventricular preexcitation will occur, producing the typical delta wave.

Preexcitation With Normal QRS Complexes (Lown-Ganong-Levine Syndrome)

It is theorized that all of the atrial impulses bypass the AV node, producing a short P–R interval, and enter the intraventricular conducting system distal to the AV node. This results in normal ventricular repolarization and depolarization, producing normal QRS complexes and normal T waves. Such patients are also prone to paroxysmal atrial arrhythmias.

Individual preexcitation beats may be seen. These may occur as isolated complexes or may occur in a regular recurring sequence.

In this syndrome, the term preexcitation refers to premature activation of the His bundle and not the ventricular myocardium.

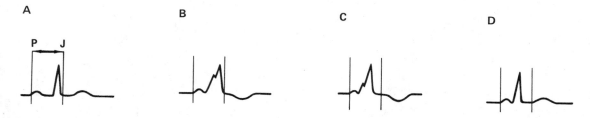

Figure 16–4. Variations in the electrocardiographic pattern of preexcitation. *A:* Normal sinus beat. *B:* Usual preexcitation beat; short P–R interval, wide and slurred QRS complex, normal P–J interval. *C:* Preexcitation beat with short P–R interval, wide and slurred QRS complex, but short P–J interval. *D:* Preexcitation beat with short P–R interval, but normal QRS–T complex and short P–J interval.

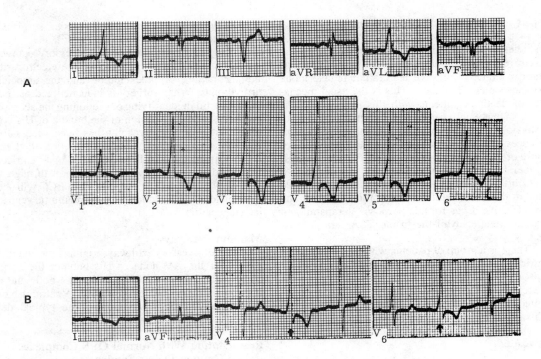

Figure 16–5. Preexcitation. *A:* Sinus rhythm; P–R = 0.14 s; QRS = 0.14 s. The major slurring of the QRS occurs in the initial portion of the R wave and is evident in I, aVL, and all precordial leads (delta wave). The ST segment and T waves are directed opposite to the major QRS deflection in each lead. The one unusual feature of this record, which otherwise is typical of preexcitation, is the relatively long P–R interval (0.14 s). The Q wave in aVF is a negative delta wave and is not indicative of inferior wall infarction. The tall R in V₁ meets the criteria for type A WPW syndrome. *B:* Two days after (A). Spontaneous reversion to normal intraventricular conduction except for the isolated beats, which are marked by arrows. The P–R interval during normal intraventricular conduction = 0.2 s. The P–R interval during preexcitation = 0.14 s. Although the latter is relatively long for this syndrome, it is appreciably shorter than the P–R interval of normally conducted beats.

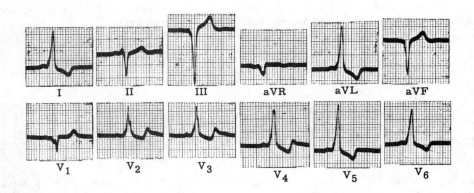

Figure 16–6. Preexcitation: Wolff-Parkinson-White syndrome. Typical electrocardiographic pattern. P–R interval = 0.1 s; QRS = 0.12 s. The initial portion of the R is slurred in leads I, aVL, and V₂₋₆. There is ST depression and T wave inversion in the latter leads. The QS complexes in leads III and aVF do not indicate inferior wall infarction. Because of the abnormal intraventricular conduction, one cannot diagnose infarction. *Clinical diagnosis:* A 26-year-old white man with no clinical evidence of organic heart disease. He did have occasional episodes of paroxysmal supraventricular tachycardia (Fig 13–23).

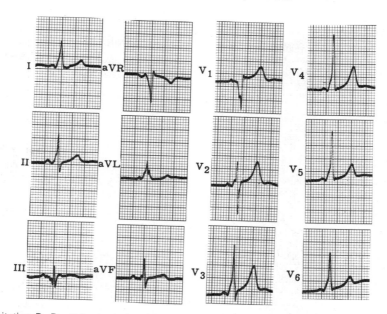

Figure 16–7. Preexcitation. P –R = 0.1 s; typical positive delta waves are seen in leads I, II, aVL, aVF, and V₂₋₆. The q wave in lead III is a negative delta wave. This ECG meets the criteria for type B WPW syndrome. *Clinical diagnosis:* Routine ECG in a clinically healthy 26-year-old man with no history of paroxysmal tachycardia.

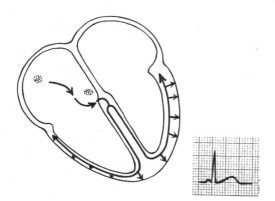

Figure 16–8. Lown-Ganong-Levine syndrome.

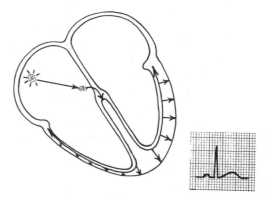

Figure 16–9. Normal regular sinus beat.

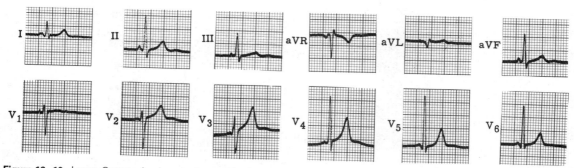

Figure 16–10. Lown-Ganong-Levine syndrome. The P waves are normal in direction, ie, upright in I, II, III, and aVF. The P –R interval = 0.1 s. The QRS –T complexes are normal. *Clinical diagnosis:* A 31-year-old healthy man with a history consistent with paroxysmal atrial tachycardia.

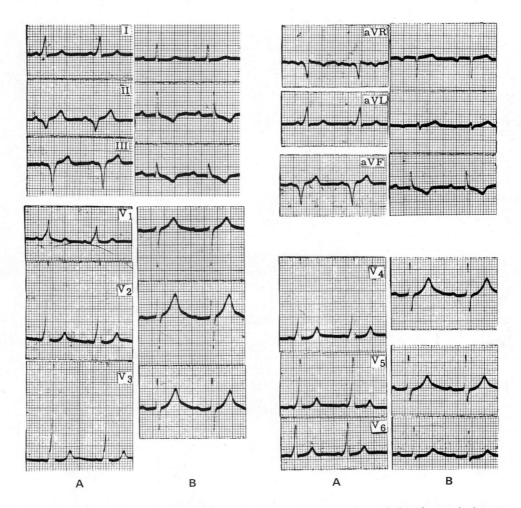

Figure 16–11. Preexcitation: Wolff-Parkinson-White syndrome. *A:* The typical characteristics of preexcitation are present: P–R = 0.1 s; QRS = 0.12 s; there is slurring of the initial upstroke of the R wave in I, aVL, and all precordial leads. Because of the abnormal intraventricular conduction, the QS complex in II, III, and aVF does not prove inferior wall infarction. From this electrocardiographic pattern alone, the diagnosis of organic heart disease cannot be made. *B:* Following conversion with quinidine. The P–R interval is now 0.24 s, the QRS interval is 0.06 s, and the QRS complexes are now normal in appearance. The T waves are inverted in II, III, and aVF. This indicates some abnormality involving the inferior wall of the left ventricle. This could be the result of inferior wall infarction but is by no means diagnostic of it. *Clinical diagnosis:* Arteriosclerotic heart disease; history of previous myocardial infarction. These tracings do not prove the acquired origin of WPW syndrome.

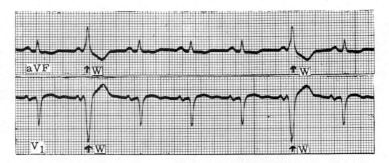

Figure 16–12. Isolated preexcitation beats. The basic rhythm is regular sinus, with a P–R interval of 0.17 s. At the arrows, there are QRS complexes (W) which have the appearance of premature ventricular contractions. However, each is preceded by a P wave. These P waves do not occur prematurely because the P–P interval is constant. The P–R interval for these beats is 0.1 s. Hence, these are preexcitation beats.

Figure 16–13. Alternating preexcitation beats. The P waves are indicated by arrows. The P–P interval is constant throughout. The regular sinus beats (R) have a P–R of 0.18 s. Each alternate beat has a very short P–R interval (0.06 – 0.08 s). The QRS complexes (W) following the short P–R interval are quite similar to those of the normal sinus beats. The P–J interval is shorter with the W beats. This record is that of alternating preexcitation, with the latter showing normal QRS complexes and a short P–J. An alternative interpretation could be the presence of AV junctional ectopic beats which fortuitously occur shortly after the sinus P wave.

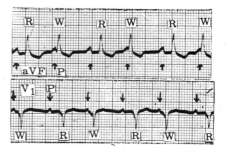

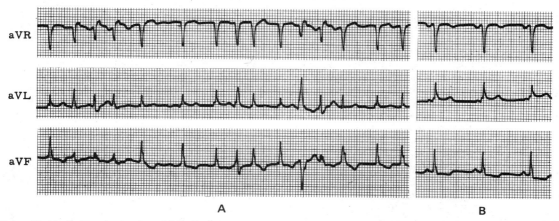

A   B

Figure 16–14. *A:* The rhythm is atrial fibrillation. Many of the QRS complexes demonstrate aberrancy of intraventricular conduction. The shortest R–R interval = 0.25 s (heart rate = 240). *B:* After DC cardioversion, sinus rhythm has been restored. The P–R interval is 0.08 s and delta waves are evident in aVL, typical of WPW syndrome.

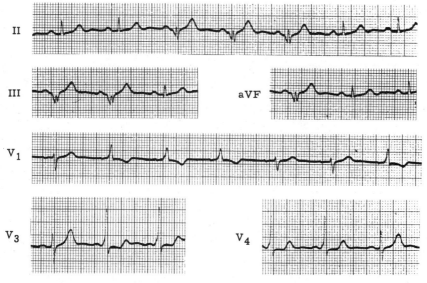

Figure 16–15. Pseudoinfarction in association with preexcitation. Leads II, III, aVF, V₁, V₃, and V₄ are illustrated. The rhythm is sinus throughout. Interspersed between entirely normal complexes are abnormal QRS complexes with deep, wide Q waves in leads II, III, and aVF and large R waves in V₁. The P–R interval of the normal complexes = 0.18 s. The abnormal complexes have a P–R = 0.12 s and a positive delta wave is evident in V₃ and V₄. This represents an intermittent preexcitation pattern (WPW type A). The pseudo Q waves in the inferior leads are negative delta waves. It can be seen that such a record (in the absence of the normal complexes) could be interpreted as inferior and posterior myocardial infarction or inferior infarction with a right ventricular conduction defect. (Courtesy of S Edwards.)

17 | Aberrancy of Intraventricular Conduction in Association With Supraventricular Arrhythmias

Wide, notched, and bizarre QRS complexes may be seen in association with any atrial or AV junctional arrhythmia and thereby simulate a ventricular arrhythmia. The abnormal QRS may be due to preexisting bundle branch block and hence will be evident in records taken during sinus rhythm (see p 262). In many instances, the aberrancy of intraventricular conduction is present only in association with the arrhythmia. Normal intraventricular conduction is present at other times.

When atrial activity is evident in the record (ie, P waves are visible), as with atrial ectopic beats, aberrancy of intraventricular conduction is easily distinguished from ventricular ectopic beats. However, when such is not evident, as in some atrial tachycardias and flutter and in the presence of atrial fibrillation, the differentiation may be exceedingly difficult. Special leads (esophageal, Lewis, or intracardiac) may clarify the atrial arrhythmia. Availability of ECGs before and after the arrhythmia will aid in differentiation. Response to vagal stimulation, such as carotid pressure, is most helpful when positive, but of little help if no response is obtained.

Features that favor aberrancy rather than ventricular ectopy are as follows: (1) rSR' in V_1. Normally, the right bundle branch has the longest refractory period of all of the fascicles of the intraventricular conduction system. Therefore, premature supraventricular impulses are more likely to be blocked in this division, resulting in the pattern of a right bundle branch block. In the presence of heart disease, conduction delay may occur in any of the fascicles. The aberrantly conducted beat may show a left bundle branch block or a left fascicular block or bifascicular block. (2) The "long-short cycle." The duration of the refractory period of the intraventricular conduction system is related to the heart rate. Increasing the R–R interval (slowing the heart rate) lengthens the refractory period of the following beat. In the presence of atrial fibrillation, a long R–R interval will prolong the refractory period of the next beat. If the latter occurs prematurely, there will be a greater chance of intraventricular conduction delay, ie, aberrancy.

Differential Diagnosis

A. Isolated Preexcitation Beats Versus Atrial Premature Contractions With Aberrant Intraventricular Conduction: Both complexes will show P waves with wide, slurred QRS complexes. The P–R interval will be shorter with the former than with the latter. However, since preexcitation is believed to be a sinus-conducted rhythm, the P waves will be normal and the P–P interval will be constant in the former. In the latter, the P' wave may have a different configuration than the normal P, and the P–P interval will not be constant, since the atrial contraction is occurring prematurely.

B. Supraventricular Tachycardia With Aberrant Intraventricular Conduction Versus Supraventricular Tachycardia With Bundle Branch Block Versus Ventricular Tachycardia: The points of differential diagnosis will be the same as those given on p 262. It may be impossible to arrive at the correct diagnosis until the arrhythmia ceases.

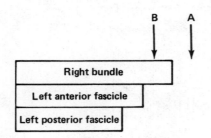

Figure 17–1. Duration of refractory periods in normal bundle branches. A premature impulse arising at arrow A will find all the bundles nonrefractory and will be conducted normally. An impulse arising at arrow B will find the right bundle refractory and will conduct with a right bundle branch block pattern.

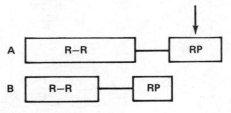

Figure 17–2. Duration of refractory period in relation to heart rate. The R–R interval is longer in A than in B. The refractory period (RP) of the beat following A will be longer than in B. A premature impulse arising at the arrow will encounter the refractory period of a portion of the intraventricular conduction system (usually the right bundle) in A and result in aberrancy of intraventricular conduction. In B, the impulse will be conducted normally.

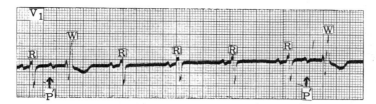

Figure 17–3. Premature atrial contractions with aberrant intraventricular conduction. The predominant rhythm is regular sinus (R). The P–R interval is 0.16 s, and the P–P interval is 0.82 s. P' waves (arrows) occur prematurely. The resulting QRS complexes (W) are wide and indicate a right ventricular conduction delay. This represents premature atrial contractions with aberrant conduction. The P'–R interval is longer (0.24 s) than the P–R interval of the sinus-conducted beats.

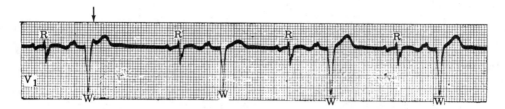

Figure 17–4. Atrial bigeminy with aberrant intraventricular conduction. Each regular sinus-conducted beat (R) is followed by a beat with a wide, bizarre QRS complex (W). This simulates a ventricular premature contraction. However, each such complex is preceded by an atrial complex that occurs prematurely and is of a different configuration than the normal P wave. This rhythm is therefore an atrial bigeminy with aberrant conduction. A notch is seen (arrow) at the termination of the first aberrantly conducted beat. This is not seen with the subsequent 3 aberrant beats. The interval between the first W and the following R is longer than similar intervals of successive cycles. This notch represents retrograde atrial depolarization following the first W which depolarizes the sinus node and thereby delays the next sinus-atrial depolarization.

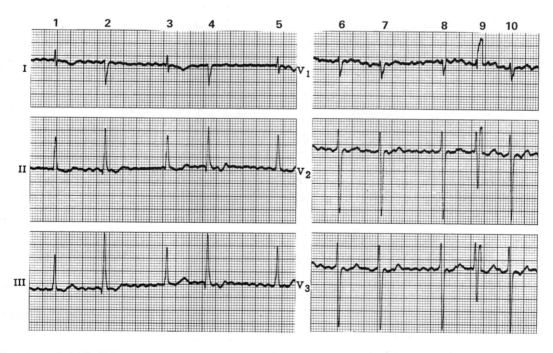

Figure 17–5. Atrial fibrillation with aberrant intraventricular conduction. The basic rhythm is atrial fibrillation. Complexes 1, 3, 5, 6, 7, 8, and 10 represent the basic QRS pattern. Complexes 2, 4, and 9 have wider QRS intervals and are oriented primarily to the right (deep S in I) and anteriorly (wide and tall R' in V_1). Superficially, these resemble ventricular ectopic beats. However, the fourth and ninth beats occur with a relatively short R–R interval preceded by a longer R–R interval. The QRS complexes have an rsR' configuration in V_1. These factors strongly favor aberrancy. The QRS orientation of these aberrantly conducted beats indicates a right bundle branch block with a left posterior fascicular block.

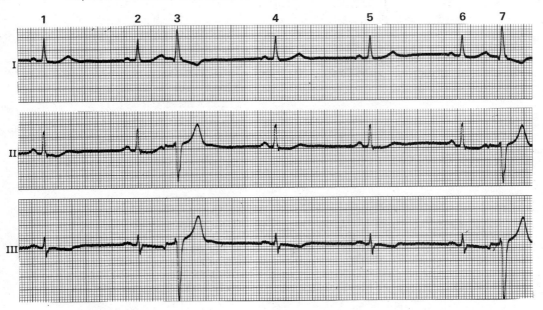

Figure 17–6. AV junctional ectopic beats with aberrancy. Complexes 1, 2, 4, 5, and 6 are sinus-conducted beats. Sinus bradycardia is present; rate = 42. Complexes 3 and 7 occur prematurely and are initiated by P waves that are inverted in II and III, indicating an AV junctional origin. The resulting QRS complexes are wider, have much greater voltage, and are oriented markedly superiorly, indicating a left anterior fascicular block in association with the junctional ectopic beats.

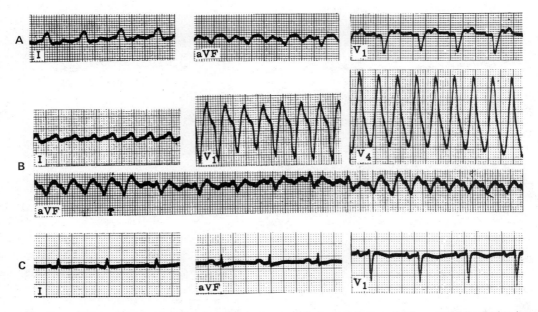

Figure 17–7. Paroxysmal atrial tachycardia with aberrant intraventricular conduction. *A:* The ventricular rhythm is regular; rate = 100. In V_1 it is evident that the atrial rate = 200, indicating atrial tachycardia with 2:1 conduction. The QRS complexes are wide, indicating aberrancy of the left bundle branch block type. *B:* Five minutes after (A). The ventricular rate is now 200. Atrial activity cannot be identified. This tracing is indistinguishable from ventricular tachycardia. Because of the diagnosis known from (A), carotid pressure was applied during the recording of aVF (arrow). The ventricular rate is reduced to 100, and atrial activity of 200 is again evident. This is therefore atrial tachycardia with 1:1 conduction and with aberrant intraventricular conduction. *C:* One day later. Although the above records of atrial tachycardia with block are strongly suggestive of digitalis toxicity, this patient had not received digitalis prior to these tracings. He was therefore treated with digitalis. The rhythm reverted to regular sinus with normal intraventricular conduction.

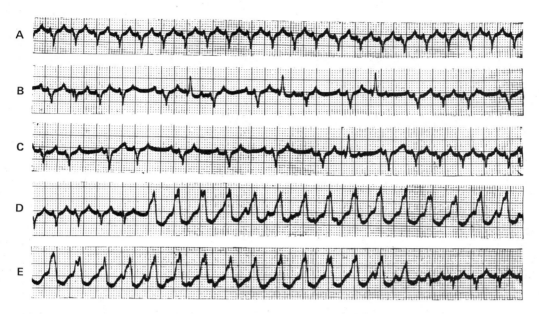

Figure 17–8. Paroxysmal atrial tachycardia, aberrant intraventricular conduction, and ventricular tachycardia (all recordings are V₁). **A:** The ventricular rate = 170; the rhythm is regular. One cannot be certain if P waves are present. Since the QRS is relatively normal, the rhythm is best identified as a supraventricular tachycardia. **B and C:** There are periods in which the ventricular rate slows to 85. Definite atrial activity is now evident, proving the presence of atrial tachycardia with periods of second degree AV block of the Wenckebach type. In addition, there are occasional QRS complexes which have an rsR' configuration. These are preceded by P waves and are, therefore, aberrantly conducted beats and not ventricular ectopic beats. **D and E:** After the first 5 beats of atrial tachycardia (rate = 170) in (D), a burst of bizarre QRS complexes appears at a rate of 150. The QRS complexes resemble the aberrant beats in (B) and (C), which could make one suspect continued atrial tachycardia with aberrancy of intraventricular conduction. However, the QRS complexes are wider, the ventricular rate is slower, independent atrial activity is evident if the P–P interval is plotted through the tachycardia, and the last 2 beats of the bizarre tachycardia in (E) show differing QRS configuration as evidence of fusion. All the above is proof of ventricular tachycardia. The above ECG is a continuous recording on a patient with idiopathic myocardiopathy and digitalis intoxication.

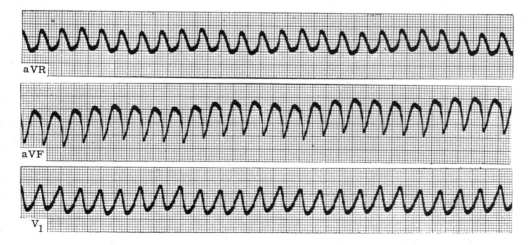

Figure 17–9. A tachycardia is present with a regular ventricular rate of 200. The QRS complexes are wide and bizarre. There is no definite evidence of atrial activity. Ventricular tachycardia is the most likely diagnosis. However, in view of the absolute regularity of the ventricular complexes, a supraventricular tachycardia with aberrant intraventricular conduction must be considered (see Fig 17–10).

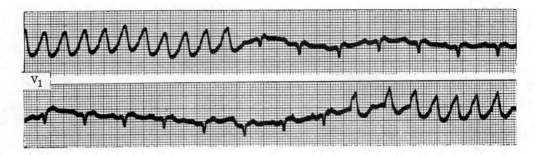

Figure 17–10. Continued record of the patient in Fig 17–9 with right carotid pressure. Carotid pressure results in the following changes: (1) slowing of the ventricular rate from 200 to 100; (2) the wide, bizarre QRS complexes of the rapid rate are changed to normal appearing complexes; and (3) an atrial rate of 200 is now evident with a constant 2:1 AV relationship. The original pattern returns when carotid pressure is released. *Interpretation:* Supraventricular tachycardia; rate = 200; 1:1 AV conduction; aberrant intraventricular conduction. With carotid pressure, a 2:1 atrial tachycardia is produced with a ventricular rate of 100 and loss of the aberrant intraventricular conduction.

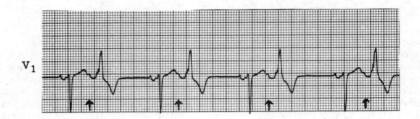

Figure 17–11. Bigeminal rhythm. Each sinus-conducted beat is followed by a premature ventricular depolarization that has the appearance of ventricular ectopy. However, each such complex is preceded by a premature atrial depolarization (arrows), indicating that the ectopics are of atrial origin with aberrancy of intraventricular conduction.

The ECG is frequently interpreted as abnormal because of ST segment and T wave changes. Because these often do not permit an etiologic diagnosis, they are referred to as "nonspecific" changes. Proper evaluation will depend upon the clinical evaluation of the patient and serial electrocardiographic studies.

PERICARDITIS

The earliest electrocardiographic evidence of pericarditis is ST segment elevation in those leads reflecting the epicardial surface of the involved area (owing to epicardial currents of injury). Typically, the ST segment elevation assumes a concave curvature in contrast to the usual convex curvature seen in myocardial infarction. Since pericarditis is usually a diffuse disease, these changes will be seen in all leads reflecting epicardial potential. A cavity lead (such as aVR) will show ST segment depression. These early segment changes can exactly simulate the normal variant described on p 81. Clinical evaluation and serial ECGs will be necessary to differentiate these 2 conditions. Occasionally, the disease process will be localized and therefore seen only in those leads reflecting the involved area.

After a period of days, the ST segments become isoelectric and the T waves begin to invert. The T wave inversion may appear while the ST segment is still elevated.

In "benign" pericarditis the ECG returns to normal within a period of weeks. In more chronic pericarditides (eg, tuberculosis), the T wave abnormalities may persist for many months.

In a mild case of "benign" pericarditis, T wave inversion may never appear. The early ST segment elevations will be seen, and these will return to the isoelectric line with normally upright T waves persisting. Conversely, T wave inversion may be seen without ST segment elevation ever being evident.

Abnormal Q waves or QS complexes are not seen in pericarditis.

In pericarditis with effusion, the QRS complexes are of low voltage. Electrical alternans may be present (see p 305).

Uremic pericarditis rarely produces a typical electrocardiographic pattern of pericarditis.

Rarely, one may see deep, symmetrically inverted T waves simulating those of infarction.

Depression of the PR segment is a common finding, usually in association with ST segment elevation. Occasionally, the former may be the only electrocardiographic abnormality in pericarditis.

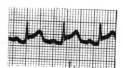

Concave ST elevation in pericarditis

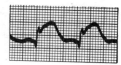

Convex ST elevation in infarction

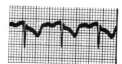

Cavity complex; pericarditis

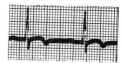

Late pattern; pericarditis

Figure 18–1. Electrocardiographic patterns in pericarditis and infarction.

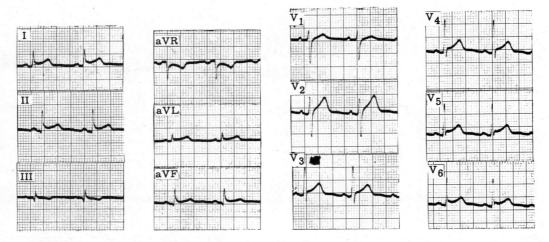

Figure 18–2. Acute pericarditis. ST segment elevation with concave upward curvature is seen in leads I, II, aVL, aVF, and V₂₋₆. Reciprocal ST segment depression is seen in cavity lead aVR. *Clinical diagnosis:* Acute "benign" pericarditis.

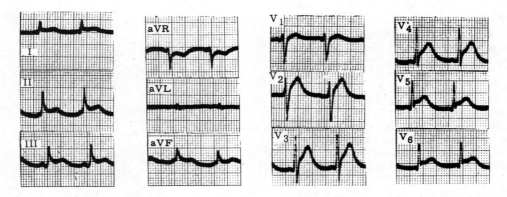

Figure 18–3. Acute pericarditis. There is ST segment elevation with a concave upward curvature in leads I, II, III, aVF, and V₂₋₆. There is reciprocal ST depression in aVR (cavity potential). The P–R interval is short, 0.1 s, and the P is upright in II, III, and aVF. This could be regular sinus rhythm or accelerated conduction. *Clinical and autopsy diagnosis:* Carcinoma of the esophagus, with rupture; secondary mediastinitis and pericarditis.

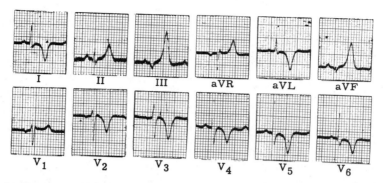

Figure 18–4. Pericarditis (late pattern). Deep, symmetrically inverted T waves in I, aVL, and V2–6. *Clinical diagnosis:* Acute rheumatic fever in a 25-year-old white man; persistent pericardial friction rub.

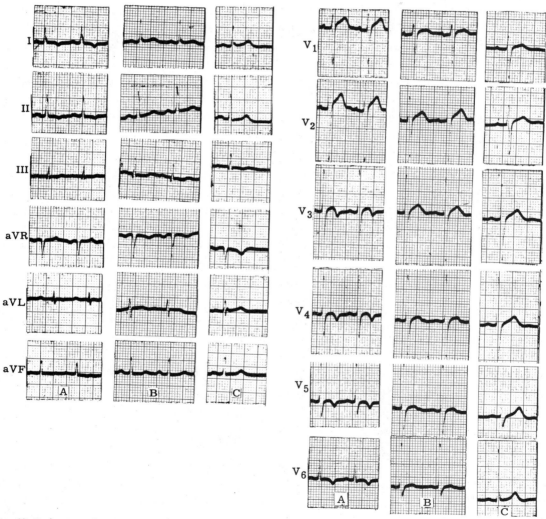

Figure 18–5. Acute pericarditis associated with serum sickness. *A:* The T waves are inverted in leads I, II, aVL, aVF, and V3–6. This pattern is consistent with pericarditis, but one could not diagnose this from the ECG. Clinically, the patient had a severe serum sickness secondary to tetanus antitoxin and had a pericardial friction rub at the time this tracing was taken. *B:* Taken 20 hours after (A). Cortisone had been given. The T waves have now become upright but are still of low voltage. *C:* Taken 48 hours after (B). Cortisone continued. The ECG is now normal. (From Goldman MJ, Lau F: *N Engl J Med* 1954;**250**:278.)

MYOCARDITIS

Almost every known acute infectious disease can involve the myocardium and thereby produce electrocardiographic abnormalities. The ECG below is an example. These may be (1) prolongation of AV or intraventricular conduction, (2) lengthening of the Q–T$_c$ interval, (3) various arrhythmias, (4) ST segment depression or T wave inversion (or both) in left ventricular epicardial leads, and (5) QRS abnormalities that may mimic myocardial infarction.

Similar nonspecific changes are seen in chronic myocarditides, beriberi, amyloidosis, etc.

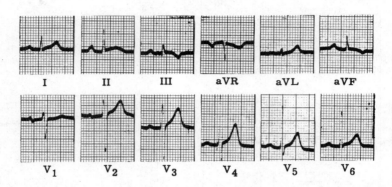

Figure 18–6. Acute rheumatic fever. The abnormalities are a prolonged P–R interval of 0.24 s and an inverted T in aVF. The ECG returned to normal when the rheumatic process became clinically inactive.

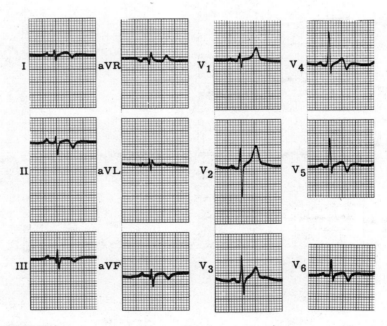

Figure 18–7. Acute viral myocarditis. The T waves are deeply and symmetrically inverted in I, II, III, and V$_{3-6}$, indicating diffuse myocardial involvement. *Clinical diagnosis:* Acute myocarditis in a 22-year-old man.

HYPERTHYROIDISM

This disease is typically characterized by tachycardia. One may also see ST segment elevation with T wave inversion in left ventricular epicardial leads. The mechanism producing this electrocardiographic change is unknown.

MYXEDEMA

Bradycardia, prolongation of the P–R interval, low voltage of the QRS complexes, and flattened T waves are the common electrocardiographic findings in myxedema.

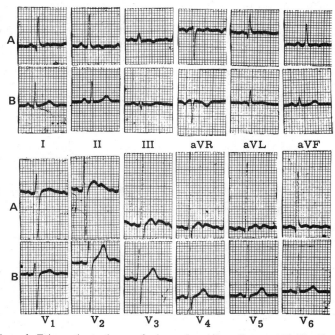

Figure 18–8. Hyperthyroidism. *A:* Taken prior to therapy for hyperthyroidism. Rate = 110. The T waves are inverted in I, II, III, aVF, and V₆, flat in aVL, and diphasic in V₂–₅. These changes are nonspecific. RV₅ + SV₁ = 40 mm. Ordinarily, this would be suggestive of left ventricular hypertrophy, but these voltage criteria are invalid in the presence of hyperthyroidism. *B:* Taken when patient was euthyroid. The ECG is now within normal limits.

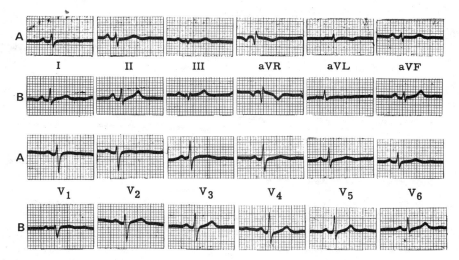

Figure 18–9. Myxedema. *A:* The QRS complexes are of low voltage and the T waves are of low amplitude in all leads. *B:* Three weeks after thyroid therapy: The T waves are now of normal amplitude, and there is a slight increase in the QRS voltage.

TRAUMATIC HEART DISEASE

This can result from penetrating or nonpenetrating injuries to the heart. The electrocardiographic abnormalities may be (1) arrhythmias of various types, (2) a pattern consistent with pericarditis, (3) nonspecific ST segment and T wave changes, and (4) an infarct pattern resulting from extensive myocardial trauma or actual traumatic coronary occlusion.

NEUROMUSCULAR DISEASES

Such diseases as myotonia atrophica, Friedreich's ataxia, and progressive muscular dystrophy may produce electrocardiographic abnormalities such as (1) prolongation of the P–R interval, (2) arrhythmias of various types, and (3) nonspecific ST segment and T wave changes.

MALIGNANCY INVOLVING THE HEART

Primary cardiac malignancy is a rare condition. However, metastatic involvement of the heart is not uncommon and is frequently not diagnosed during life.

An arrhythmia may be a manifestation of cardiac malignancy. The sudden appearance of atrial flutter, atrial tachycardia, or atrial fibrillation in a patient with known extracardiac malignancy should arouse suspicion of pericardial or atrial metastatic disease.

Diffuse malignant involvement of the pericardium can produce a pattern of pericarditis.

Extensive but localized involvement can produce a pattern indistinguishable from myocardial infarction.

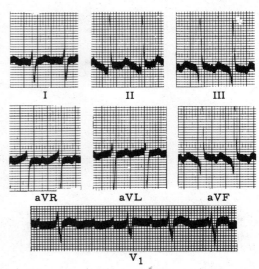

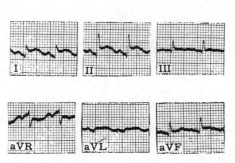

Figure 18–10. Cardiac trauma. The above individual sustained a gunshot wound of the chest. The bullet traumatized the epicardial half of the myocardium at the apex of the heart (as visualized at surgery). Precordial leads could not be taken because of the chest injury. Marked concave ST segment elevation and PR segment depression are seen in leads I, II, aVL, and aVF; reciprocal ST depression is present in aVR. Such a pattern is consistent with either early myocardial infarction or pericarditis, but in this instance it was due to trauma.

Figure 18–11. Myotonia atrophica. The patient was a 46-year-old man. The ECG reveals an atrial flutter with 2:1 AV block in standard and extremity leads and a changing block in V_1.

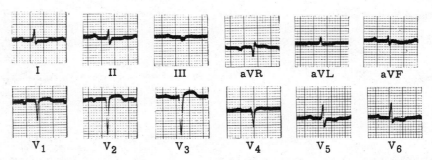

Figure 18–12. Tumor of the heart. Complexes are of low voltage in frontal plane leads. QS complexes are present in V_{1-2}; there are minute r waves in V_{3-4}; there is slight ST elevation of V_{2-3}; the T waves are inverted in V_{5-6}. The above findings are typical of anterior wall infarction, but in this case they were the result of metastatic bronchogenic carcinoma to the anterior wall of the left ventricle. The ECG records the electrically "dead" or "silent" area and of course cannot differentiate between death of heart muscle due to infarction and replacement and death of heart muscle due to tumor.

HYPOTHERMIA

With the clinical use of total body hypothermia or cold cardioplegia it is essential that one be aware of untoward effects as evidenced in the ECG. Similar abnormalities occur in individuals accidentally exposed to cold. Sinus bradycardia, AV junctional rhythm, and prolongation of the Q–T interval are common findings. With more extreme degrees of hypothermia, an intraventricular conduction delay develops that is characterized by prominent notching of the terminal portion of the QRS complex (Osborn wave) followed by ST segment elevation. When the rectal temperature falls below 28 °C, ventricular fibrillation may occur.

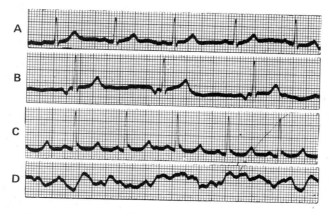

Figure 18–13. Effect of surgical hypothermia. *A:* Before hypothermia. *B –D:* During hypothermia. All illustrations are lead II. *A:* Q–T$_c$ = 0.41 s. *B:* AV junctional rhythm; rate = 45. *C:* Q–T$_c$ = 0.52 s. *D:* Ventricular fibrillation.

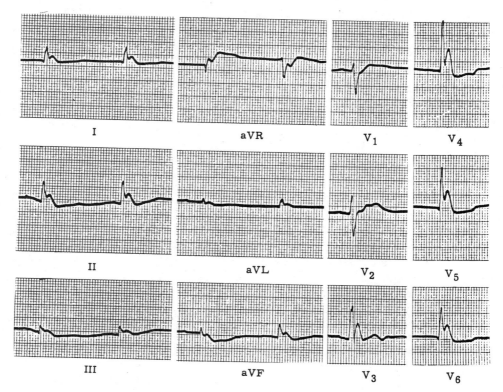

Figure 18–14. Hypothermia. Sinus bradycardia, rate = 50; notching of the terminal portion of the QRS with ST segment elevation (Osborn waves); prolonged Q–T interval. This individual had been exposed to a cold environment for an unknown period of time. Rectal temperature = 27 °C (81 °F) at the time of this record. (Courtesy of R Brindis.)

EFFECTS OF DRUGS ON
THE ELECTROCARDIOGRAM

DIGITALIS

This is by far the most commonly used drug that produces electrocardiographic abnormalities.

Digitalis Effect

Digitalis commonly produces ST segment depression in ventricular epicardial leads. Characteristically, the ST segment assumes a rounded, concave ("scooped") configuration or an oblique line descending from the ST junction. Because of the ST segment depression, the T wave may be "dragged" downward, giving the appearance of T wave inversion. In addition, there is a shortening of the Q–T interval resulting from a shortening of electrical systole. It must be emphasized that the above findings will be seen in most individuals who are adequately digitalized. This represents digitalis effect but not digitalis toxicity.

Digitalis Toxicity

Any arrhythmia may result from overdigitalization. The most common arrhythmias are sinus bradycardia, first degree AV block, isolated ventricular premature beats arising from single or multiple foci, and ventricular bigeminy.

Associated with the injudicious dosages of purified digitalis preparations and the frequent administration of potent diuretic agents that can cause hypokalemia, digitalis toxicity as manifested by serious arrhythmias is unfortunately being observed more frequently. In addition to the arrhythmias mentioned above, paroxysmal atrial tachycardia, usually with block and an atrial rate of 200 or less, is quite common. Less common are atrial flutter (atrial rate over 250) and atrial fibrillation. It is important to realize that the appearance of these 3 rhythms in a patient who has been in regular sinus rhythm and has received adequate doses of digitalis (and especially if diuretics have also been given) is more an indication of digitalis toxicity than an indication for further digitalis therapy.

Less common arrhythmias resulting from digitalis intoxication are second and third degree AV block, AV junctional rhythm, AV dissociation, ventricular tachycardia, and ventricular fibrillation.

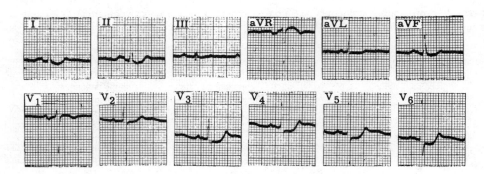

Figure 18–15. Digitalis effect. Note the typical rounded ST segment depression in I, II, aVF, and V_{2-6}. There is reciprocal ST elevation in aVR. These changes are characteristic of digitalis effect but do not indicate digitalis toxicity. Note also the notched P waves, the typical "P mitrale." This patient has mitral stenosis.

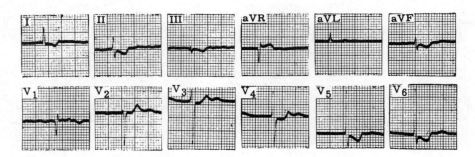

Figure 18–16. Digitalis effect. Note the ST segment depression. This produces an oblique downward configuration of the first portion of the ST in leads I, II, III, aVF, and V_{5-6}. There is a rounded ST segment depression in V_{3-4}. As a result, the T waves are "dragged" downward. There is reciprocal ST elevation in aVR. The above changes are indicative of digitalis effect but do not indicate digitalis toxicity. The rhythm is atrial fibrillation.

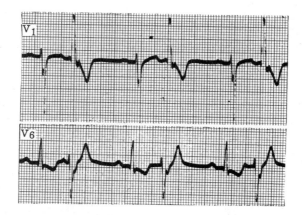

Figure 18–17. Digitalis toxicity. Ventricular bigeminy. Regular sinus rhythm alternating with ventricular premature contractions (left ventricular origin). ST segment depression and T wave inversion in the sinus-conducted beats are seen in V_6. The latter could also be the result of digitalis.

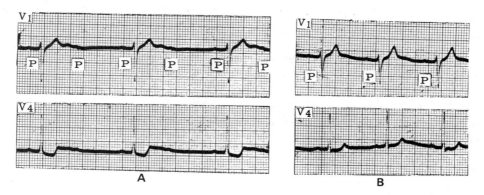

Figure 18–18. Digitalis toxicity. Second degree 2:1 AV block. *A:* The atrial rhythm is regular at a rate of 86. The ventricle responds to every second atrial beat, resulting in a ventricular rate of 43. There is ST segment depression in V_4. This rhythm has resulted from digitalis intoxication. *B:* Digitalis discontinued. The rhythm is now regular sinus. There is much less ST segment depression in V_4.

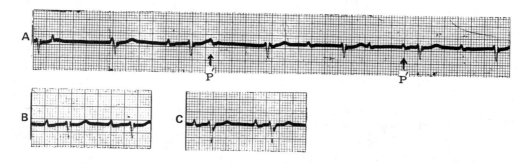

Figure 18–19. Digitalis toxicity. Complete heart block. The patient had been in regular sinus rhythm. He then received increasing doses of digitalis. *A:* Complete heart block: The atrial rate is 66 and the ventricular rate is 52. The QRS complexes are of normal configuration, indicating that the second pacemaker is in the AV junction. In addition, there are blocked atrial premature contractions (indicated by the arrows). *B:* Four days after (A) (digitalis discontinued): First degree heart block; P–R = 0.3 s. *C:* One week after (B): P–R has been reduced to 0.24 s. (All recordings are lead V_1.)

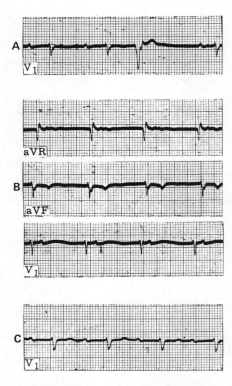

Figure 18–20. Digitalis toxicity. AV junctional rhythm. *A:* First degree AV block (P–R = 0.32 s). One ventricular premature beat is seen. The P–R interval of the first sinus beat after the ectopic beat is shorter, 0.24 s. *B:* Increasing doses of digitalis have been given. The rhythm is now AV junctional. P' waves are seen. These are upright in aVR and inverted in aVF, indicating a reverse spread through the atrium. This results from retrograde atrial stimulation secondary to the AV junctional rhythm. *C:* Six days after (B). Digitalis withheld. The rhythm is again regular sinus (P–R = 0.32 s).

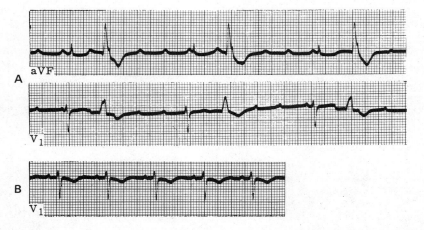

Figure 18–21. Digitalis toxicity. Atrial tachycardia, complete heart block, and ventricular bigeminy. The patient had been in regular sinus rhythm and received large doses of digitalis. *A:* An atrial tachycardia is now present with a regular atrial rate of 164. The ventricular rhythm exclusive of the premature ventricular contractions is perfectly regular at a rate of 31. There is no constant relation between the QRS and the preceding P' wave, indicating a complete heart block. The QRS complexes are of normal configuration, indicating that the second pacemaker is in the AV junction. Ventricular bigeminy is present. All of the above resulted from digitalis intoxication. *B:* Five days after (A). Digitalis has been discontinued and potassium given. The rhythm is again regular sinus.

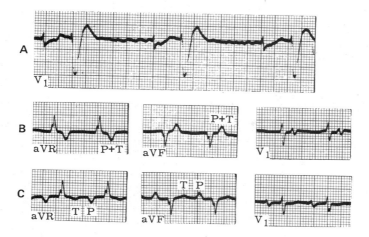

Figure 18–22. Digitalis toxicity, atrial fibrillation, complete AV block, and ventricular bigeminy. Prior to (A) the rhythm had been regular sinus. The patient was receiving increasing doses of digitalis in an attempt to improve the degree of congestive failure. **A:** The atrial rhythm is that of fibrillation. The ventricular rhythm is regular; the rate exclusive of the premature ventricular beats is 37. Since the ventricular rhythm is regular, the ventricles are responding not to the atrial fibrillation but to an independent pacemaker in the AV junction. A premature ventricular contraction follows each junctional beat, ie, ventricular bigeminy is present. All of the above has been produced by digitalis intoxication. **B:** Four days after (A); digitalis withheld. The rhythm is now a first degree AV block with a P–R interval of 0.52 s. The P waves are fused with the T waves. This is not a junctional rhythm since the P waves are inverted in aVR and upright in aVF, ie, the pattern is normal, indicating sinus origin. **C:** Three days after (B); digitalis still withheld. First degree AV block; the P–R interval reduced to 0.25. P and T waves are now separated and prove the interpretation made in (B).

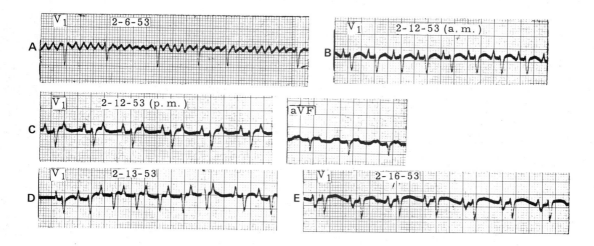

Figure 18–23. Digitalis toxicity producing atrial tachycardia. **A:** 2-6-53: Atrial fibrillation. The patient is receiving digitalis. **B:** 2-12-53 a.m.: An atrial tachycardia with 1:1 conduction has appeared; the rate is 160. This sudden appearance of an atrial tachycardia during digitalis therapy for atrial fibrillation (in the absence of quinidine therapy) should always make one suspicious of digitalis intoxication. This was not appreciated, and more digitalis was given. **C:** 2-12-53 p.m.: Four hours after the last dose of digitalis. The extra digitalis has increased the AV block, producing atrial tachycardia with 2:1 block. The direct effect of digitalis on atrial conduction has increased the atrial rate to 200. The P' waves are upright in aVF, indicating a high atrial ectopic focus. **D:** 2-13-53: Digitalis has been discontinued and potassium and quinidine therapy begun. The atrial rhythm remains regular at a rate of 177, but the ventricular response is irregular. One notices a progressive increase in the P'–R interval and finally a failure of ventricular response. Thus, this is an atrial tachycardia with a Wenckebach type of AV block. **E:** 2-16-53: Further quinidine therapy. The rhythm has been reverted to regular sinus. The sinus P waves are diphasic in contrast to the tall, upright P' waves of the tachycardia.

QUINIDINE

Quinidine produces ST segment depression and flattening of the T waves in leads reflecting a left ventricular epicardial complex. These changes are similar to those produced by digitalis. However, in contrast to digitalis, quinidine produces a lengthening of the Q–Tc interval. The major therapeutic action of quinidine in the treatment of ectopic atrial tachyarrhythmias is initially a slowing of the rate of the ectopic discharge and then elimination of the ectopic dis-

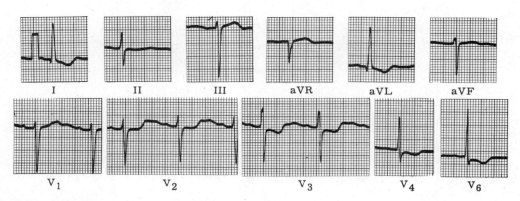

Figure 18–24. Effect of quinidine. The rhythm is regular sinus, P–R = 0.2 s. The R in aVL = 14 mm. There is ST depression and T wave inversion in I, aVL, and V$_{2-6}$. The measured Q–T interval (see V$_{2-3}$) = 0.6 s (Q–T$_c$ = 0.65 s). *Clinical diagnosis:* Aortic stenosis; quinidine therapy for previous ventricular arrhythmias. The R voltage in aVL and some of the ST–T changes are due to left ventricular hypertrophy. The long Q–T interval is due to quinidine. Although there are no quantitative data to differentiate quinidine effect from quinidine toxicity by Q–T measurement, the marked prolongation in this case favors toxicity.

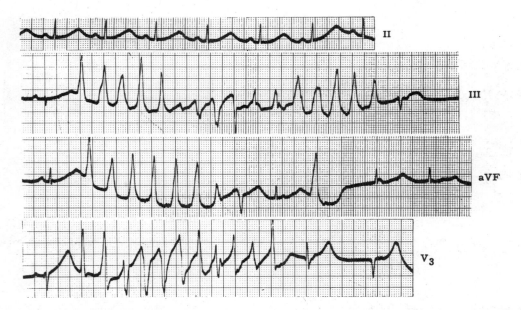

Figure 18–25. Toxic effect of quinidine. The above ECG strips were taken during treatment for cardiac arrest in a hospital emergency room. There are periods of sinus rhythm in which the P–R interval = 0.18 s, QRS = 0.06 s, and Q–T$_c$ exceeds 0.6 s. Interspersed are periods of bizarre ventricular tachycardia. Note that the QRS complexes change from upright to inverted during the tachycardia. This has been called "torsade de pointes" and is most commonly associated with clinical conditions manifested by Q–T prolongation. *Clinical features:* The patient had been taking excessive doses of quinidine. Serum quinidine level was 19 mg/L (average therapeutic level = 4–8 mg/L). The above was not known at the time of initial emergency therapy. The very long Q–T interval was a clue to the possibility of quinidine toxicity which initially was confirmed by the history obtained from the patient's wife. If this had not been appreciated, the patient could have been treated with quinidine (this occurred in 1955) with an almost certain fatal outcome. He was successfully treated with molar sodium lactate.

charge, allowing a resumption of normal rhythm. In addition, quinidine has a vagolytic action, thus increasing the ability of the AV node to conduct impulses. When quinidine is administered to a patient with atrial fibrillation, the initial slowing of the ectopic atrial rhythm results in atrial flutter and tachycardia. This slower and more regular atrial rhythm combined with increased conductivity through the AV node produces a "paradoxic" increase in the ventricular rate. This explains the necessity for prior administration of digitalis in order to achieve the vagotonic (ie, blocking) action of digitalis on the AV node. With continued quinidine effect, the atrial ectopic discharge is completely eliminated, allowing for resumption of sinus rhythm. Quinidine is equally efficacious in the elimination of ventricular ectopic rhythms, ie, ventricular premature contractions and ventricular tachycardia.

Toxic manifestations of quinidine are as follows: (1) first degree AV block, (2) second degree AV block, (3) third degree (complete) AV block, (4) AV dissociation, (5) AV junctional rhythm with any associated atrial rhythm including atrial standstill, (6) marked prolongation of the $Q-T_c$ interval, (7) widening of the QRS complex to 50% or more of the prior QRS interval, (8) idioventricular rhythm, (9) ventricular premature beats, (10) ventricular tachycardia, (11) ventricular fibrillation, and (12) cardiac standstill. With the exception of a first degree heart block, the appearance of any of the above is an absolute contraindication to continuation of quinidine therapy.

OTHER DRUGS

Emetine

Emetine occasionally produces the following electrocardiographic changes: (1) ST segment depression or T wave inversion (or both) in epicardial leads and (2) prolongation of the P–R interval.

These changes may persist for days to weeks after emetine is discontinued. They do not necessarily contraindicate continuation of emetine if clinically necessary. More serious toxic effects can produce intraventricular conduction disturbances.

Tartar Emetic

All patients receiving a full course of this drug (as in the therapy of schistosomiasis) will develop electrocardiographic abnormalities. Most commonly this is T wave inversion in epicardial leads. These electrocardiographic changes alone are not a contraindication to continuation of therapy.

Phenothiazines & Related Drugs

The phenothiazines and the antidepressant group of drugs—eg, imipramine, amitriptyline, and related compounds—are myocardial depressants and impair conduction. With excessive dosages, ST depression, T wave flattening or inversion, prolongation of the $Q-T_c$ interval or prominent U waves, and AV and intraventricular conduction disturbances may occur. These changes are similar to those that result from quinidine toxicity. Because of the widespread use of these drugs, the physician must be aware of this potential toxicity.

Anthracyclines

Two congeners of anthracycline antibiotics—doxorubicin (Adriamycin) and daunorubicin (Cerubidine)—used in chemotherapy of cancer are potentially cardiotoxic, and once this becomes manifest it may be irreversible. Care must be exerted to limit the total dose of these drugs and monitor the patient for evidence of cardiotoxicity. Unfortunately, electrocardiographic evidence of toxicity, which is usually diffuse T wave inversion, is often a late sign (Fig 18–29).

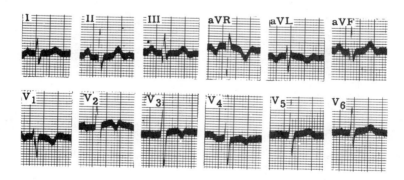

Figure 18–26. Effect of emetine on the ECG. *Standard leads:* Frontal plane QRS axis = +80 degrees. *Extremity leads:* Vertical heart. The standard and extremity leads are normal. *Precordial leads:* Clockwise rotation; the T waves are inverted in V_{1-4}. These changes are nonspecific, but they could be the result of coronary artery disease or right heart strain. *Clinical diagnosis:* Amebiasis treated with emetine. The ECG became normal after treatment had been discontinued.

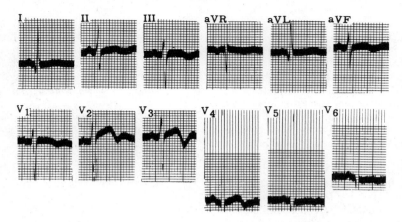

Figure 18–27. Effect of tartar emetic on the ECG. *Standard leads:* Frontal plane QRS axis = 0 degrees; low amplitude T in I. *Extremity leads:* Horizontal heart; low amplitude T in aVL. *Precordial leads:* Inverted T waves in V_{2-4} and flat T waves in V_{5-6}. These changes are nonspecific and could result from coronary artery disease. *Clinical diagnosis:* Schistosomiasis. The changes seen in the ECG invariably occur as a result of therapy with tartar emetic. The ECG became normal after therapy had been discontinued.

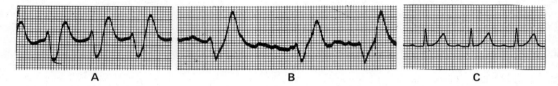

Figure 18–28. Amitriptyline toxicity. (All are lead II.) The patient had ingested about 2 g of this drug in a suicide attempt. *A:* On admission: Patient comatose and in shock. The ECG shows extremely wide QRS complexes, indicating an idioventricular rhythm; rate = 95. There is no definite evidence of atrial activity. *B:* One hour after admission: Patient receiving supportive treatment. A slow and irregular ventricular rhythm is present with persisting wide QRS complexes. Irregular atrial activity is seen, probably indicating atrial fibrillation. *C:* Six hours after admission: Regular sinus rhythm is now present with normal intraventricular conduction; P–R = 0.2 s; the $Q-T_c$ is prolonged to 0.46 s, indicating prolonged repolarization.

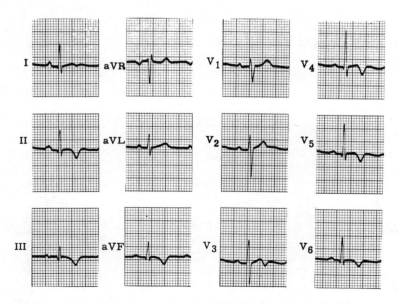

Figure 18–29. Effect of daunorubicin. There are deeply inverted T waves in leads II, III, aVF, and V_{4-6}, indicating diffuse myocardial abnormality. *Clinical features:* A 31-year-old man receiving daunorubicin for acute myelogenous leukemia. The ECG was normal before the above drug therapy and reverted to normal 1 week after discontinuation of the drug.

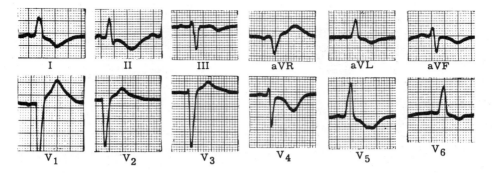

Figure 18–30. Cerebral hemorrhage. This tracing was taken on a patient with a massive intracerebral hemorrhage. He was known to have hypertensive cardiovascular disease. Previous ECGs had revealed a typical left bundle branch block. New electrocardiographic findings are the broad negative T waves in leads I, II, aVL, aVF, and V$_{4-5}$. The serum electrolytes and arterial oxygen saturation were normal. *Autopsy findings:* Left ventricular hypertrophy; no myocardial infarction. It is assumed that the bizarre ST–T changes and markedly prolonged Q–T$_c$ interval were the result of the cerebral disease.

EFFECTS OF CEREBRAL DISEASE ON THE ELECTROCARDIOGRAM

Abnormal ECGs may be seen in association with cerebral disease, especially cerebral and subarachnoid hemorrhage. These changes are ST depression, flat to inverted T waves, marked prolongation of the Q–T$_c$ interval, and prominent U waves in leads that reflect a left ventricular epicardial complex (I, aVL, V$_{4-6}$). In such cases, autopsy examination has shown the absence of myocardial disease.

EFFECTS OF ELECTROLYTE DISTURBANCES ON THE ELECTROCARDIOGRAM

HYPERKALEMIA

The first electrocardiographic evidence of an elevated extracellular potassium level is the appearance of tall, slender, ''tented'' T waves, usually best seen in precordial leads. Although this pattern strongly suggests hyperkalemia, it is not absolutely diagnostic since patients with posterior wall infarction and even normal individuals may show a similar pattern.

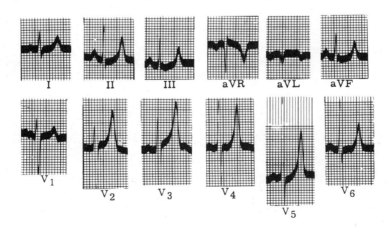

Figure 18–31. Hyperkalemia (chronic glomerulonephritis with uremia). Tall slender T waves are seen in I, II, III, aVF, and V$_{2-6}$. The rhythm is regular sinus; QRS interval = 0.09 s. Serum potassium = 7.2 mEq/L.

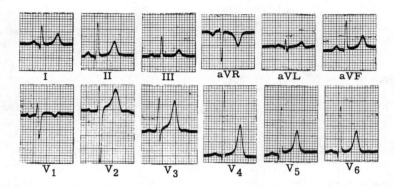

Figure 18–32. Normal ECG simulating a hyperkalemia pattern. Note the tall slender T waves in leads I, II, aVF, and V_{2-6}. This finding is strongly suggestive of hyperkalemia. However, this record was taken on a normal young adult with no clinical evidence of heart disease or electrolyte disturbance. The serum potassium at the time of this record was 4.7 mEq/L. Serial ECGs over the course of many months showed no change.

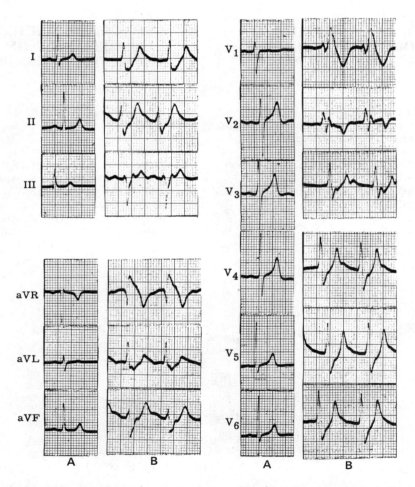

Figure 18–33. Hyperkalemia. The above tracings were taken on a patient with glomerulonephritis. *A:* Taken one year before death. The tracing is normal. Serum potassium = 5 mEq/L. *B:* Taken terminally; serum potassium = 8.9 mEq/L. There is no definite evidence of regular atrial activity. The QRS interval has increased to 0.16 s. The QRS complexes simulate a right bundle branch block. The T waves are tall and peaked in I, II, and V_{4-6}. (These tracings were recorded prior to the advent of dialysis therapy.)

With further elevation of the serum potassium level, atrial activity disappears and wide, slurred, bizarre QRS complexes develop that simulate an idioventricular rhythm. However, experimental studies with multiple intramyocardial electrodes indicate that the sinus node continues to fire and its impulse is transmitted via the internodal pathways to the AV node and the ventricles. No atrial complex is recorded because the atrial myocardium is not activated. This is known as sinoventricular rhythm. As the serum level rises, ventricular fibrillation or asystole may result.

ST segment elevation may be seen in association with hyperkalemia. In experimental studies in which the surface of the heart is bathed with a potassium solution, ST segment elevation is produced. It is likely that one reason for ST segment elevation in acute myocardial infarction is the leakage of potassium from damaged myocardial cells into the interstitial fluid, resulting in ''localized'' hyperkalemia. However, the clinical finding of ST elevation in association with hyperkalemia is uncommon.

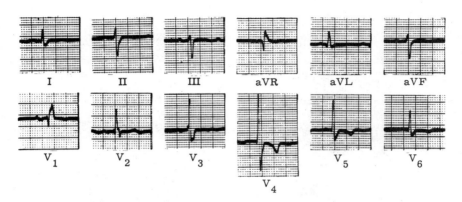

Figure 18–34. Hyperkalemia. This tracing was taken on a 70-year-old man with carcinoma of the prostate and coronary artery disease. A right bundle branch block is present—as evidenced by a QRS interval of 0.12 s, wide s waves in leads I and V_{5-6}, and wide R' in V_1. The vector of the initial 0.04 s QRS in the frontal plane is −50 degrees, indicating a left anterior fascicular block. This with the right bundle branch block is evidence of bilateral bundle branch disease. The T wave inversion in V_{4-6} indicates additional anterior wall disease. At this time the serum potassium = 4.6 mEq/L. (See Fig 18–35.)

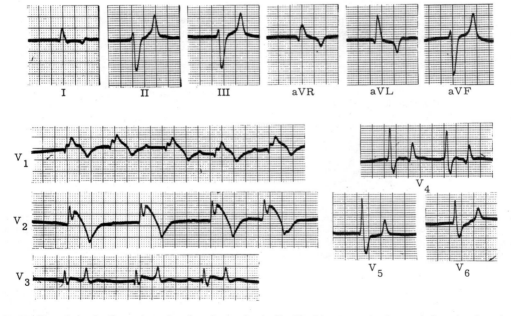

Figure 18–35. Hyperkalemia. Several weeks after the tracing in Fig 18–34 was made. Azotemia has developed; serum potassium = 9.3 mEq/L. Only occasional P waves are seen, and the rhythm is probably an incomplete AV dissociation. The QRS interval has widened to 0.14 s. The T waves are tall and peaked in II, III, aVF, and V_{3-6}. Marked ST elevation is seen in V_{1-2} and to a lesser degree in V_3. The patient was given hypertonic glucose and insulin intravenously, and 20 minutes later the ECG reverted to that seen in Fig 18–34, at which time the serum potassium equaled 6.1 mEq/L.

HYPOKALEMIA

Typically, one may see prolongation of the P–R interval and ST segment depression in epicardial leads. Formerly, it was stated that prolongation of the Q–T interval was a significant electrocardiographic finding. This is now known to be incorrect. Owing to prolonged repolarization of ventricular Purkinje fibers, a prominent U wave occurs in hypokalemia. This is frequently superimposed upon the T wave and therefore produces the appearance of a prolonged Q–T interval.

The electrocardiographic findings are therefore ST segment depression and, at times, T wave inversion in epicardial leads, prominent U waves, and prolongation of the P–R interval. These findings are not pathognomonic of hypokalemia. Myocardial ischemia, quinidine, procainamide, phenothiazines, and the tricyclic antidepressants can prolong ventricular repolarization and result in similar electrocardiographic abnormalities.

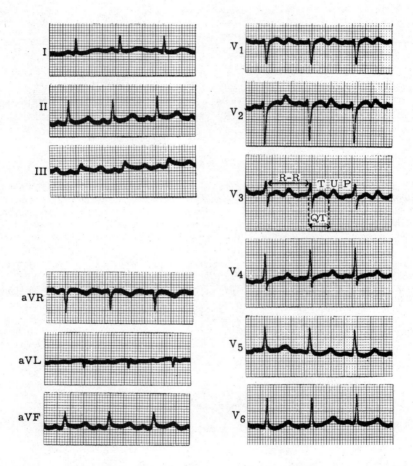

Figure 18–36. Hypokalemia. An apparently upright T wave is seen in leads II, III, aVF, and V₅₋₆. If this deflection were the T wave, the Q–T interval would be 0.4 s (corrected for R–R interval of 0.66 s, the Q–T$_c$ = 0.5 s) and therefore prolonged. In leads V₁₋₄ separate T and U waves are clearly evident. The true Q–T interval in V₃ is 0.29 s (Q–T$_c$ = 0.36 s), which is normal. The above tracing was taken on a 51-year-old man who had had persistent vomiting. The serum potassium = 2.3 mEq/L.

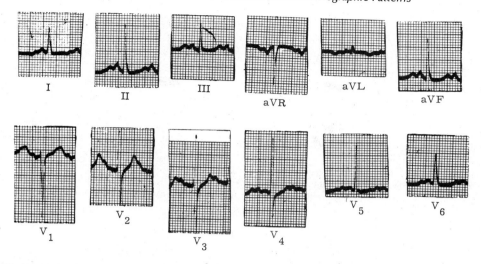

Figure 18–37. Hypokalemia. In the precordial leads a clear distinction can be made between T and U waves. The Q–T$_c$ interval is normal. The U wave is more prominent than the T in V$_{4-6}$, and slight ST depression is present in V$_{4-6}$. In the frontal plane leads only a single wave is seen between the QRS and P. If this were interpreted as a T wave, it would lead to a mistaken determination of a long Q–T interval. Instead, it is a U wave. This patient had been on corticosteroid therapy for rheumatoid arthritis, with more recent thiazide administration for attempted control of edema. The serum potassium = 2.6 mEq/L.

Postextrasystolic U Wave

On occasion, the normal sinus (basic) beat that follows a ventricular ectopic beat will show an abnormal U wave when such a wave is not evident in other complexes. In the illustration below, the sinus beat that follows the first ventricular ectopic beat shows a large, abnormal U wave. U waves are visible in the other sinus beats, but these are small and normal. The postextrasystole U wave was therefore the only electrocardiographic clue to hypokalemia in this patient, who was on digitalis and thiazide therapy. Serum potassium = 3.1 mEq/L.

ELECTROCARDIOGRAM AS GUIDE TO POTASSIUM LEVELS

The ECG serves as a reasonably satisfactory guide to serum potassium levels when actual determination of the serum potassium is not available. At times, the ECG will be more helpful than the serum potassium level. The ECG is a reflection of the potassium gradient across the cell membrane and hence indicates the ratio of extracellular to intracellular potassium.

HYPERCALCEMIA

Elevated serum calcium levels (above 12 mg/dl) produce a shortening of the Q–T$_c$ interval. This is correlated with a shortening of phase 2 of the intracellular action potential curve. Such an electrocardiographic finding has obvious diagnostic and therapeutic implications.

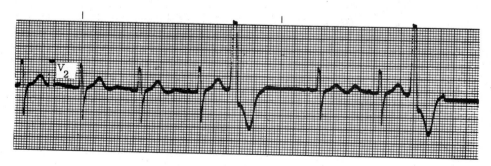

Figure 18–38. Postextrasystolic U wave.

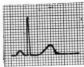

Normal tracing (serum potassium 4–5.5 mEq/L): P–R interval = 0.16 s; QRS interval = 0.06 s; Q–T interval = 0.4 s (normal for an assumed heart rate of 60).

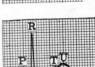

Hypokalemia (serum potassium ±3.5 mEq/L): P–R interval = 0.2 s; QRS interval = 0.06 s; ST segment depression. A prominent U wave is now present immediately following the T wave. The actual Q–T interval remains 0.4 s. If the U wave is erroneously considered a part of the T, a falsely prolonged Q–T interval of 0.6 s will be measured.

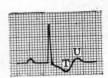

Hypokalemia (serum potassium ±2.5 mEq/L): The P–R interval is lengthened to 0.32 s; the ST segment is depressed; the T wave is inverted; a prominent U wave is seen. The true Q–T interval remains normal.

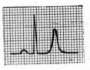

Hyperkalemia (serum potassium ±7 mEq/L): The P–R and QRS intervals are within normal limits. Very tall, slender, peaked T waves are now present.

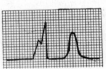

Hyperkalemia (serum potassium ±8.5 mEq/L): There is no evidence of atrial activity; the QRS complex is broad and slurred, and the QRS interval has widened to 0.2 s. The T waves remain tall and slender. Further elevation of the serum potassium will result in ventricular tachycardia and ventricular fibrillation.

Figure 18–39. Correlation of serum potassium level and the ECG. (Assuming serum calcium is normal.) The diagrammed complexes are left ventricular epicardial leads.

HYPOCALCEMIA

A low serum calcium level results in a prolongation of the Q–Tc interval. There is no abnormality of the T wave. The Q–T prolongation results from a lengthening of the ST segment, and this is evidenced by a prolongation of phase 2 of the intracellular action potential curve. A similar pattern may be seen in patients with severe liver disease without reduction in the serum calcium. This may be a result of hypomagnesemia.

Hypocalcemia may be associated with hypokalemia, in which case epicardial leads will show ST segment depression, T wave inversion, prominent U waves, and a prolonged Q–Tc interval.

Hypocalcemia with hyperkalemia is commonly seen in patients with renal insufficiency.

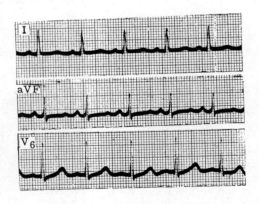

Figure 18–40. Hypocalcemia. The T waves are upright, but the Q–T interval is prolonged. This is 0.4 s (corrected for R–R of 0.66 s, Q–Tc = 0.48 s) and is abnormal. The lengthening of the Q–T interval is due to a lengthening of the ST segment and not to any abnormality in the T wave itself. Blood calcium at time of above record was 6.8 mg/dL.

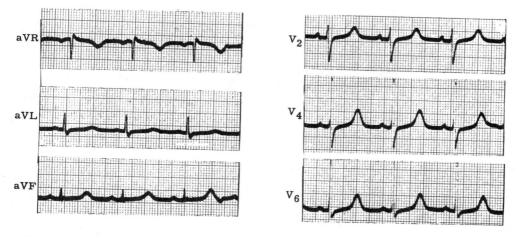

Figure 18–41. Hypocalcemia and hyperkalemia. The ST segment is prolonged, resulting in a $Q-T_c$ of 0.52 s. Although not diagnostic, the T waves are tall in aVF and V_{2-6}. *Clinical diagnosis:* Chronic glomerulonephritis; serum calcium = 7 mg/dL; serum potassium = 7.1 mEq/L.

ELECTRICAL ALTERNANS

This produces an electrocardiographic pattern in which the height of the R wave (and at times also the T) alternates every other beat. Except when associated with paroxysmal atrial tachycardia, it is an indication of organic heart disease. Pericardial effusion is a common clinical cause. Electrical alternans should not be confused with the clinical sign of pulsus alternans; the 2 have no relationship.

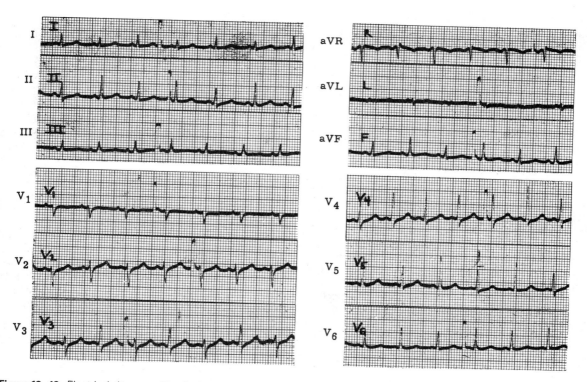

Figure 18–42. Electrical alternans. The rhythm is sinus. The QRS morphology and polarity alternate in an absolutely regular fashion. It is most obviously seen in lead V_3. *Clinical diagnosis:* Pericardial effusion with tamponade.

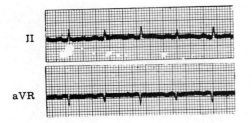
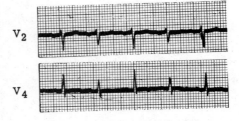

Figure 18–43. Electrical alternans. The rhythm is regular sinus. The QRS complexes are of 2 differing amplitudes. This occurs in an alternating pattern. *Clinical diagnosis:* Arteriosclerotic heart disease.

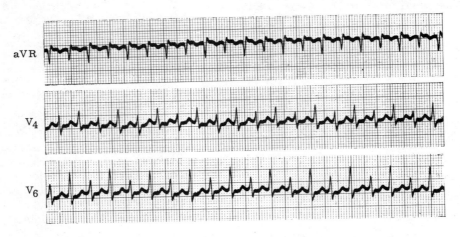

Figure 18–44. Electrical alternans. The rhythm is a paroxysmal atrial tachycardia with a rate of 200. There is an alternating amplitude of the QRS complexes. In the presence of paroxysmal tachycardia, electrical alternans has no special clinical significance.

HEREDITARY Q–T INTERVAL PROLONGATION

In addition to the more common causes of Q–T interval prolongation (electrolyte abnormalities, drug effects, ischemic heart disease, cerebral disease), there are rare hereditary syndromes characterized by sudden death, episodes of syncope associated with ventricular arrhythmias, and Q–T prolongation. Jervell-Lange-Nielsen syndrome is associated with congenital deafness and maintained by autosomal recessive inheritance. Romano-Ward syndrome is autosomal dominant but not associated with deafness. Although the causes of these syndromes are not known, there is experimental and clinical evidence that asymmetric sympathetic stimulation of the heart may be responsible. Surgical interruption of the left stellate ganglion combined with sympathectomy has been of value in some patients.

NEGATIVE U WAVES

Negative U waves are occasionally seen and represent an abnormality in the late phase of ventricular repolarization. This finding is most commonly associated with coronary artery disease and left ventricular hypertrophy.

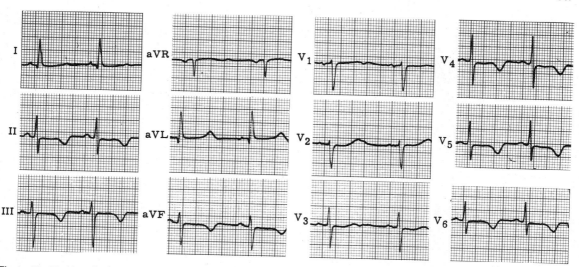

Figure 18–45. Hereditary QT syndrome. The striking feature of this ECG is the marked prolongation of the Q–T interval, which = 0.58 s with a heart rate = 68. The patient was a 62-year-old man who was asymptomatic. Clinical evaluation revealed no evidence of heart disease. He was not taking any medication. All measured serum electrolytes were normal. Similar ECGs were recorded over a 4-year period. A 25-year-old daughter who is asymptomatic has a similar ECG. Neither individual has hearing loss. This is an example of the Romano-Ward syndrome.

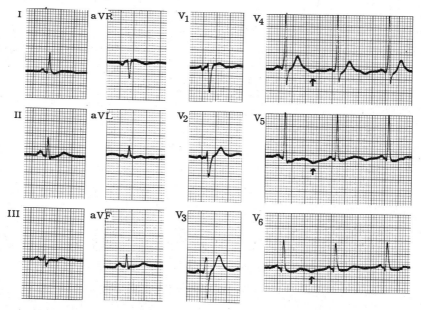

Figure 18–46. Negative U waves. The ECG reveals ST depression in I, II, aVL, and V$_{4-6}$. The T waves are of low amplitude in I, aVL, and V$_{5-6}$. The QRS voltage is insufficient to meet the criteria for left ventricular hypertrophy. Inverted U waves (arrows) are seen in V$_{4-6}$. *Clinical diagnosis:* Aortic insufficiency with left ventricular enlargement.

LIQUID PROTEIN–MODIFIED FAST (LPMF) DIETS

In recent years, such diets became fashionable as a means of weight reduction. Liquid protein was the only source of caloric intake. Between July 1977 and January 1978, at least 60 deaths were reported in users of this diet. In cases clinically evaluated, there was a prolongation of the Q–T interval and frequent episodes of ventricular tachycardia. No specific cause could be found to explain the Q–T prolongation, and the ventricular tachycardia was often refractory to all modalities of therapy. (Isner JM: *Circulation* 1979;**60:** 1401.)

19 | Cardiac Pacing & Defibrillation

Electrical depolarization of the heart is a valuable clinical means of therapy which by now has become commonplace. Its major uses include (1) cardiac pacing for control of rate and rhythm and (2) countershock for correction of an arrhythmia. It is beyond the scope of this text to discuss this field in detail, but it will suffice to outline the indications and techniques and the appearance of the electrocardiographic tracings of the patient before and after electrical depolarization.

Electrical Pacing of the Heart

This is indicated in any situation when an uncontrolled reduction in heart rate diminishes cardiac output sufficiently to result in syncope or other serious symptoms. The prime example is the patient with Stokes-Adams syndrome. Three methods of pacing are the following:

A. External pacing is effective in an emergency situation but becomes ineffective after several hours. It is painful to the conscious patient.

B. Internal pacing with the power source external to the body can be accomplished by inserting an electrode into the heart by way of a neck or arm vein or by direct puncture of the myocardium through the chest wall. These techniques are effective for emergency situations and short-term therapy.

C. Internal pacing with power source implanted in body:

1. Left ventricular epicardial pacemaker–The electrodes are sutured into the myocardium via thoracotomy or a subxiphoid approach. The power source is imbedded in the abdominal wall.

2. Right ventricular endocardial pacemaker–An electrode is introduced into the apex of the right ventricle via an axillary, subclavian, or neck vein, and the power unit is implanted in the pectoral-axillary area. Because of the relative simplicity of the procedure and its efficacy, this type of pacemaker insertion is preferable.

Types of Pacemaker Units

A. **Ventricular Asynchronous Pacemaker:** The pacemaker fires continuously and regularly at a preselected rate. If sinus rhythm and AV conduction are still possible, the ventricles may respond to both the patient's sinus pacemaker and the artificial electri-

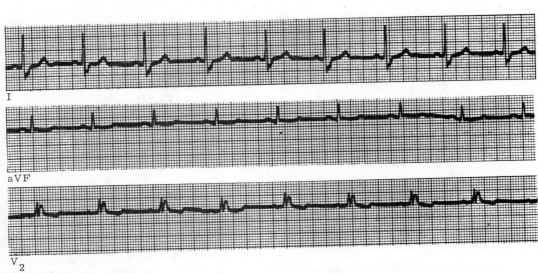

I

aVF

V₂

Figure 19–1. The above ECG is that of a 75-year-old man with repeated episodes of syncope. This tracing reveals a right bundle branch block. The rhythm is normal sinus; the rate = 65. (See Figs 19–2, 19–3, and 19–4.)

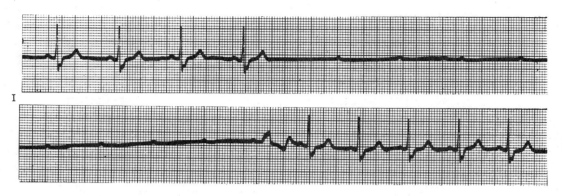

Figure 19–2. The above is a continuous recording of lead I in the same patient as in Fig 19–1. Ventricular asystole (with continuing atrial activity) is present for 8.3 s.

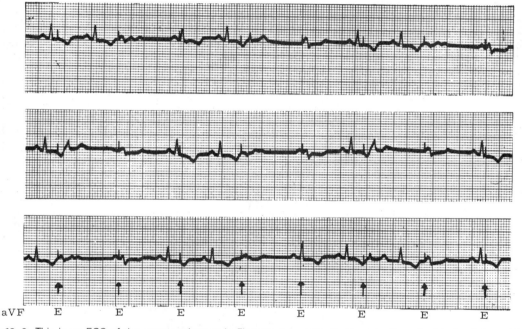

Figure 19–3. This is an ECG of the same patient as in Figs 19–1 and 19–2 after insertion of a bipolar, left ventricular epicardial asynchronous (fixed rate) pacemaker. The electrical pace (E) discharges regularly at a rate of 65. A parasystolic rhythm is present. The ventricle responds to the normal sinus pacemaker or the electrical pacemaker.

cal pacemaker, thereby producing a parasystolic rhythm (see p 268). Also, the electrical pacemaker could discharge during the supernormal period of the heart cycle (see pp 17 and 256) and produce a serious ventricular arrhythmia.

B. Ventricular Demand Pacemaker: Both sensing and firing circuits are present. A spontaneous ventricular depolarization, either sinus-conducted or ectopic in origin, is sensed by the unit and prevents the pacemaker from firing for a preset interval, usually 1 s. Therefore, if the patient's intrinsic heart rate exceeds this value (over 60/min), there will be no pacer discharge. At all other times, the pacemaker functions as a fixed rate unit. This prevents the possibility of competition, ie, iatrogenic parasystole. It is the most popular type of pacemaker in current use. The sensing rate need not be the same as the paced rate. The former can be set at a slower rate (hysteresis) to permit a slower sinus rhythm without pacemaker turnover. This can afford greater patient comfort, but the lengthened hysteresis escape interval may permit the emergence of ventricular ectopy.

One potential hazard exists. An external signal (eg, from a diathermy unit, electric razor, or electronic oven) can inactivate the demand circuitry and lead to asystole in the patient with complete heart block. Cur-

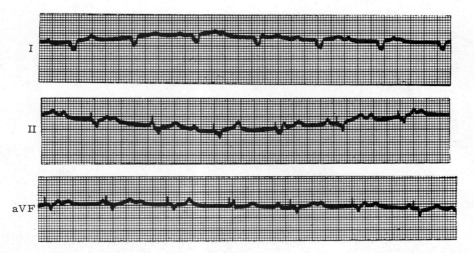

Figure 19–4. This is an ECG of the same patient as in Figs 19–1, 19–2, and 19–3 several weeks later. Ventricular activation is now completely controlled by the pacemaker, which is firing at a rate of 65. Independent atrial activity continues at a rate of 85 but never results in ventricular capture. QS complexes in leads I and aVF indicate that the ventricular activation wave (ie, vector) is oriented toward the right and superiorly owing to the electrode placement in the lower portion of the left ventricle. The small size of the pace artifact is indicative of a bipolar unit.

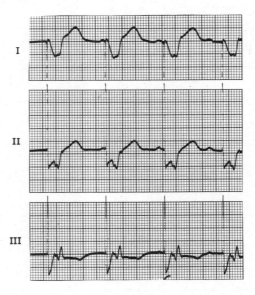

Figure 19–5. Unipolar left ventricular epicardial pacemaker. Very large pace spikes are seen which are the result of a unipolar pacemaker. The spike is negative in lead I (rightward) and positive in leads II and III (inferior). Therefore, if the anode is on the power unit, the unit is to the right and inferior to the heart. The unit was implanted in the right upper abdominal wall. The QRS is negative in lead I (rightward), consistent with a left ventricular epicardial pacemaker. Inverted P waves are seen following the paced QRS complexes, indicating retrograde ventriculoatrial conduction.

rent pacemaker units are so constructed as to eliminate this risk.

Since spontaneous cardiac rhythm at a rate more rapid than that set for the demand unit will inhibit the pacemaker, no pace artifact will be seen in the ECG. Therefore, one cannot tell if the demand unit is functioning normally or if the pacemaker is incapable of assuming its function. Externally applied devices are available to make this determination. An external magnet is placed on the body over the site of the implanted unit. This converts the demand mode into a fixed rate pacemaker. The pace artifact is then seen and will result in ventricular capture whenever the impulse falls in a nonrefractory period. There is always the danger, as with fixed rate pacemakers, that an impulse firing in the supernormal period could set off a serious

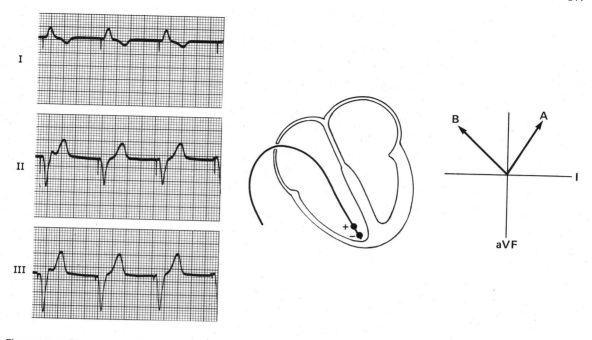

Figure 19–6. Diagrammatic illustration of a bipolar right ventricular endocardial pacemaker located in the proper apical position. The distal pole is the cathode and the proximal pole is the anode. The pace artifact will be small; it will be oriented rightward and superiorly (arrow B), producing small negative spikes in leads I, II, and III. The myocardium is depolarized leftward and superiorly (arrow A), producing upright QRS complexes in lead I and negative complexes in leads II and III.

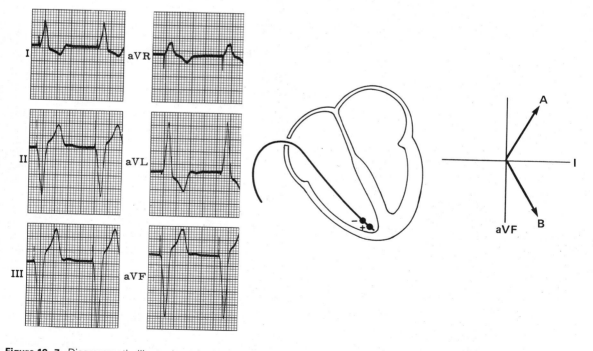

Figure 19–7. Diagrammatic illustration of a bipolar right ventricular endocardial pacemaker located in the proper apical position. The distal pole is the anode and the proximal pole is the cathode. The pace artifact is now oriented leftward and inferiorly (arrow B), resulting in positive spikes in leads I, II, and aVF. The myocardium is depolarized leftward and superiorly (arrow A), producing upright QRS complexes in leads I and aVL and negative complexes in leads II, III, and aVF.

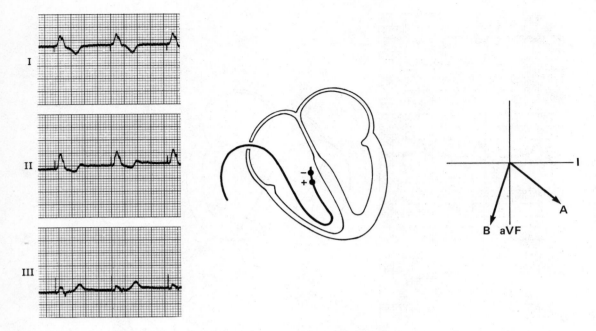

Figure 19–8. Diagrammatic illustration of a bipolar right ventricular endocardial pacemaker which has become dislodged from the apex and is in the right ventricular outflow tract. The distal pole is the cathode. The pace artifact is directed rightward and inferiorly (arrow B), producing a negative spike in lead I and positive spikes in leads II and III. The myocardium is being depolarized to the left and inferiorly (arrow A), resulting in upright QRS complexes in leads I, II, and III.

ventricular arrhythmia. However, this theoretical risk has rarely, if ever, been documented.

The paced rate with the magnet need not be the same as the set spontaneous rate of the pacemaker. Some models produce a more rapid rate. Other models purposely introduce an initial series of rapid paces associated with a progressive reduction in the milliamperage. This serves as a check for the stimulus threshold (Fig 19–18).

C. Ventricular Synchronous Pacemaker: During sinus-conducted rhythm (or other spontaneous rhythm), the pacemaker discharges approximately 0.04–0.08 s after the onset of the QRS complex. Thus, it can be seen in the ECG and indicates pacemaker function but plays no role in ventricular depolarization because the artifact constantly falls in the absolute refractory period of the ventricle. Whenever spontaneous rhythm falls below a preset rate, the pacemaker assumes a fixed rate function.

D. Atrial Synchronous Pacemaker: In the past, this unit required insertion via thoracotomy. Electrodes were sutured into the right atrium and left ventricle. In the presence of sinus rhythm, the P wave is detected by the electronic circuitry and after an interval of 0.16–0.2 s (simulating average P–R intervals) triggers the ventricular pacemaker. Such a unit has the physiologic advantage of permitting atrial contraction to contribute to ventricular filling and allows the ventricular rate to vary with the atrial rate in a more normal fashion. If the sinus rate falls below a certain preset value or if sinus rhythm ceases, the ventricular

pacemaker fires in a fixed rate manner. If atrial tachycardia or atrial flutter develops, the circuitry is designed to permit a certain maximum ventricular rate, usually not to exceed 140/min. Such units are currently available that can be inserted transvenously. One electrode is imbedded in the right atrial appendage and the other into the right ventricular apex (as in any transvenous ventricular pacemaker).

E. Atrial Pacemaker: If the patient's problem requiring pacing is due to SA node or atrial disease and AV nodal and distal His-Purkinje conduction are normal, a transvenously inserted atrial pacemaker is effective. However, since more distal conduction problems may develop thereafter, it is safer to have an additional standby ventricular pacemaker inserted at the same time (modification of D above) (Fig 19–11).

F. Programmable Pacemaker: Advancements in the manufacture of many of the above pulse generator systems permit modifications of many of the functions of the unit by external means, thereby sparing the need for an invasive procedure. Changes can be made in the pacing rate, sensing interval (rate hysteresis), pulse width, amplitude, and milliamperage.

G. Identification Code: The Intersociety Commission for Heart Disease has recommended the following 5-letter code system to identify (1) the chamber paced, (2) the chamber sensed, (3) the mode of pacemaker response, (4) programmable functions, and (5) special tachyarrhythmia functions. (*Circulation* 1981;**64**:60A.)

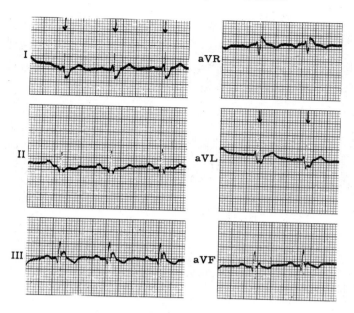

Figure 19–9. Ventricular synchronous pacemaker. The rhythm is regular sinus, rate = 80, P–R = 0.18 s. The QRS morphology indicates a right bundle branch block. A pace artifact is seen within each QRS complex (arrows) occurring 0.07 s after the beginning of each QRS. It represents the firing of the ventricular synchronous unit. The artifact appears during the refractory period of the ventricle and therefore cannot result in ventricular capture. Its only purpose is to indicate that the pacer is functional.

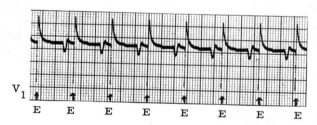

Figure 19–10. Atrial synchronous pacemaker. Regular pacemaker activity (E) is seen at a rate of 79. Each pace artifact follows the onset of the P wave by 0.18 s. The pace is triggered by the P, which in turn activates the ventricles.

1. Chamber paced:
   V = Ventricle.
   A = Atrium.
   D = Atrium and ventricle ("double").
2. Chamber sensed:
   V = Ventricle.
   A = Atrium.
   D = Atrium and ventricle ("double").
   O = None.
3. Mode of response:
   T = Triggered (ventricular synchronous).
   I = Inhibited (ventricle demand).
   D = Double response modes to a sensed signal (atrial triggered and ventricular inhibited).
   O = None.
   R = Reverse function. The pacemaker is silent at slow rates and activated by fast rates.

4. Programmable functions:
   P = Programmable for rate or output (or both).
   M = Multiprogrammable.
   O = None.
5. Special tachyarrhythmia functions:
   O = None.
   B = Bursts of impulses.
   N = Normal rate competition (such as in the dual demand pacemaker).
   S = Scanning response.
   E = External control (activated by magnet or radiofrequency).

The minimum code designation is the first 3 letters. If positions 4 and 5 are O, they need not be indicated.
   Examples:
   VVI: A ventricular pacemaker that senses a spontaneous ventricular depolarization and inhibits the

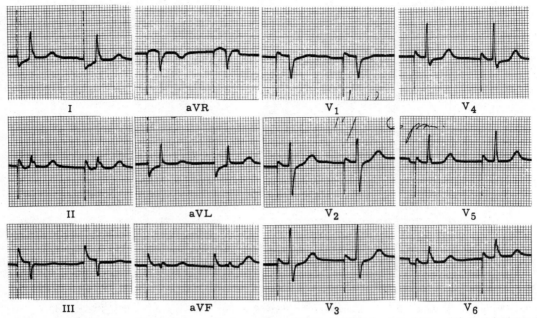

Figure 19–11. Atrial pacemaker. Unipolar pace artifacts are seen with a pace interval = 1.0 s (rate = 60). Each initiates atrial depolarization followed by ventricular depolarization after a P–R interval of 0.18 s. This unit was inserted in a patient with sick sinus syndrome who had normal A–H and H–V intervals.

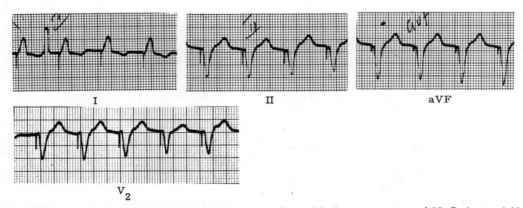

Figure 19–12. Ventricular demand pacemaker. Regular pacemaker activity is seen at a rate of 95. Each pace initiates a ventricular response. The QRS is oriented leftward (upright in I), superiorly (downward in II and aVF), and posteriorly (downward in V_2), indicating an origin in the apex of the right ventricle. This patient had a transvenous demand pacemaker inserted into the right ventricle. From the ECG it would be impossible to differentiate this from an asynchronous pacemaker.

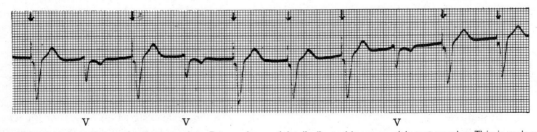

Figure 19–13. Ventricular demand pacemaker. Pacemaker activity (indicated by arrows) is not regular. This is a demand pacemaker which has been set at a rate of 75 (interval = 0.8 s). Spontaneous discharges (V) are occurring 0.76 s after the preceding pace. This inactivates the next pacemaker discharge and therefore does not permit competition between spontaneous and pacemaker activity.

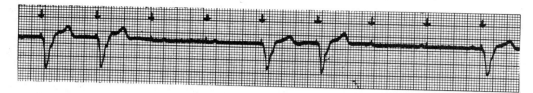

Figure 19–14. Example of pacemaker failure. Regular pacemaker activity (indicated by arrows) is seen at a rate of 73. However, each pace does not produce ventricular activation. The third, fourth, seventh, and eighth paces do not excite the ventricle. In this patient there were also longer periods of ventricular asystole with resulting syncope. This was corrected by replacement of the power unit.

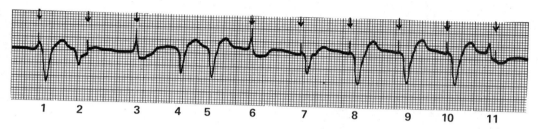

Figure 19–15. Failure of proper ventricular demand pacemaker function. Pacemaker activity is indicated by the arrows. Beats 7, 8, 9, and 10 are initiated by the pacemaker. Beats 4 and 5 are spontaneous discharges which properly prevent the demand pacemaker from firing. However, because of malfunction, beats 1, 2, 3, 6, and 11 do not prevent pacemaker discharge. Such competition could permit pacemaker firing during a vulnerable period (this is approximated in beat 11) and thereby result in a serious ventricular arrhythmia.

pacer for a given preset interval (a ventricular demand pacemaker). The absence of letters in the fourth and fifth positions indicates absence of such functions.

VVIMB: Similar to above (VVI) and is multi-programmable with pacing bursts for tachyarrhythmia.

DVIM: An atrioventricular pacemaker that paces both the atrium and ventricle, is ventricular inhibited, and is multiprogrammable.

DDD: An atrioventricular pacemaker that paces and senses both the atrium and ventricle, is not programmable, and has no special tachyarrhythmia functions.

AOOOE: An atrial pacemaker that is activated only by an externally applied radiofrequency unit.

Unipolar & Bipolar Pacing

All pacemaker units mentioned can function in a unipolar or bipolar manner. The unipolar circuitry consists of the cathode inserted in the myocardium (either right ventricular endocardial or left ventricular epicardial) and the anode at a remote site (usually on the surface of the implanted power unit). The bipolar pacemaker has both the cathode and anode within the heart, usually 1–2 cm apart.

Electrocardiographic Pattern

The ventricular complex (QRS) which results from electric pacing will be wide, slurred, or notched, similar to spontaneous ventricular ectopic beats. Therefore, the recognition of specific disease states by ECG analysis during pacing is usually impossible. However, the ECG is of value in confirming the location of the site of electrode placement and detecting a change in the position of the electrode.

With a left ventricular epicardial pacemaker, the heart will be depolarized from left to right, producing negative QRS complexes in lead I and simulating a right bundle branch block.

With a right ventricular apical endocardial pacemaker, the heart will be depolarized from right to left and from apex to base. The resulting QRS therefore will be oriented to the left and superiorly, producing an upright QRS complex in lead I and mainly negative QRS complexes in leads II, III, and aVF. If the electrode is displaced from the right ventricular apex, it tends to float into the right ventricular outflow tract. In this instance, the heart is still depolarized from right to left but is now depolarized from base to apex. The QRS remains upright in lead I but now becomes upright in leads II, III, and aVF.

A right ventricular apical endocardial demand pacemaker, in association with atrial-conducted beats which have a right bundle branch block pattern, will not sense the latter until the depolarization wave arrives at the right ventricular apical area. This is represented by the R′ wave of the right bundle branch complex. Therefore, the pacer can fire within the rsR′ complex and does not indicate failure of the sensing mechanism (Fig 19–17).

In the interpretation of serial ECGs in patients

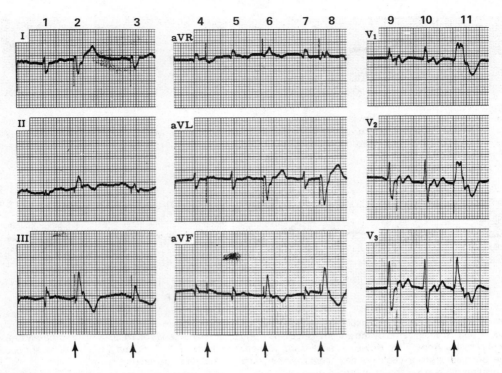

Figure 19–16. Effect of external magnet on demand pacemaker. A transvenous demand pacemaker was inserted in this patient and was thought to be positioned in the apex of the right ventricle. Following insertion, the patient's own intrinsic rate exceeded that which had been set for the pacemaker and therefore no pacemaker artifacts were seen. A magnet was then placed on the chest wall over the implanted unit. This converted the pacemaker into a fixed rate mode. Regular pacemaker spikes (arrows) appear regularly at an interval of 0.86 s (rate = 70). Beats 1, 4, 5, 7, 9, and 10 are the patient's spontaneously conducted beats. These complexes are indicative of inferior wall infarction, incomplete right bundle branch block, and left posterior fascicular block. Beats 2, 3, 6, 8, and 11 are pacemaker captures. The QRS complexes resemble a right bundle branch block and left posterior fascicular block. This would be expected if the pacemaker were in the left ventricle but should not result from a right ventricular pacemaker. Fluoroscopy proved that the pacemaker wire had inadvertently been passed into the coronary sinus and peripherally into a distal coronary vein which overlay the epicardial surface of the left ventricle and therefore was functioning as a left ventricular epicardial pacemaker.

with functioning pacemakers, it is essential to accurately measure the pacemaker rate. Any change in rate should alert the physician to early battery failure.

When pacing in a patient with a right ventricular endocardial pacemaker is either purposely discontinued or overridden by a more rapid spontaneous rhythm, the ECG will commonly show T wave inversions that were not present in the record obtained before insertion of the pacemaker. These inversions do not prove the presence of new myocardial disease, however, since such abnormalities have been documented in normal individuals. These findings are analogous to similar changes that occur following (1) reversion of paroxysmal supraventricular tachycardia or (2) spontaneous reversion of left bundle branch block to normal intraventricular conduction.

The distance between cathode and anode in a bipolar unit is short, whereas this distance in a unipolar unit is relatively long. Therefore the magnitude of the pacemaker artifact in the ECG will be relatively small with a bipolar unit and quite large with a unipolar unit.

The spatial orientation of the pace artifact can be determined and is of clinical significance in detecting a change in pacemaker position. This is especially applicable to a bipolar right ventricular endocardial pacemaker. The cathode is usually distal to the anode, and, as a result of its position in the right ventricular apex, the electric artifact will be oriented to the right and superiorly, producing negative artifacts in leads I, II, and aVF. If the electrode becomes detached and floats into the right ventricular outflow tract, the artifact vector will be directed inferiorly, producing upright signals in II, III, and aVF. The anode-cathode relation in the right ventricular pacemaker may be reversed, ie, the distal pole is the anode. In this instance, the pace artifact with the pacer in the right ventricular apex will be oriented to the left and inferiorly, producing upright signals in leads I, II, and aVF.

Ventricular pacing has been used successfully to prevent recurrent ventricular tachycardia and ventricular fibrillation when anti-arrhythmia drug therapy has failed. This is of value even in the absence of as-

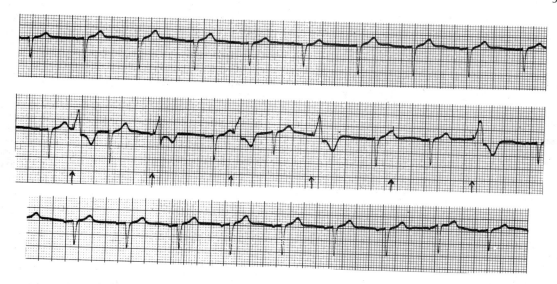

Figure 19–17. Effect of external magnet on demand pacemaker. This is a continuous recording of lead V$_1$. The upper and lower strips indicate regular sinus rhythm, rate = 72. A left ventricular demand pacemaker had been inserted but is being suppressed in a normal fashion by the more rapid intrinsic rhythm. In the middle strip an external magnet has been placed over the implanted power unit. The pacemaker now functions in a fixed rate (50/min), asynchronous mode. The first 4 and the sixth paces result in ventricular capture. The fifth is occurring on the summit of the T wave of the sinus beat and does not activate the ventricle.

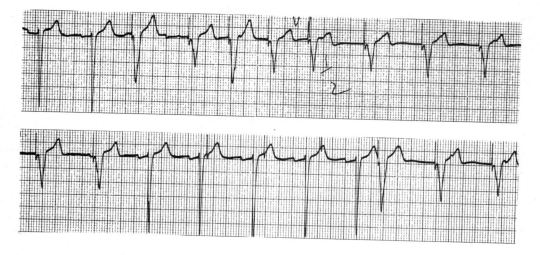

Figure 19–18. Effect of magnet on a demand ventricular pacemaker (continuous recording of lead V$_1$). The first 2 complexes are sinus-conducted with an R–R interval = 0.8 s. The magnet then converts the demand unit, which was being overridden by the more rapid sinus-conducted rhythm, into a fixed rate mode. The first 2 paced spikes appear at an interval = 0.86 s. The next 3 paces appear at intervals = 0.6 s, and all result in ventricular capture. This unit is purposely programmed to do so in order to test threshold response with progressive reduction in the milliamperage. The pace interval then returns to 0.86 s and competes with the sinus rhythm for ventricular capture.

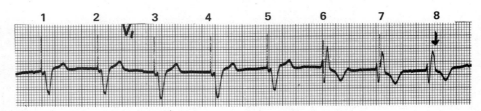

Figure 19–19. Right ventricular demand pacemaker in the presence of spontaneously conducted beats with right bundle branch block. Beats 1, 2, 3, 4, and 5 are pacer-induced. Beats 6, 7, and 8 are atrial-conducted with right bundle branch block. The pace artifact is seen within the rsR' complex of beats 6 and 7 because the depolarization wave has not reached the right ventricular apex and is not sensed. The R' of beat 8 is recorded before the next pacing spike is due (arrow), is appropriately sensed, and therefore does not fire.

sociated heart block. The rationale of pacing is as follows: Prolonged ventricular repolarization can result in ventricular arrhythmias (see Chapter 14), especially if repolarization is asynchronous in areas of the myocardium, leading to local potentials with resulting ectopic discharge. By pacing the heart at rates of 120–150, ventricular repolarization may become synchronous throughout the entire myocardium, thereby eliminating local potentials and the resulting arrhythmia. This type of pacing is known as "overdriving." In the treatment of refractory ventricular tachycardia, ventricular pacing at rates slower than the tachycardia ("underdrive pacing") may abolish the arrhythmia by interrupting the reentry circuit that causes the tachycardia.

Intermittent atrial pacing has been successful in the treatment of paroxysmal atrial tachycardia and flutter. Atrial impulses are introduced at a rate of 300–400/min. Within seconds, one of these impulses will interrupt the reentry pathway of the tachycardia, permitting reversion to sinus rhythm. When clinically indicated, such a unit can be implanted surgically and activated when needed by placement of a radiofrequency transmitter over the implanted unit.

Atrial Mechanism During Ventricular Pacing

Various atrial rhythms are present during continuous ventricular pacing: (1) Regular sinus rhythm with complete atrioventricular dissociation. This can result in a reduction in ventricular filling and cardiac output due to asynchrony of atrial and ventricular contractions. It is especially evident when the sinus and ventricular paced rates are fortuitously the same and the sinus P wave occurs immediately after the paced QRS complex. When clinically significant, it may be partially corrected by changing the rate of the ventricular pacemaker or completely corrected by use of an atrioventricular sequential pacemaker. (2) Independent atrial fibrillation, flutter, or tachycardia. (3) Retrograde ventriculoatrial conduction, in which the atria are activated in a retrograde direction from the

ventricular pacemaker and will be evidenced by inverted P waves in leads II, III, and aVF, which immediately follow the paced QRS complex (Fig 19–5). This can result in a significant increase in left atrial and pulmonary capillary pressures, with resultant pulmonary edema, and is known as the pacemaker syndrome. It may be partially corrected by altering the rate or output of the ventricular pacemaker or completely corrected by use of an atrioventricular sequential pacemaker.

Electrical Countershock

An electrical charge can be introduced into the myocardium which is sufficient to depolarize the entire heart and permit the normal cardiac rhythm to be reestablished. This countershock is usually delivered externally, but it can be applied internally during intrathoracic surgery. Its major lifesaving function is in the elimination of ventricular fibrillation as part of the resuscitation therapy of cardiac arrest. It is also of great value in the treatment of ventricular tachycardia. When clinical judgment indicates the need for reversion of atrial flutter or atrial fibrillation, countershock may be preferable to drug therapy. Two types of units for the administration of countershock follow:

(1) The AC defibrillator introduces a charge for approximately 0.25 s. Because of this relatively long duration, the charge could fall within the supernormal phase of excitability in any rhythm other than ventricular fibrillation and thereby produce a serious ventricular arrhythmia, eg, fibrillation.

(2) The DC defibrillator introduces a charge for 0.0025 s. Most units are now coupled with a synchronizing device that prevents discharge in the critical phase of the heart cycle and thus largely eliminates the danger of producing a more serious arrhythmia.

Caution must be used in countershock therapy for elective reversion of arrhythmias (ie, atrial) in patients who are receiving digitalis, since serious ventricular arrhythmias can follow its use.

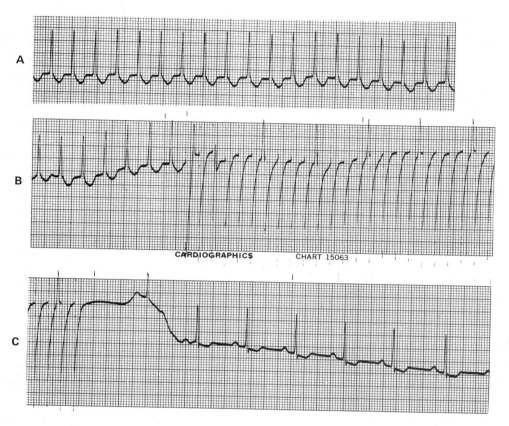

Figure 19–20. Reversion of paroxysmal atrial tachycardia by atrial pacing. This is a continuous recording of lead II. *A:* Atrial tachycardia, rate = 187. *B:* A previously implanted right atrial pacemaker is activated by an external radiofrequency transmitter. This introduces stimuli into the right atrium at a rate of 300/min, which interrupts the reentry pathway and results in reversion to sinus rhythm, *C.*

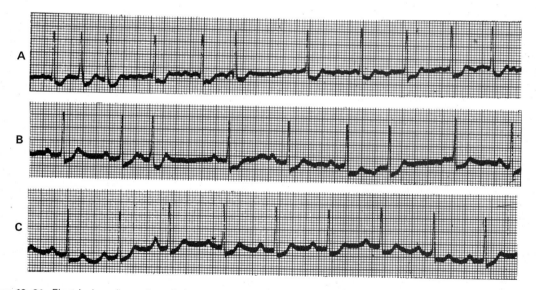

Figure 19–21. Electrical cardioversion of chronic atrial fibrillation in a patient with mitral stenosis. This is a continuous recording of lead II. *A:* Immediately prior to cardioversion. The rhythm is atrial fibrillation. Digitalis therapy had been purposely withheld for 3 days. *B:* Immediately after delivery of a 200 watt-second charge from a synchronized DC defibrillator. *C:* Five minutes later. (B) and (C) indicate reversion to sinus rhythm, with occasional atrial premature beats.

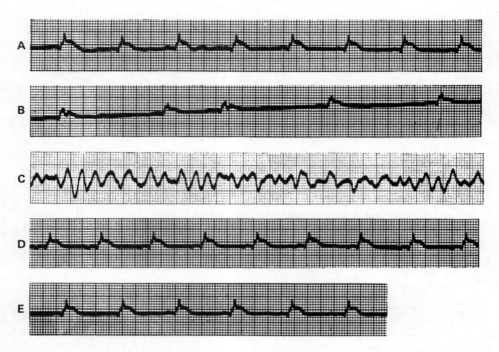

Figure 19–22. Therapy of ventricular fibrillation. The above are selected strips of lead II taken during constant oscilloscopic monitoring of a patient with acute myocardial infarction. *A:* Vital signs stable; sinus rhythm, rate = 72; small q and marked ST elevation indicate recent infarction. *B:* One minute after (A). The blood pressure has fallen; the ventricular rhythm has become irregular and slower; atrial activity cannot be identified. *C:* One minute after (B). Cardiac arrest has occurred; ventricular fibrillation is present. Immediate measures for cardiac resuscitation are instituted (cardiac compression, ventilation, and intravenous sodium bicarbonate). A DC countershock of 400 watt-seconds is given. (This is not recorded on the ECG.) *D:* Fifteen seconds after defibrillation. A regular ventricular rhythm has been restored; the rate = 78; QRS–T complexes are similar to (A). The P waves are inverted, indicating a low atrial or AV junctional pacemaker. *E:* Two minutes after (D). Reversion to sinus rhythm. Following this, the patient made an uneventful recovery.

Vectorcardiography and electrocardiography must not be considered different sciences. They are both methods of recording the varying electrical potentials that result during the cardiac cycle. With the use of cathode ray oscilloscopes, the spatial vectorcardiogram can be recorded stereoscopically or in its projection in the frontal, sagittal, and horizontal planes. Whereas any electrocardiographic lead records the electrical potentials (ie, the instantaneous vectors) in one single axis (see p 30), a loop recording (ie, vectorcardiogram) records the same electrical events simultaneously in 2 perpendicular axes. The frontal plane loop records simultaneous events in the right-to-left (X) axis and the head-to-foot (Y) axis. The sagittal plane loop records simultaneous events in the head-to-foot (Y) axis and the anteroposterior (Z) axis. The horizontal plane loop records simultaneous events in

the right-to-left (X) axis and the anteroposterior (Z) axis.

In a simplified fashion, the derivation of the spatial vectorcardiogram can be illustrated by the following diagrams. (The propagation of the electrical impulse through the ventricular myocardium has been described on p 38.)

The major problem in electrocardiography and vectorcardiography is to determine the most accurate method by which the electrical potentials of the heart (ie, the cardiac vector) can be recorded from the surface of the body. Vector analysis, based initially on the Einthoven triangle and modified to include unipolar electrocardiography (see p 30), is based on the following hypotheses: (1) The heart "generator" acts as a dipole; (2) this generator is centrally located in the chest; (3) the standard leads (I, II, and III) are all

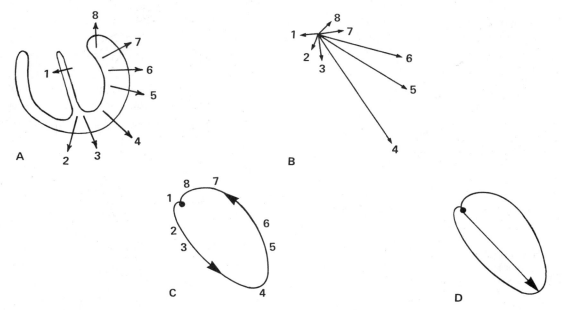

Figure 20-1. The derivation of the spatial vectorcardiogram. *A:* The initial vector (1) is the septal activation from left to right. Next (2) is the activation of the anteroseptal region of the myocardium. Then follows the activation of the remainder of the myocardium (3 –8). *B:* By connecting all the vectors to one starting point the diagram above can be constructed. *C:* A loop can now be drawn connecting the tips of all the vectors. This represents the vectorcardiogram in the frontal plane. *D:* The average direction and magnitude of all the instantaneous QRS vectors is the mean QRS vector. The maximal QRS vector is drawn from the starting point to the farthest point of the loop.

equidistant from the center of the heart generator; (4) the shape of the human torso can be assumed to be a sphere; and (5) all body tissues are homogeneous electrical conductors. At the present time the dipole hypothesis is accepted, at least as a means of explaining 95% of the electrical potentials of atrial and ventricular depolarization as recorded from the body surface, and all advances now being made in modern vectorcardiography are based on acceptance of the dipole hypothesis. However, it is now known that the other hypotheses listed above are unwarranted: The origin of electrical activity is not centrally located in the chest, the standard and unipolar leads are not all equidistant from the center of electrical activity, the human torso is by no means a perfect sphere, and all body tissues are not equally good conductors. If all this were true, electrocardiographic recording would be simple: Lead I would represent the horizontal axis (right-to-left axis or X axis); VF would represent the long axis (head-to-foot axis or Y axis); and V_2 would approximate the transverse axis (anteroposterior axis, or Z axis).

The diagrams below show X, Y, and Z axes in a theoretically perfect sphere, homogeneous in conductivity with the origin of electrical activity in the center of the sphere.

Primarily as a result of the interdisciplinary cooperation of physiologists, physicists, mathematicians, electrical engineers, and physicians in electrocardiographic research, electronic techniques and equipment have been devised in an attempt to compensate for the errors in these hypotheses. The result has been the development of the *"corrected" orthogonal lead systems* of which the systems of Frank and Schmitt are most popular at the present time.

The vectorcardiograms to be illustrated in this chapter have been recorded with the Frank system. The anterior pole of the Z axis is positive to conform with conventional unipolar precordial leads. Although it is felt by many that the Schmitt system is slightly superior, the Frank system has the advantage of being easier to use on a patient since it requires fewer electrodes.

One result of the greater mathematical accuracy of a corrected orthogonal lead system is that it is necessary to modify the space relationships of the axes of the frontal plane electrocardiographic leads to conform to the corrected lead system. For the Frank system, the frontal planes can be illustrated in the following diagrams: (The necessary corrections for the horizontal plane remain to be accurately described in a similar fashion.)

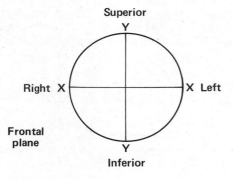

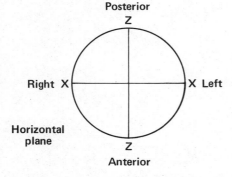

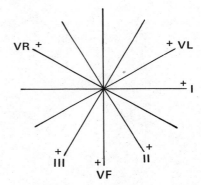

Figure 20–2. Hexaxial reference system used in conventional electrocardiography.

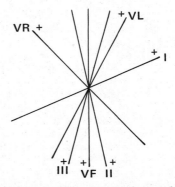

Figure 20–3. Corrected reference lead system for the Frank technique.

The tetrahedron vector system utilizes the standard leads with a fourth lead placed on the back; the cube vector system utilizes 4 different electrode positions. However, neither of these systems offers major revisions of the invalidated hypotheses discussed above and so neither is mathematically accurate.

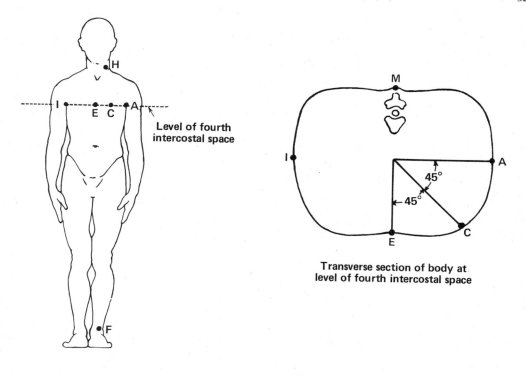

Level of fourth intercostal space

Transverse section of body at level of fourth intercostal space

Figure 20–4. Electrode positions for the Frank system.

Technique of the Frank System

Seven electrodes, designated as H, F, I, E, C, A, and M are applied to the body at the following locations:

H: Forehead or neck.

F: Left leg.

I, E, C, A, and M are located along the same transverse level: the fourth intercostal space if the patient is supine; the fifth intercostal space if the patient is sitting.

I: Right anterior axillary line.

E: Center of sternum.

A: Left anterior axillary line.

C: At a 45-degree angle between E and A.

M: Center of spine.

For detailed information on the electronic circuitry and resistance networks of this system, the reader is referred to Frank's original articles.

The beam visualized on the oscilloscope screen is interrupted by an electrical tuning fork at a fixed rate of 500 cps. This produces a series of dashes, each representing 2 ms (0.002 s). Each dash is comma-shaped, the head or tail (depending on the design of the machine) indicating the direction in which the beam is traveling. The direction of inscription of the loop is described as either clockwise or counterclockwise in the usual meaning of these terms. (This description is not to be confused with the electrocardiographic terminology used in reference to rotation on the long axis. See p 59.)

The Value of Spatial Vectorcardiography in Clinical Medicine

At present, spatial vectorcardiography is used only in medical centers and by specialty medical groups. For routine clinical practice its value is limited (1) because of the expense of the equipment and the time involved; (2) because definite standards for the normal and abnormal vectors are only now being established; and (3) because no complete uniformity of opinion exists as to the best lead system to be used.

Vectorcardiography is of little value in the recording of arrhythmias unless moving photographic equipment is used or independent scalar X, Y, and Z leads are recorded. It is of distinct value in the study and diagnosis of the hypertrophies, bundle branch blocks, and myocardial infarction.

Vectorcardiography serves its most useful purpose in the teaching and understanding of electrocardiography.

Utilizing a corrected orthogonal lead system, such as the Frank system, computer programs have been developed for vectorcardiographic interpretation. Extensive spatial measurements that are impossible for the human to perform can be made by a computer. The analysis is accomplished within seconds. Physician time is spared and human error is avoided. Of greater importance is the fact that computer analysis has resulted in a greater degree of accuracy than has resulted from human interpretation (see bibliography at end of book). It is to be expected that computer analysis will replace physician interpretation in the near future.

This chapter has been entitled "An Introduction to Spatial Vectorcardiography" because it is beyond the scope of this text to present the many theoretical, mathematical, and electrophysical principles involved. The limited discussion offered here is intended only to give the beginner an insight into the subject and its present place in the field of clinical medicine.

ORIENTATION OF THE VECTORCARDIOGRAPHIC ILLUSTRATIONS

The vectorcardiographic illustrations, as recorded in the frontal, sagittal, and horizontal planes, are oriented in space as shown in the following diagrams:

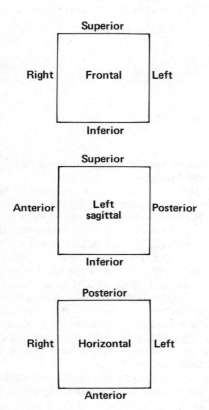

Thus, right-to-left movement is seen in the frontal and horizontal views; superior-inferior movement is seen in the frontal and sagittal views; and anteroposterior movement is seen in the sagittal and horizontal views.

If accurate records are obtained, only 2 views are necessary (eg, frontal and horizontal) to envision the spatial orientation. However, the third view is of value in checking the accuracy of the other 2 views.

The direction of the vector is defined by the angle it forms with an imaginary 360-degree circle surrounding each projection. The left sagittal rather than the right sagittal view was selected by the Committee on Electrocardiography of the American Heart Association. This explains the discrepancy in the degree markings of the sagittal in comparison with the frontal and horizontal views.

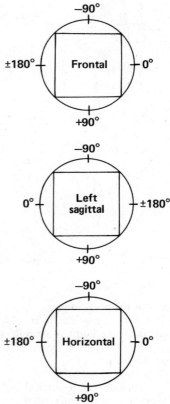

THE NORMAL ADULT SPATIAL VECTORCARDIOGRAM

Each spatial vectorcardiogram consists of 3 loops:

A. The P Loop: Depolarization of the atria produces a small initial loop, the P vector. It is oriented inferiorly, to the left, and slightly anteriorly.

B. The QRS Loop: Depolarization of the ventricles produces the large QRS vector loop. Most of the studies in spatial vectorcardiography to date have been devoted to this vector. The normal spatial orientation of the mean QRS vector in the adult is to the left, inferiorly, and posteriorly.

1. Frontal plane–A small initial deflection may be seen extending to the right and occasionally superiorly. The major portion of the loop is oriented downward and to the left in the 0–85 degree range. The loop may be inscribed in either a clockwise or counterclockwise direction or may be a "figure-of-eight."

2. Left sagittal plane–A small initial deflection appears anteriorly and occasionally superiorly, with the major portion of the loop extending inferiorly and posteriorly. The normal QRS loop is always inscribed in a counterclockwise direction.

3. Horizontal plane–An initial small deflection is inscribed anteriorly and to the right. The major portion of the loop extends to the left and posteriorly. The normal loop is always inscribed in a counterclockwise direction.

C. The T Loop: Repolarization of the ventricles produces a small final loop, the T vector. It is usually larger than the P loop but is considerably smaller than the QRS loop. The normal T vector is usually slightly anterior, inferior, and to the right of the QRS vector by 0–40 degrees.

The periods in the cardiac cycle during which there is no electrical activity (corresponding to the isoelectric P–R, S–T, and T–P intervals of the ECG) will not be evident in the stationary record of the spatial vectorcardiogram.

SEQUENCE DIAGRAM SHOWING CORRELATION OF THE NORMAL ADULT SPATIAL VECTORCARDIOGRAM & THE RESULTING ELECTROCARDIOGRAM*

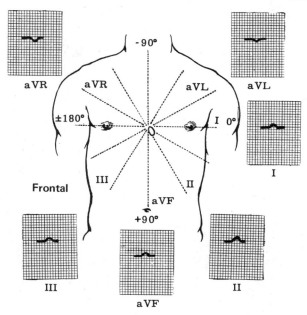

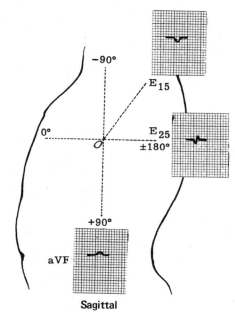

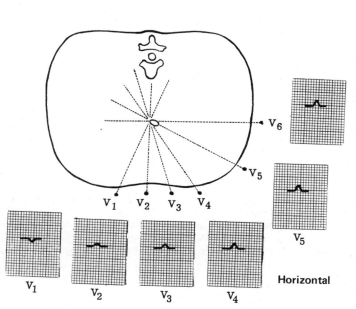

Figure 20–5. Correlation of P loop and P wave. The P loop: This is produced by atrial depolarization. Since the spread of excitation in the atria is in a head-to-foot direction (Fig 5–16), the vector is directed inferiorly. It is also oriented to the left and anteriorly.

*The conventional hexaxial reference system is being diagrammed with the realization that it is inaccurate for a corrected orthogonal lead system. However, because it is simpler to understand and is more conventionally used, it seems preferable in an introductory discussion of spatial vectorcardiography.

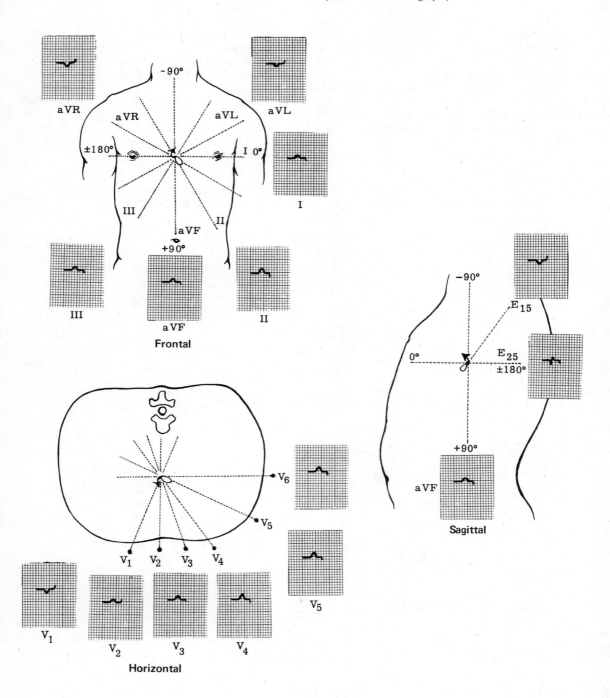

Figure 20–6. Correlation of initial septal depolarization. Ventricular depolarization: Initial spatial QRS loop. Initial septal depolarization results in a QRS vector that is oriented to the right and anteriorly (Fig 5–18). The early activation of the anteroseptal region of the myocardium (Fig 5–19) contributes to the initial right and anterior force. This initial force may be directed superiorly or inferiorly. It is more commonly inferior when the mean frontal plane QRS axis is horizontal and may be superior with a vertically directed mean frontal plane QRS axis. The duration of a normal initial superior vector never exceeds 0.025 s.

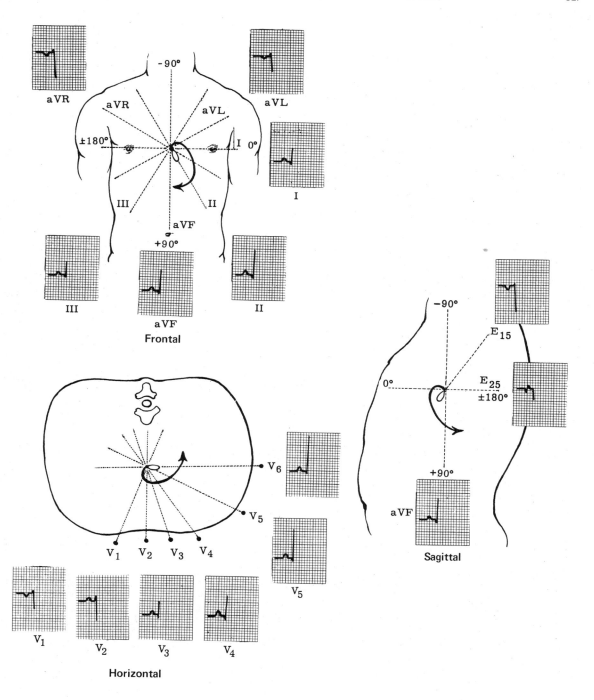

Figure 20–7. Correlation of major ventricular depolarization. Ventricular depolarization: Major activation of the left and right ventricles. Since the major electromotive forces are generated in the larger muscle mass of the left ventricle (Fig 5–20), the major portion of the QRS vector is directed to the left, inferiorly, and posteriorly.

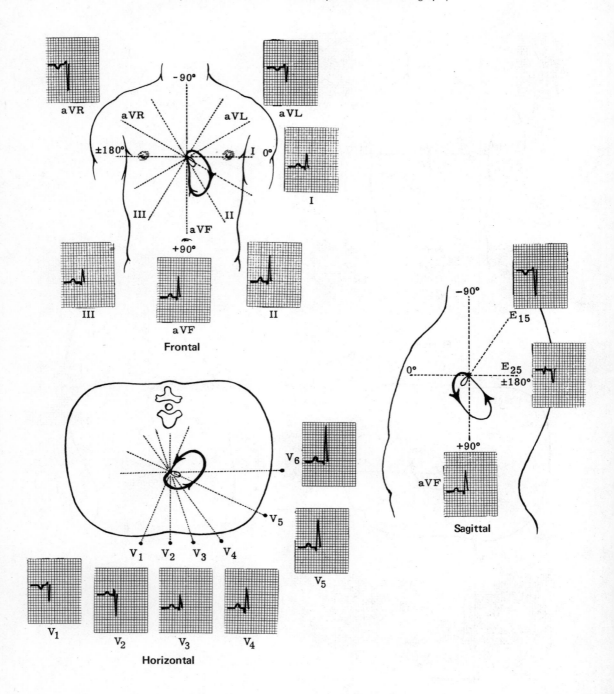

Figure 20–8. Correlation of completion of ventricular depolarization. Ventricular depolarization: Completion of ventricular depolarization. The loop returns to the center point. It is usually inscribed in a clockwise direction in the frontal plane when the mean frontal plane QRS axis is vertical (as in the above illustration) and is counterclockwise with horizontal mean frontal plane QRS axes; counterclockwise in the sagittal plane, and counterclockwise in the horizontal plane. The direction of inscription in the sagittal and horizontal planes is an absolute feature of the normal QRS loop. ¶In this illustration the mean QRS vector is approximately +80 degrees in the frontal plane, +110 degrees in the sagittal plane, and −20 degrees in the horizontal plane.

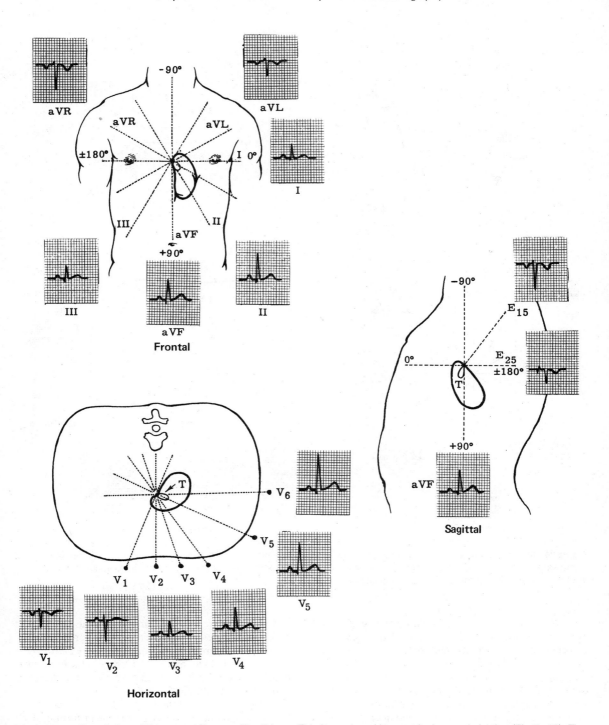

Figure 20–9. Correlation of T loop and T wave. The T loop: This is produced by ventricular repolarization (Fig 5–22). The mean T vector is oriented to the left, inferiorly, and anteriorly. The angle between the mean QRS vector and the mean T vector should not exceed 40 degrees in the frontal plane and 90 degrees in the horizontal plane. (The P loops are not illustrated.)

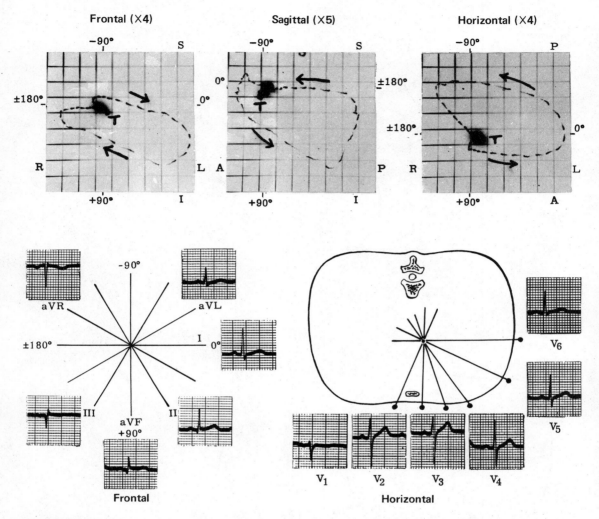

Figure 20–10. Normal adult vectorcardiogram. S = superior; I = inferior; R = right; L = left; A = anterior; P = posterior. The symbols (×2), (×2.8), (×4), (×5), and (×8) in this and subsequent illustrations indicate the photographic magnification of the vector loop, (×8) being the greatest magnification.

The P loop is not readily identified since it is small and buried in the larger T loop. The initial QRS vector is oriented to the right (see frontal and horizontal views), anteriorly (see sagittal and horizontal views), and superiorly (see frontal and sagittal views). The major portion of the QRS loop is then inscribed inferiorly (frontal and sagittal), to the left (frontal and horizontal), and at first anteriorly and later posteriorly (sagittal and horizontal). The last portion of the QRS vector is oriented to the right (frontal and horizontal) and posteriorly (sagittal and horizontal). The loop is inscribed in a clockwise direction in the frontal plane

and in a counterclockwise direction in the sagittal and horizontal planes. The major QRS vector is approximately +40 degrees in the frontal plane, +120 degrees in the sagittal plane, and −20 degrees in the horizontal plane. The T loop is oriented to the left and inferiorly and anterior to the QRS loop.

The ECG is within normal limits. There is no abnormal axis deviation since the mean frontal plane QRS vector is +15 degrees; the heart position is intermediate. The small s waves in leads I and aVL and the small r' wave in aVR are due to the late right orientation of the QRS vector.

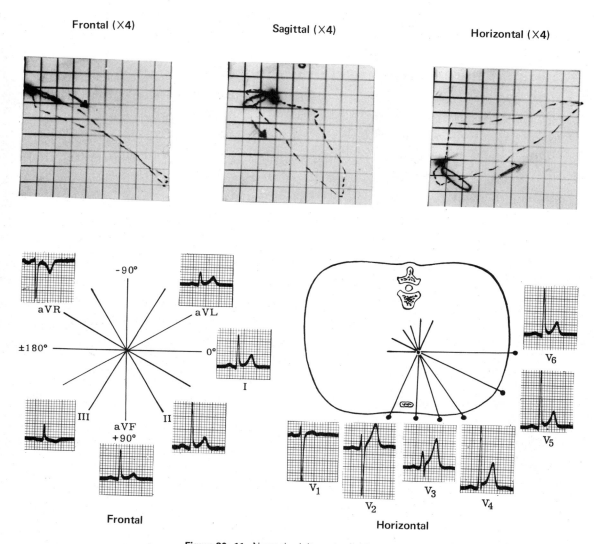

Figure 20–11. Normal adult vectorcardiogram.

The P loop is best seen in the frontal plane as a small loop oriented inferiorly and to the left. The initial QRS vector is oriented to the right and anteriorly (see horizontal view) and slightly superiorly (see sagittal view). The main portion of the QRS is oriented left and inferiorly (see frontal view) and initially anteriorly and then mainly posteriorly (see horizontal view). The end of the QRS does not return to the beginning point (see horizontal view), but ends to the left and anterior of the beginning point, resulting in an ST vector oriented to the left and anteriorly. The T loop is oriented to the left and inferiorly, in the same direction as the mean QRS in the frontal plane, but normally anterior to the QRS (see sagittal and horizontal views).

The ECG is within normal limits. There is ST segment elevation in leads I, II, and V_{3-6}. This is the scalar representation of the ST vector described above. It is a normal variant resulting from early repolarization in this clinically normal 22-year-old man (see p 82).

LEFT VENTRICULAR HYPERTROPHY

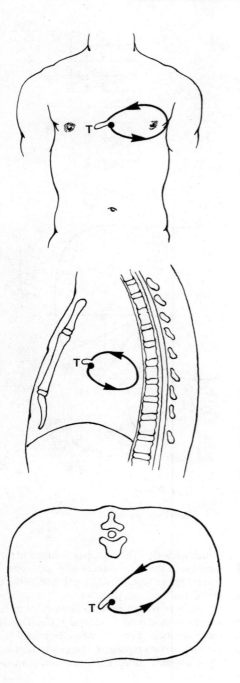

Frontal

There is the normal initial orientation of the QRS loop to the right. The major portion of the loop is then oriented to the left and is usually inscribed in a counterclockwise direction. There may be superior orientation of the loop, resulting in a mean QRS angle of −30 degrees or more. The QRS loop may fail to close (ie, return to the center point before inscription of the T loop), thus explaining the ST segment change seen in the ECG. The ST and T vectors are opposite the mean QRS vector.

Sagittal

The QRS loop is inscribed in a normal counterclockwise direction. There is a small initial anterior deflection; then the major portion of the QRS loop is oriented posteriorly and, at times, superiorly. The QRS loop fails to close, and the ST and T vectors are opposite the mean QRS vector.

Horizontal

The QRS loop is inscribed in the normal counterclockwise direction. There is the normal initial deflection to the right and anteriorly. The major portion of the loop is oriented to the left and posteriorly, the mean axis being posterior, usually in the −30 to −60 degree range. The QRS loop may fail to close, and the ST and T vectors are opposite the mean QRS vector.

In approximately 10% of patients with left ventricular hypertrophy (usually severe), there will be a marked reduction or loss of the normal left and anterior forces, simulating anterior wall infarction. The counterpart in the ECG is the finding of QS complexes in V_{1-3} (or V_{1-4}). (See p 190.)

Typical Features

The major abnormality of the QRS vector is an increase in magnitude (voltage). The QRS loop is inscribed in a normal direction but is oriented more posteriorly than normal and occasionally is oriented superiorly. The horizontal plane loop may inscribe a "figure-of-eight" instead of an entirely counterclockwise loop. The ST and T vectors are opposite the mean QRS vector. (The P loops are not illustrated.)

Figure 20–12. Vector loops in left ventricular hypertrophy.

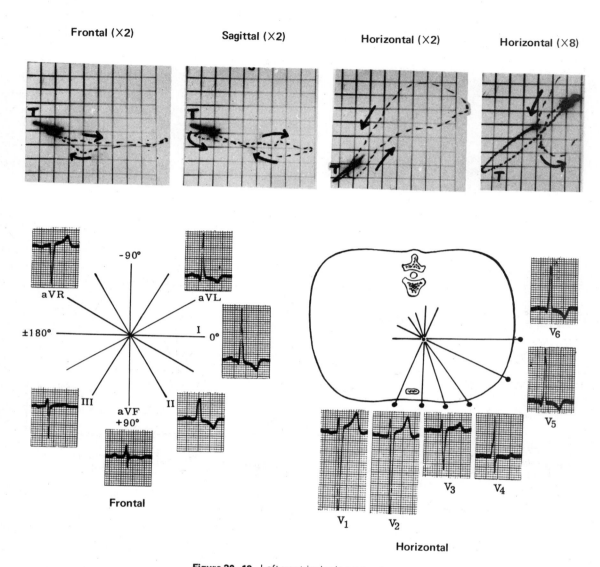

Figure 20–13. Left ventricular hypertrophy.

The initial portion of the QRS vector is normally oriented to the right, anteriorly, and slightly inferiorly. The major portion of the QRS loop is oriented to the left and posteriorly. The magnitude is greater than normal as indicated by the large size of the loops in a ×2 magnification. The QRS loop is inscribed in a clockwise direction in the frontal plane, in a "figure-of-eight" in the sagittal plane, and in the normal counterclockwise direction in the horizontal plane. The terminus of the QRS loop fails to return to the zero point before the T loop is inscribed (best seen in horizontal ×8). This results in an open ST vector that is oriented to the right and anteriorly. The T loop is oriented to the right, anteriorly, and slightly superiorly.

The ECG reveals a typical pattern of left ventricular hypertrophy. The frontal plane axis = 0 degrees; the heart position is horizontal. The QRS interval = 0.1 s; VAT = 0.07 s; the R in aVL = 19 mm; and there is ST depression and T wave inversion in leads I, aVL, aVF, and V_{5-6}.

Clinical and autopsy diagnosis: Rheumatic heart disease with aortic incompetency.

Frontal (×4)   **Sagittal (×5)**   **Horizontal (×4)**   **Horizontal (×8)**

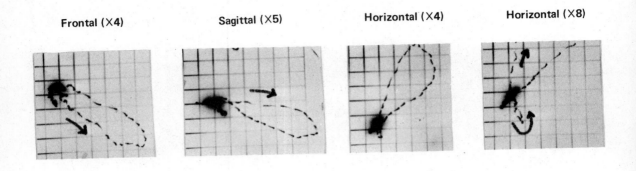

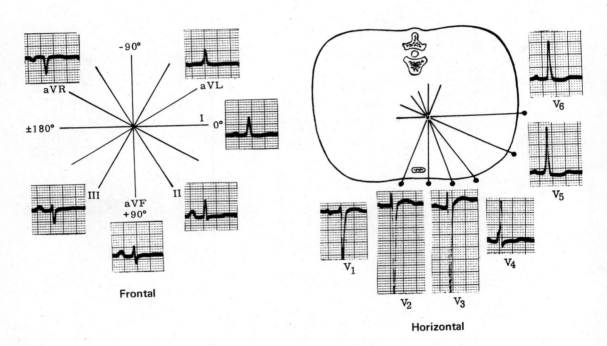

Figure 20-14. Left ventricular hypertrophy.

The initial portion of the QRS is oriented to the left, inferiorly, and anteriorly. The major portion of the QRS is oriented to the left and posteriorly and is inscribed in an abnormal clockwise direction in the horizontal plane. This is not an uncommon finding in the advanced stages of left ventricular hypertrophy. The T loop is oriented to the right and anteriorly.

The ECG reveals a first degree AV block (P–R interval = 0.24 s). $SV_1 + RV_5 = 37$ mm; there is slurring of the R waves, the ST segments are depressed, and the T waves flattened in left precordial leads.

Clinical and autopsy diagnosis: Hypertensive cardiovascular disease; left ventricular hypertrophy.

LEFT BUNDLE BRANCH BLOCK

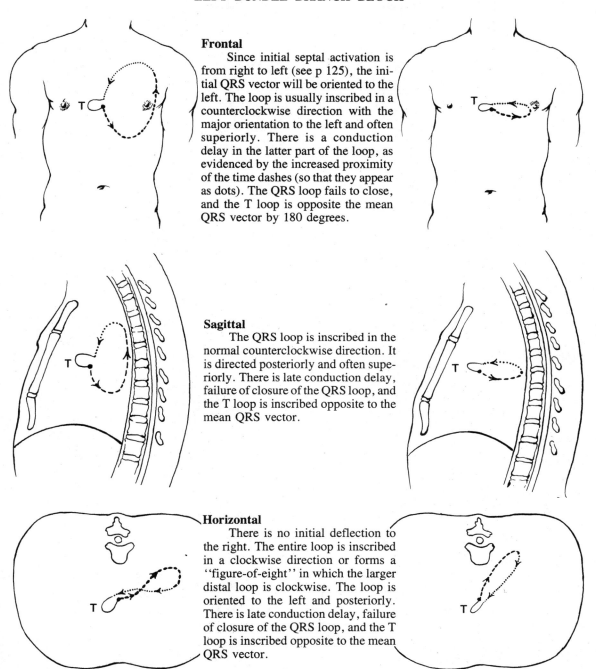

Frontal

Since initial septal activation is from right to left (see p 125), the initial QRS vector will be oriented to the left. The loop is usually inscribed in a counterclockwise direction with the major orientation to the left and often superiorly. There is a conduction delay in the latter part of the loop, as evidenced by the increased proximity of the time dashes (so that they appear as dots). The QRS loop fails to close, and the T loop is opposite the mean QRS vector by 180 degrees.

Sagittal

The QRS loop is inscribed in the normal counterclockwise direction. It is directed posteriorly and often superiorly. There is late conduction delay, failure of closure of the QRS loop, and the T loop is inscribed opposite to the mean QRS vector.

Horizontal

There is no initial deflection to the right. The entire loop is inscribed in a clockwise direction or forms a "figure-of-eight" in which the larger distal loop is clockwise. The loop is oriented to the left and posteriorly. There is late conduction delay, failure of closure of the QRS loop, and the T loop is inscribed opposite to the mean QRS vector.

Typical Features

The QRS loop is oriented to the left and posteriorly; the normal initial orientation to the right does not occur; the entire loop in the horizontal plane is inscribed in a clockwise direction or forms a "figure-of-eight" in which the distal loop is clockwise. There is evidence of conduction delay in the latter portion of the loop, as evidenced by increased proximity of the time markings. The QRS loops fail to close, and the T loops are opposite the mean QRS vector. (The P loops are not illustrated.)

Figure 20–15. Vector loops in left bundle branch block.

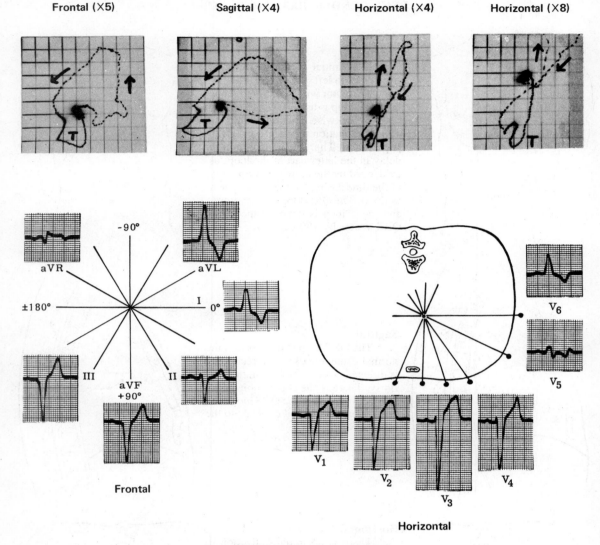

Figure 20–16. Left bundle branch block.

There is no initial deflection of the QRS loop to the right. The major portion of the QRS loop is directed superiorly, to the left, and posteriorly. There is increased proximity of the time markings in the latter portion of the loop. In the horizontal plane the typical "figure-of-eight" loop is seen in which the distal loop is inscribed in a clockwise direction. The QRS loop fails to close, resulting in an open ST vector to the right and anteriorly. The T loop is oriented inferiorly, anteriorly, and to the right.

The ECG reveals the typical pattern of a left bundle branch block: left axis deviation; QRS = 0.16 s; VAT = 0.1 s; wide slurred R waves in I, aVL, and V_6; and ST depression in I, aVL, and V_{5-6}.

Clinical diagnosis: Arteriosclerotic heart disease.

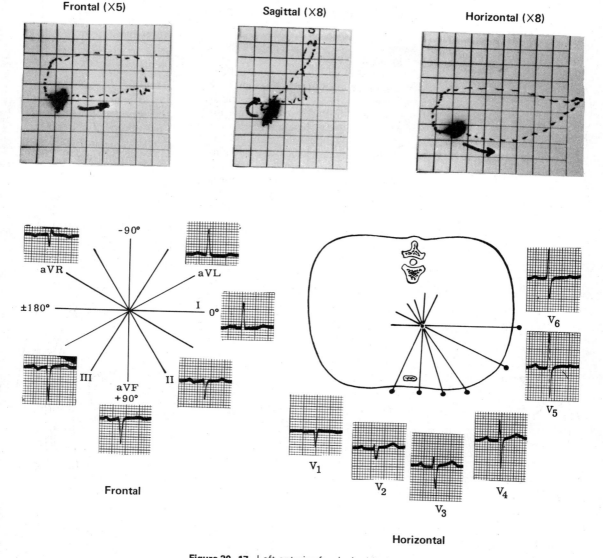

Figure 20–17. Left anterior fascicular block.

The initial portion of the QRS loop is oriented to the left, anteriorly, and minimally inferiorly. The major portion of the QRS is directed leftward, posteriorly, and superiorly. The mean QRS vector in the frontal plane = −30 degrees. This is abnormal for the Frank lead system, the upper limit of normal being −9 degrees. The T loop is indistinct but can be seen to be directed inferiorly, anteriorly, and slightly leftward.

The ECG reveals a first degree AV block (P–R interval = 0.23 s). The mean frontal plane QRS axis = −45 degrees. The deep S waves in V_{5-6} (clockwise rotation) are the result of the superior orientation of the QRS. The T waves are of low amplitude in I, aVL, aVF, and V_{5-6}.

Clinical diagnosis: Arteriosclerotic heart disease.

RIGHT VENTRICULAR HYPERTROPHY

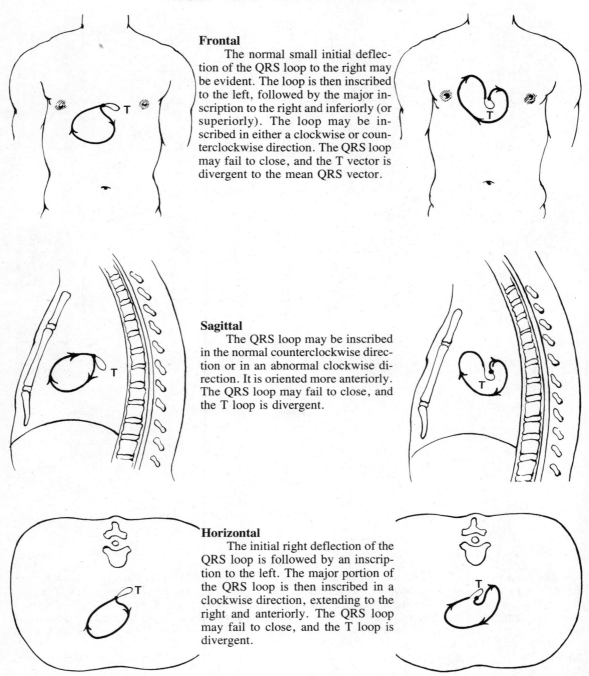

Frontal
 The normal small initial deflection of the QRS loop to the right may be evident. The loop is then inscribed to the left, followed by the major inscription to the right and inferiorly (or superiorly). The loop may be inscribed in either a clockwise or counterclockwise direction. The QRS loop may fail to close, and the T vector is divergent to the mean QRS vector.

Sagittal
 The QRS loop may be inscribed in the normal counterclockwise direction or in an abnormal clockwise direction. It is oriented more anteriorly. The QRS loop may fail to close, and the T loop is divergent.

Horizontal
 The initial right deflection of the QRS loop is followed by an inscription to the left. The major portion of the QRS loop is then inscribed in a clockwise direction, extending to the right and anteriorly. The QRS loop may fail to close, and the T loop is divergent.

Typical Features
 The spatial orientation of the QRS loop is to the right, anteriorly, and inferiorly (occasionally superiorly). The loop is inscribed in a clockwise direction in the horizontal plane and may be inscribed in a clockwise direction in the sagittal plane. The QRS loop may fail to close, and the T loop is divergent.

Figure 20–18. Vector loops in right ventricular hypertrophy.

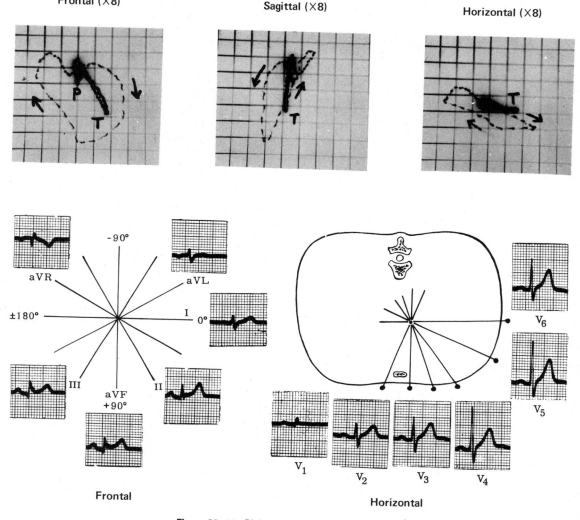

Figure 20—19. Right ventricular hypertrophy.

The initial portion of the QRS loop is oriented to the left, anteriorly, and slightly superiorly. The major portion of the QRS loop is oriented abnormally anteriorly, and the latter half is deviated to the right. The loop is inscribed in a clockwise (abnormal) direction in the horizontal plane. The T loop is oriented to the left and inferiorly.

The ECG is indicative of right ventricular hypertrophy. The frontal plane axis is +90 degrees, which is normal. The only definite electrocardiographic evidence of right ventricular hypertrophy is the qr complex in V_1 (see p 101).

Clinical diagnosis: Cor pulmonale.

RIGHT BUNDLE BRANCH BLOCK

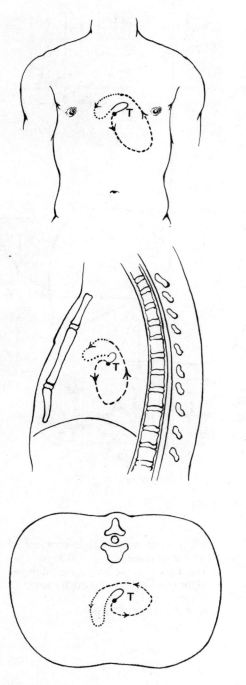

Frontal

The major portion of the QRS loop is inscribed in a normal fashion, with initial orientation to the right and inferiorly followed by inscription to the left and inferiorly. A terminal deflection is present which is oriented to the right and shows increased proximity of the time markings as evidence of the intraventricular conduction delay. The QRS loop may fail to close, and the T loop is opposite the terminal QRS deflection.

Sagittal

The major portion of the QRS loop is inscribed in a normal manner and in a counterclockwise direction. A terminal QRS deflection is present which is oriented anteriorly and has increased proximity of the time markings. The QRS loop may fail to close, and the T loop is opposite the terminal QRS deflection.

Horizontal

The major portion of the QRS loop is inscribed in a normal fashion, with initial deflection to the right and anteriorly followed by inscription in a counterclockwise direction to the left. The characteristic vectorcardiographic feature of right bundle branch block is a terminal deflection oriented to the right and anteriorly which shows increased proximity of the time markings. The QRS loop may fail to close, and the T loop is opposite the terminal QRS deflection.

Typical Features

The major portion of the QRS loop is inscribed in a normal direction. An abnormal terminal deflection is present that is oriented to the right and anteriorly. This terminal deflection is inscribed slowly (increased proximity of time markings), indicating the intraventricular conduction delay. The QRS loop may fail to close, and the T loop is opposite the direction of the terminal QRS deflection. (The P loops are not illustrated.)

Figure 20–20. Vector loops in right bundle branch block.

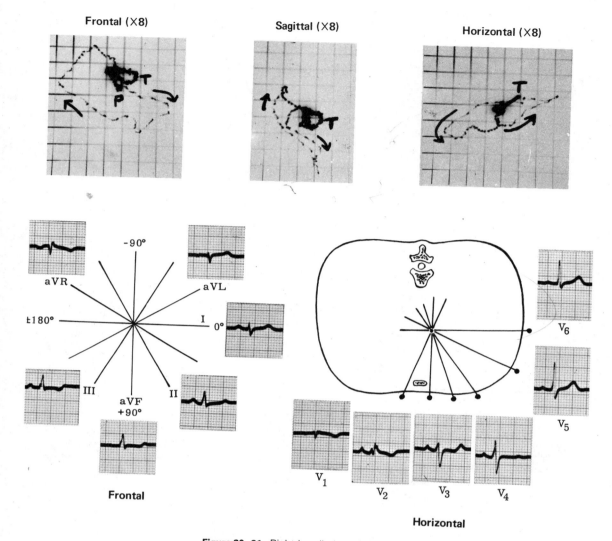

Figure 20–21. Right bundle branch block.

The first half of the QRS loop is inscribed in a normal fashion with its major orientation being to the left, inferiorly, and slightly posteriorly. However, the latter half of the QRS loop is oriented to the right, anteriorly, and superiorly. The terminal portion demonstrates conduction delay as evidenced by the increased proximity of the time markings. The loop is inscribed in a normal counterclockwise direction in the horizontal plane. The T loop is oriented to the left, posteriorly, and slightly inferiorly, ie, opposite to the terminal portion of the QRS loop.

The ECG reveals a right bundle branch block: QRS = 0.12 s (in V_2); rsR′ with wide R′ in V_2; inverted T waves in V_{1-2}.

Clinical diagnosis: Interatrial septal defect.

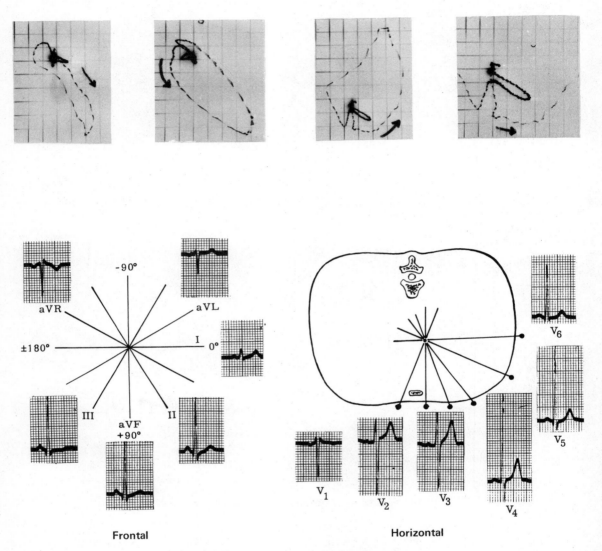

Figure 20–22. Incomplete right bundle branch block.

The initial portion of the QRS loop is oriented anteriorly and superiorly. The major portion of the QRS is directed leftward and inferiorly (+75 degrees in the frontal plane) and posteriorly. The terminal portion of the QRS is oriented to the right and anteriorly. The dashes are small and close together, indicating slowing of conduction. The QRS ends anterior to the beginning point. The T loop is normally directed to the left, anteriorly, and slightly inferiorly.

The ECG reveals a frontal plane QRS axis of +80 degrees (vertical heart position); QRS = 0.08 s; rSr' complex in V_1, and ST elevation in V_{2-3}. The record meets the criteria for incomplete right bundle branch block but in itself does not indicate clinical abnormality. The above vectorcardiogram and ECG are tracings taken on a 27-year-old normal man.

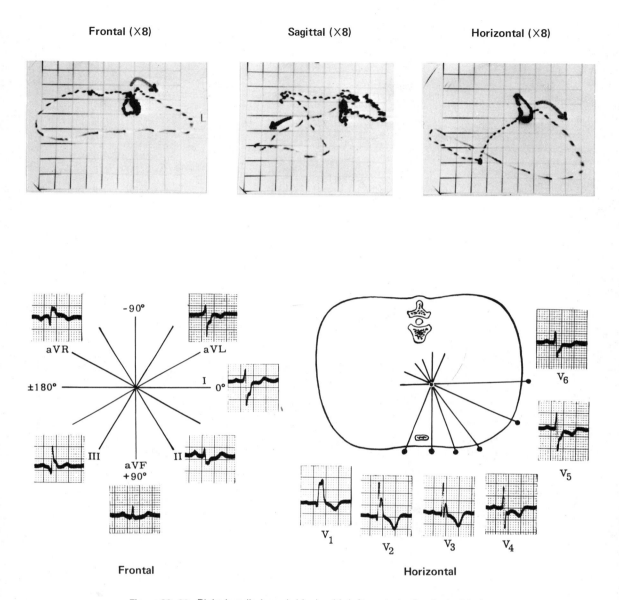

Frontal (×8)   **Sagittal (×8)**   **Horizontal (×8)**

Frontal

Horizontal

Figure 20–23. Right bundle branch block with left posterior fascicular block.

The initial portion of the QRS is oriented to the left, superiorly, and posteriorly. The loop is then directed to the left, inferiorly, and anteriorly. The terminal and major portion of the QRS is oriented to the right, inferiorly, and anteriorly, with the last portion showing evidence of conduction delay. The mean frontal plane QRS vector = +120 degrees. The ST and T vectors are directed inferiorly, posteriorly, and slightly rightward.

The ECG reveals a right bundle branch block: QRS = 0.14 s; wide notched R waves in V_{1-3} and wide S wave in I. There is ST depression and T wave inversion in precordial leads. The mean frontal plane QRS axis = +120 degrees, indicative of a left posterior fascicular block. The small q waves in V_{1-3} are not diagnostic of infarction in the presence of the bilateral bundle branch block.

Clinical diagnosis: Arteriosclerotic heart disease; old myocardial infarction.

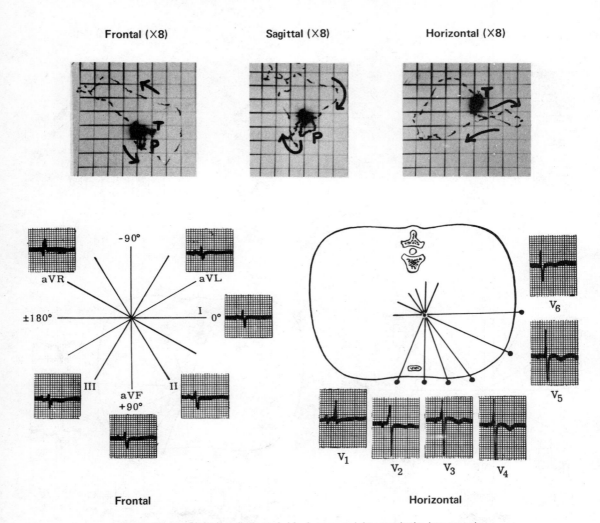

Figure 20-24. Right bundle branch block versus right ventricular hypertrophy.

A readily visible large P loop is seen oriented inferiorly, at a 90-degree angle in the frontal plane. This is consistent with right atrial hypertrophy. The initial portion of the QRS loop is oriented to the left, inferiorly, and anteriorly. The major portion of the QRS loop is then oriented to the right, superiorly, and at first anteriorly and then posteriorly in the terminal stage. The loop is inscribed in a clockwise (abnormal) fashion in the horizontal plane, and there is no terminal conduction delay. The vectorcardiogram is therefore indicative of right atrial and right ventricular hypertrophy.

The ECG reveals the following: the spiked, diphasic P wave in V_1 is suggestive of right atrial hypertrophy (however, the P waves are not abnormal in frontal plane leads); right axis deviation (frontal plane axis = +110 degrees); an rsR' complex in V_1; QRS = 0.09 s. The pattern is that of an incomplete right bundle branch block and is only indirectly suggestive of right ventricular hypertrophy.

Clinical and autopsy diagnosis: Right atrial and right ventricular hypertrophy secondary to chronic pulmonary disease.

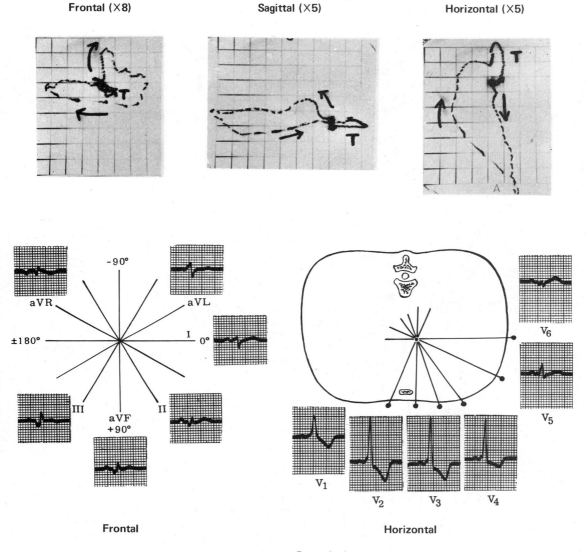

Figure 20–25. Preexcitation.

The initial portion of the QRS loop is oriented superiorly and anteriorly. The time markings are very closely recorded, indicating a conduction delay in the early phase of the QRS cycle. The major portion of the QRS loop is oriented anteriorly, at first to the left and then to the right. The ST vector and the T loop are oriented posteriorly.

The ECG is typical of preexcitation (WPW syndrome). The P–R interval = 0.09 s; QRS = 0.14 s; a wide q wave is seen in leads II, III, and aVF. However, in the presence of abnormal intraventricular conduction, as exists in this condition, a diagnosis of inferior wall infarction must not be made from this finding. The slurring of the q waves in II, III, and aVF and of the R waves in I, aVL, and V_{1-4} is due to the early QRS conduction delay.

ANTERIOR MYOCARDIAL INFARCTION

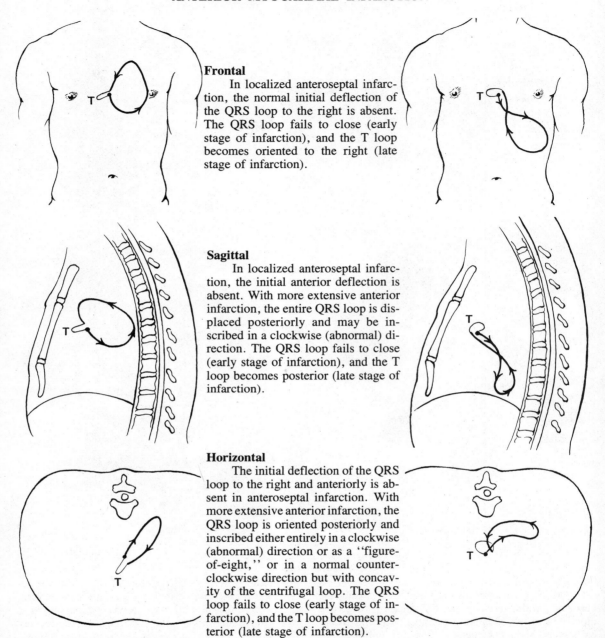

Frontal

In localized anteroseptal infarction, the normal initial deflection of the QRS loop to the right is absent. The QRS loop fails to close (early stage of infarction), and the T loop becomes oriented to the right (late stage of infarction).

Sagittal

In localized anteroseptal infarction, the initial anterior deflection is absent. With more extensive anterior infarction, the entire QRS loop is displaced posteriorly and may be inscribed in a clockwise (abnormal) direction. The QRS loop fails to close (early stage of infarction), and the T loop becomes posterior (late stage of infarction).

Horizontal

The initial deflection of the QRS loop to the right and anteriorly is absent in anteroseptal infarction. With more extensive anterior infarction, the QRS loop is oriented posteriorly and inscribed either entirely in a clockwise (abnormal) direction or as a "figure-of-eight," or in a normal counterclockwise direction but with concavity of the centrifugal loop. The QRS loop fails to close (early stage of infarction), and the T loop becomes posterior (late stage of infarction).

Typical Features

The loss of electromotive forces resulting from anterior myocardial infarction causes the QRS loop to be deviated posteriorly. In localized anteroseptal infarction, the normal initial deflection to the right and anteriorly does not occur. Instead, the initial deflection is to the left and posteriorly. With more extensive anterior infarction, the QRS loop may be inscribed in a clockwise direction in the sagittal plane. In the horizontal plane the QRS loop, in addition to being oriented posteriorly, is inscribed either entirely in a clockwise direction or as a "figure-of-eight," or entirely counterclockwise but with a marked concavity of the centrifugal limb. The QRS loop will remain open in the early stage of infarction (ST change), and the T loop will become posterior in the later stage. (The P loops are not illustrated.)

Figure 20–26. Vector loops in anterior myocardial infarction.

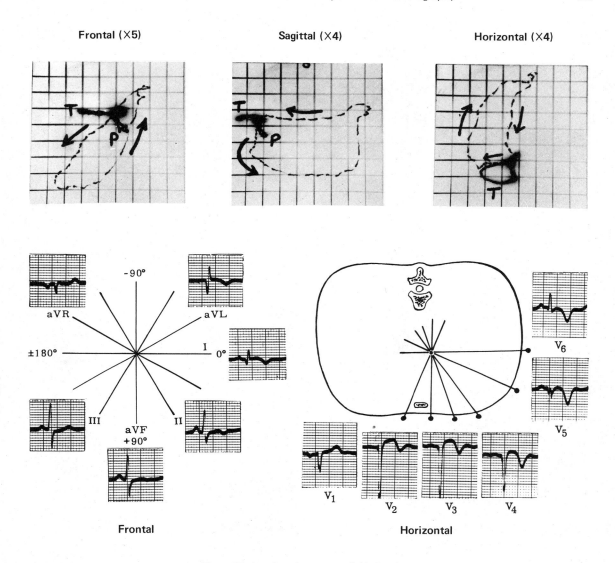

Figure 20–27. Anterior myocardial infarction.

A normal P loop can be seen in the frontal and sagittal views. It is normally oriented to the left and inferiorly. The QRS loop is inscribed in a grossly abnormal direction. The initial portion is oriented far to the right and inferiorly. Almost the entire loop is oriented posteriorly, and in the horizontal plane the QRS loop is inscribed in a clockwise (abnormal) direction. The T loop is oriented to the right and anteriorly.

The ECG is indicative of anterior myocardial infarction: deep Q waves in I and aVL; QS complexes from V_{2-5}; inverted T waves in I, aVL, and V_{2-6}.

Autopsy diagnosis: Extensive anterior wall infarction.

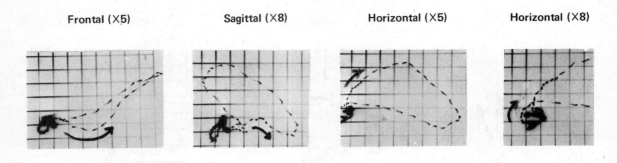

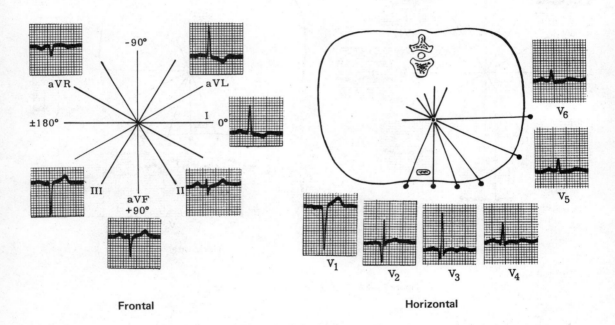

Figure 20—28. Anterior myocardial infarction with left anterior fascicular block.

The initial portion of the QRS is oriented to the left, inferiorly, and posteriorly. The major portion of the QRS is directed leftward, superiorly, and posteriorly. Terminally, the QRS becomes anterior and the loop is inscribed in an abnormal clockwise direction in the horizontal plane. The mean QRS vector in the frontal plane = −30 degrees. The T loop is oriented to the right, inferiorly, and anteriorly.

The ECG reveals a mean frontal plane QRS axis = −40 degrees. This is consistent with left anterior fascicular block. The Q waves in V_{2-3} are indicative of anterior myocardial infarction. There is ST depression and T wave inversion in I, aVL, and left precordial leads.

Autopsy diagnosis: Anterior wall infarction.

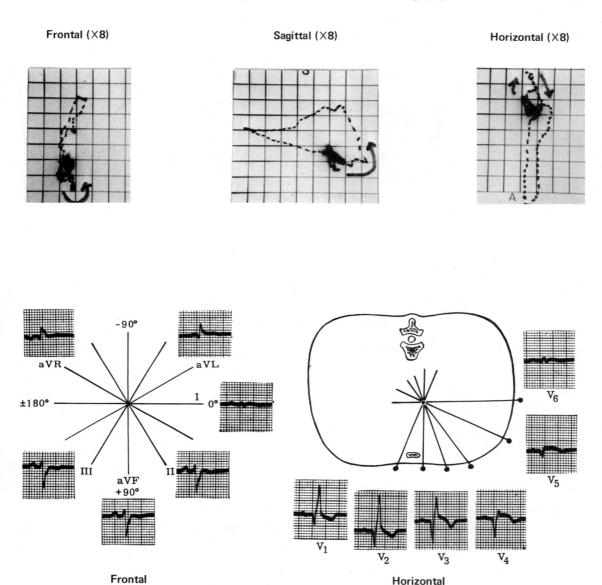

Frontal (×8)   Sagittal (×8)   Horizontal (×8)

Frontal   Horizontal

Figure 20–29. Anterior myocardial infarction with right bundle branch block and left anterior fascicular block.

The initial portion of the QRS loop is oriented slightly to the left and inferiorly and posteriorly (best seen in sagittal view): The major portion of the QRS is then directed superiorly, anteriorly, and terminally rightward. The mean frontal plane QRS vector = −90 degrees. The increased number of time markings indicates an intraventricular conduction defect. The T vector is oriented rightward, inferiorly, and posteriorly.

The ECG reveals a right bundle branch block: QRS interval = 0.14 s and late R waves in V_{1-3}. The Q waves in V_{1-5} indicate anterior myocardial infarction. The mean frontal plane QRS axis = −90 degrees and represents a left anterior fascicular block. The ST segment elevation in precordial leads is consistent with recent infarction.

Autopsy diagnosis: Extensive recent anterior and septal infarction.

INFERIOR MYOCARDIAL INFARCTION

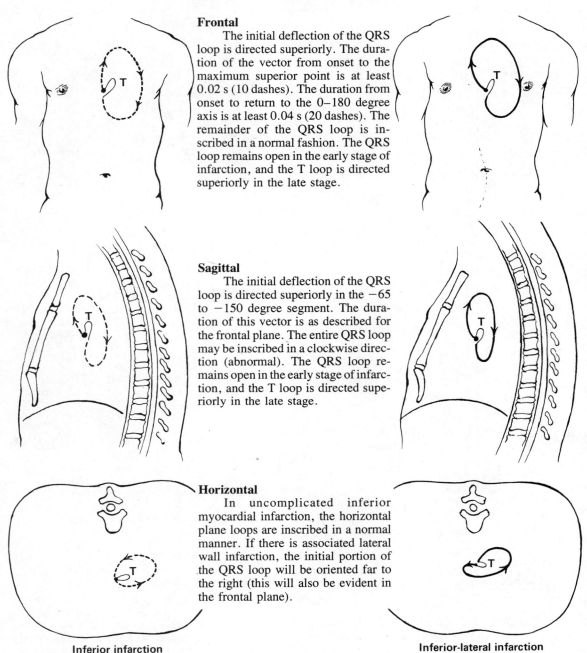

Frontal

The initial deflection of the QRS loop is directed superiorly. The duration of the vector from onset to the maximum superior point is at least 0.02 s (10 dashes). The duration from onset to return to the 0–180 degree axis is at least 0.04 s (20 dashes). The remainder of the QRS loop is inscribed in a normal fashion. The QRS loop remains open in the early stage of infarction, and the T loop is directed superiorly in the late stage.

Sagittal

The initial deflection of the QRS loop is directed superiorly in the −65 to −150 degree segment. The duration of this vector is as described for the frontal plane. The entire QRS loop may be inscribed in a clockwise direction (abnormal). The QRS loop remains open in the early stage of infarction, and the T loop is directed superiorly in the late stage.

Horizontal

In uncomplicated inferior myocardial infarction, the horizontal plane loops are inscribed in a normal manner. If there is associated lateral wall infarction, the initial portion of the QRS loop will be oriented far to the right (this will also be evident in the frontal plane).

Inferior infarction   Inferior-lateral infarction

Typical Features

As a result of the loss of electromotive forces caused by inferior myocardial infarction, the QRS loop is deviated superiorly. This will be evident in the frontal and sagittal planes. The initial vector in these 2 planes is oriented superiorly (in the −65 to −150 degree segment in the sagittal plane) and to a magnitude much greater than normal. The duration of this initial superior orientation is at least 0.02 s (10 dashes), and the total duration before the inscription returns to the 0–180 degree axis is at least 0.04 s (20 dashes). The QRS loop will remain open in the early stage of infarction, and the T loop will be directed superiorly in the late stage. (The P loops are not illustrated.)

Figure 20–30. Vector loops in inferior myocardial infarction.

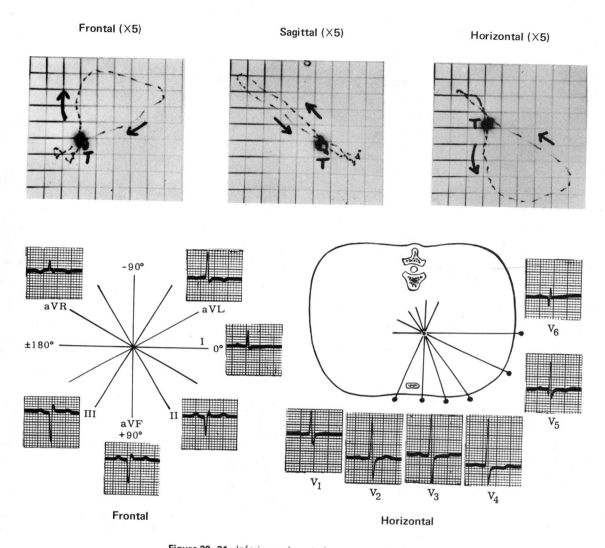

Figure 20–31. Inferior and posterior myocardial infarction.

There is a marked superior orientation of the QRS loop. There are 22 dashes from the onset of the QRS loop (in the frontal and sagittal planes) to the point where the QRS loop recrosses the 0–180 degree axis ($22 \times 0.002 = 0.044$ s; this should equal the width of the Q wave in aVF). This is diagnostic of inferior wall infarction. In addition, practically the entire QRS loop is oriented markedly anteriorly, with only a very small terminal orientation posteriorly (and to the right and inferiorly). This unusual degree of anterior displace-ment is indicative of true posterior wall infarction.

The ECG reveals deep and wide (0.04 s) Q waves in II, III, and aVF, indicative of inferior wall infarc-tion. The prominent q wave in V_6 indicates associated lateral wall infarction. Abnormally tall R waves are seen in V_{1-3}. This is the result of the marked anterior orientation of the QRS vector as the result of posterior wall infarction.

Autopsy diagnosis: Extensive infarction involv-ing the inferior and posterior portions of the left ventri-cle.

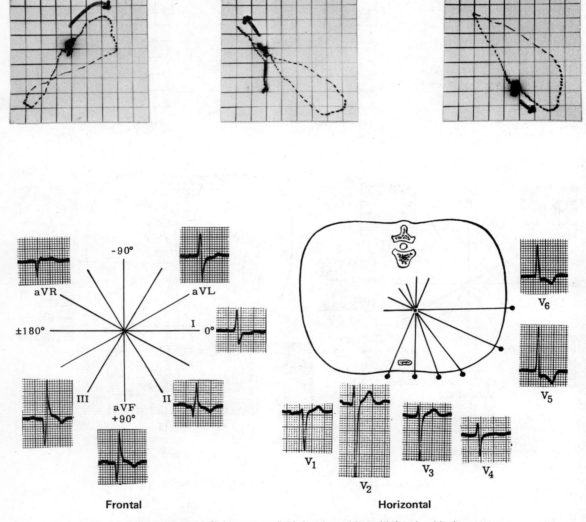

Figure 20–32. Inferior myocardial infarction with peri-infarction block.

The initial portion of the QRS is oriented to the left, superiorly, and anteriorly. The terminal portion of the QRS is directed rightward, inferiorly, and posteriorly. The increased proximity of the time markings both initially and terminally is indicative of a widened QRS duration. Small T loops are directed superiorly and anteriorly.

The ECG reveals wide Q waves with inverted T waves in II, III, and aVF as evidence of inferior myocardial infarction. The QRS interval = 0.13 s, and the S wave in I, R wave in aVF, and S wave in V_2 represent the terminal orientation to the right, inferiorly, and posteriorly. This is consistent with left posterior fascicular block, but because of the widened QRS interval it is indicative of a peripheral, intramural conduction delay which is called peri-infarction block.

Clinical diagnosis: Arteriosclerotic heart disease; old myocardial infarction.

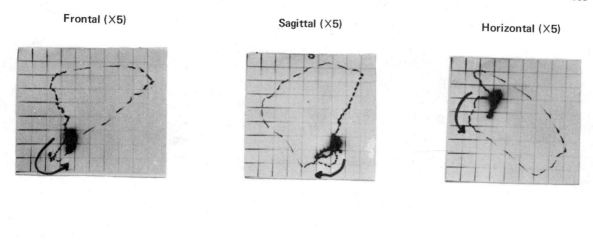

Frontal (X5)   Sagittal (X5)   Horizontal (X5)

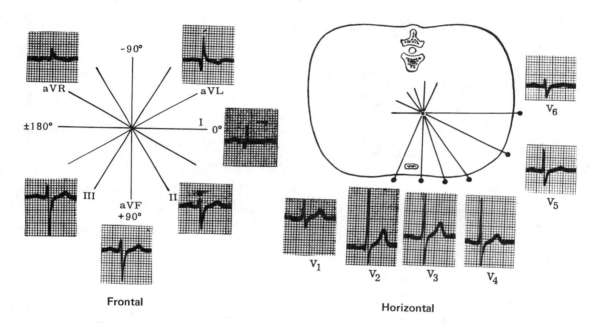

Frontal

Horizontal

Figure 20–33. Posterior-lateral myocardial infarction with left anterior fascicular block.

The initial portion of the QRS is oriented to the right, inferiorly, and anteriorly. The major portion of the QRS is directed superiorly, leftward, and anteriorly. The mean frontal plane QRS vector = −70 degrees. The T loop is oriented to the right, inferiorly, and anteriorly.

The ECG reveals significant q waves in I and aVL, indicating lateral wall infarction. The tall R waves and upright T waves in V_{1-2} indicate posterior wall infarction. The mean frontal plane QRS axis = −70 degrees, which represents a left anterior fascicular block. The latter should not occur with posterior-lateral infarction and therefore is indicative of a separate myocardial lesion. The S waves in V_{5-6} (clockwise rotation) are the result of the superiorly directed QRS vector.

Clinical diagnosis: Arteriosclerotic heart disease; old myocardial infarction.

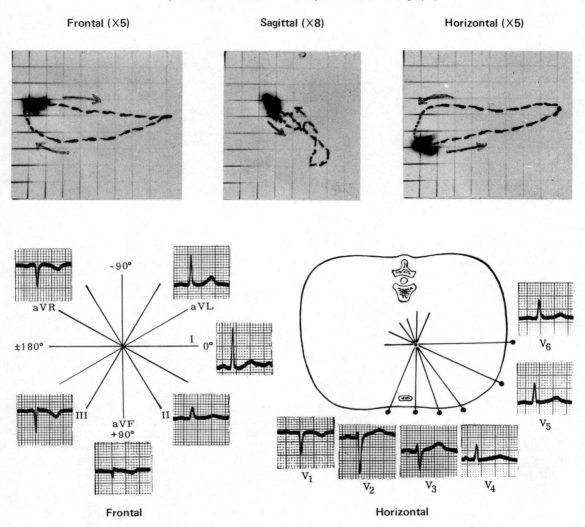

Figure 20–34. Inferior wall infarction versus normal record.

The ECG reveals a prominent Q wave and inverted T in aVF. This is strongly suggestive of inferior wall infarction. A deep Q is seen in III, but the absence of a Q in II could be reason to question the diagnosis of inferior wall infarction.

The vectorcardiogram reveals no evidence of any superior orientation in the frontal and sagittal planes. The vectorcardiogram reveals no evidence of infarction.

Clinical findings: The patient had Laennec's cirrhosis. There was no clinical evidence of heart disease. Five ECGs and vectorcardiograms taken over a 1-year period remain unchanged from those illustrated.

Autopsy findings: Normal heart; death due to cirrhosis.

In this instance, the vectorcardiogram offered more correct information than the ECG.

VENTRICULAR GRADIENT

As explained in Chapter 2, the activation of a myocardial cell involves 2 major phases: depolarization and repolarization. If repolarization begins at the same point as depolarization and spreads in the same direction and at the same uniform rate as depolarization (see pp 19–22), the area of the wave of repolarization (T wave) will equal the area of the wave of depolarization (R wave) but will be of opposite polarity. Expressed as vectors, these 2 forces will be equal but 180 degrees apart. This does not hold true when one analyzes the waves of depolarization (QRS) and repolarization (T) of the entire ventricular myocardium. It is apparent that the R wave and the T wave are normally in the same direction in lead I (an approximate right-to-left axis) and that the area of the QRS does not necessarily equal the area of the T wave. The vector that represents the net effect of the QRS vector and the T vector is the ventricular gradient. By definition, this vector has magnitude, polarity, and direction in space (3-dimensional). In clinical unipolar electrocardiography, the determination of the ventricular gradient has been limited to the frontal plane. The determination is quite time-consuming and is not popular as a routine measurement in clinical electrocardiography.

The ventricular gradient in the frontal plane can be determined in the following manner: The net areas of the QRS complexes and T waves are measured in 2 frontal plane leads, such as I and III (see p 32). The QRS and T vectors are thereby determined and plotted. The resultant of the QRS and T vectors can be geometrically determined by the law of the parallelogram and will represent the frontal plane ventricular gradient. Since this is a reflection of the QRS vector and the T

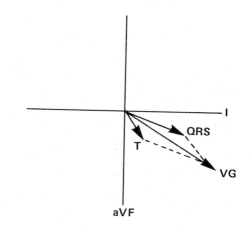

Figure 20–35. Diagram of ventricular gradient (VG) in frontal plane.

vector, the concept of primary and secondary T wave changes has been proposed. When the changes in repolarization (T wave) are associated with changes in depolarization (QRS complex), as in bundle branch block and infarction, the T changes are termed secondary. T wave changes are termed primary if there are changes in repolarization with apparently normal depolarization.

With the advent of corrected orthogonal leads, an accurate determination of the spatial ventricular gradient is possible. It is quite time-consuming, and it is questionable that this determination will offer valuable information that cannot be obtained by the more routine evaluation of the record.

21 | Interpretation of the Electrocardiogram

Ideally, the person best qualified to read and interpret the ECG is the physician who is taking care of the patient. Since this is not always possible, the individual reading the record must have the following data as a minimum:

History Accompanying Record

A. Age: Remember that the normal pattern in infants or children is considerably different from that in adults.

B. Race: Young adult blacks may show a pattern that would be abnormal in a white person of the same age.

C. Height, Weight, and Body Build: Obese and thick-chested individuals will have reduced amplitude of the complexes.

D. Associated Pulmonary Disease: Marked emphysema, pleural effusion, and previous chest surgery may affect the heart position and voltage of the complexes.

E. Medication, Especially Digitalis: Remember that digitalis leaf and digitoxin can affect the electrocardiographic pattern for as long as 3 weeks after the drug has been discontinued.

F. Blood pressure and clinical impression.

G. Tentative diagnosis or pertinent cardiorespiratory findings (or both).

Technique of Reading the Record

It is preferable to read the tracing before it is cut and mounted since in arrhythmias it is frequently essential to study long strips of any one lead in order to reach the proper diagnosis (see, for example, pp 268 and 271). Furthermore, isolated abnormalities may be present that are unintentionally omitted when small segments of the tracing are mounted. One sequence that can be followed is given below.

A. Scan the entire record to make sure it is technically good, ie, free of electrical interference, with good skin contact, and leads properly taken. Check the standardization; this should be 10 mm.

B. Determine the rhythm. If an arrhythmia is present, check the leads that best illustrate it (usually V_1).

C. Determine the heart rate. If the rhythm is not of sinus origin, determine both the atrial and ventricular rates.

D. Determine the P–R, QRS, and Q–T_c inter-

vals. By custom, this is done from the standard leads, but this is not essential.

E. Study of Frontal Plane Leads (I, II, III, aVR, aVL, aVF): Determine the frontal plane QRS axis; note any abnormalities of the P wave, QRS complex, ST segment, and T wave. If there are questionable T wave abnormalities, determine the mean T vector and thereby the QRS–T angle.

F. Study of Precordial Leads: Note the degree of rotation on the long axis; note any abnormalities of the P and T waves, QRS complexes, and ST segments.

Electrocardiographic Interpretation

The following types of conclusions can be made.

A. The tracing is normal.

B. Borderline record; there are minor changes (enumerate) the significance of which will depend on the clinical findings and serial ECGs if clinically indicated.

C. Abnormal record typical of (name of condition).

D. Abnormal record consistent with (names of conditions).

E. Abnormal record not characteristic of any specific entity.

In all the above instances, one must remember that a normal ECG does not imply a normal heart and that an abnormal ECG does not necessarily imply organic heart disease. The tracing must be interpreted in the light of clinical findings and serial tracings and additional leads taken as indicated.

ELECTROCARDIOGRAMS FOR INTERPRETATION

In order that the reader of this text might gain some practical experience in the interpretation of the ECG, the following ECGs are included. It is suggested that the readers interpret these tracings themselves before reading the text, and then compare interpretations with that of the author.

In most of the following ECGs, it will not be possible to determine the heart rate and the Q–T_c since only single complexes are shown. However, in the tracings selected this does not affect the interpretation.

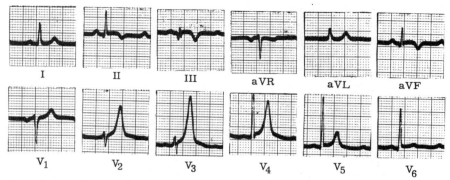

Regular sinus rhythm; P–R = 0.14 s; QRS = 0.06; small q waves with ST elevation and T wave inversion in leads II, III, and aVF. There are very tall symmetric T waves in V_{2-4}.

Interpretation: (See p 177.) Inferior-posterior myocardial infarction.

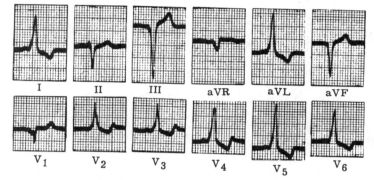

Regular sinus rhythm; P–R = 0.1 s; QRS = 0.12 s. The frontal plane QRS axis = −45 degrees. The initial portion of the R is slurred in leads I, aVL, and V_{2-6}. There is ST depression and T wave inversion in the latter leads. The voltage of the R in lead aVL = 15 mm. Ordinarily this would indicate left ventricular hypertrophy, but in the presence of the abnormal conduction pattern, this is invalid.

Interpretation: (See p 276.) Preexcitation syndrome (Wolff-Parkinson-White syndrome).

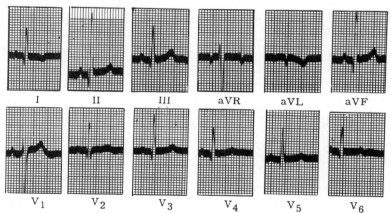

Regular sinus rhythm; P–R = 0.16 s; QRS = 0.08 s. There is no abnormal axis deviation. The T in lead I is inverted. The heart position is vertical. The T is inverted in aVL as a manifestation of normal left ventricular cavity potential. Precordial leads show counterclockwise rotation.

Interpretation: (See p 78.) Abnormal ECG as evidenced by inverted T in lead I. No clinical diagnosis can be made from the ECG. In view of the clinical finding of dextroversion and the absence of other evidence of cardiovascular disease, one is justified in considering this ECG normal for this individual. The counterclockwise rotation is also consistent with the clinical diagnosis. *Clinical diagnosis:* Heart displaced to the right; bronchiectasis; sinusitis.

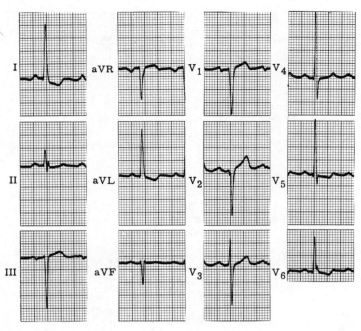

Regular sinus rhythm; P–R = 0.18 s; QRS = 0.1 s; frontal plane QRS axis = −15 degrees. R in aVL = 18 mm, $RV_5 + SV_1$ = 38 mm. There is notching of the QRS complexes in II and V_6. The ST segment is depressed and the T wave inverted or diphasic in I, aVL, and V_{5-6}.

Interpretation: (See p 91.) Left ventricular hypertrophy. *Clinical diagnosis:* Hypertensive cardiovascular disease.

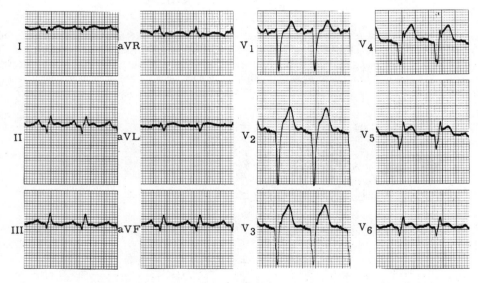

Regular sinus rhythm; rate = 98; P–R = 0.18 s; QRS = 0.12 s. The P waves are notched in all leads with a wide, late negative deflection in V_1. There is a notched qs complex in I, QR complexes in II, III, and aVF, an rS in V_1, QS in V_{2-3}, and QR complexes in V_{4-6}. The ST segments are elevated in V_{2-5} and the T waves inverted in II, III, aVF, and V_6.

Interpretation: (See p 207.) The P waves are indicative of a left atrial conduction defect. Although this is consistent with left atrial hypertrophy, it is not pathognomonic of such. There is evidence of extensive infarction, involving inferior, anterior, and lateral walls. The wide QRS interval is indicative of peri-infarction block. The ST segment elevation in precordial leads is consistent with recent anterior wall infarction. *Clinical diagnosis:* Myocardial infarction (inferior), 1 year old; myocardial infarction (anterior and lateral), 4 months old. The ST elevations have persisted for 4 months and are indicative of an anterior and lateral ventricular aneurysm. This was confirmed by angiography.

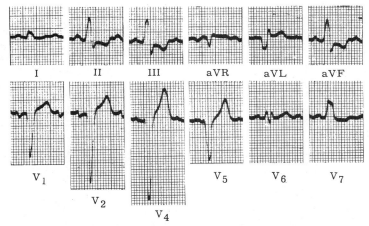

Regular sinus rhythm; P–R = 0.16 s; QRS = 0.15; depressed ST with T wave inversion in leads II and III; vertical heart position; wide R with depressed ST and inverted T in aVF. There is an rsr' complex in V_6 and a wide, notched R in V_7. VAT = 0.1 s in V_6.

Interpretation: (See p 127.) Left bundle branch block. *Clinical and autopsy diagnosis:* Hypertensive and arteriosclerotic heart disease; no evidence of myocardial infarction.

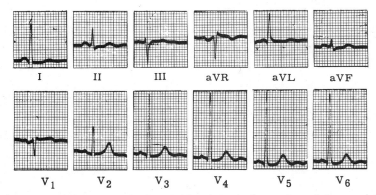

Regular sinus rhythm; P–R = 0.14 s; QRS = 0.08 s; frontal plane axis = 0 degrees; slight ST depression with low amplitude T in lead I. The heart position is semihorizontal: the T is of low amplitude in aVL. Precordial leads reveal counterclockwise rotation. There are tall R waves in V_{3-6}; R in V_5 = 28 mm.

Interpretation: (See p 97.) Left ventricular hypertrophy. *Clinical diagnosis:* Hypertensive cardiovascular disease.

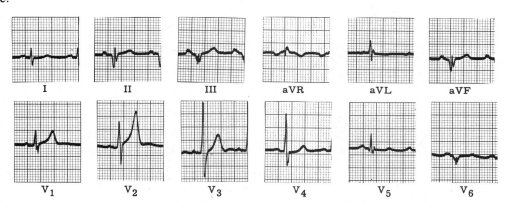

Regular sinus rhythm; rate = 86; P–R = 0.16 s; QRS = 0.1 s. There are deep, wide Q waves in II, III, and aVF. A QS complex is present in V_6. A tall R with an Rs ratio of 4:1 is seen in V_1. The T waves are upright in V_{1-3}.

Interpretation: (See p 178.) Inferior-posterior-lateral myocardial infarction, clinically 1 year old.

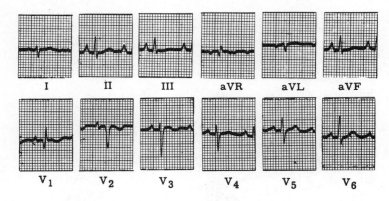

Regular sinus rhythm; P–R = 0.14 s; QRS = 0.06 s; frontal plane QRS axis = +115 degrees; tall slender P waves in leads II and III. The heart position is vertical; tall slender P in aVF. A qR complex is seen in V_1; the T waves are inverted in V_{1-3}.

Interpretation: (See p 103.) Right ventricular hypertrophy; right atrial hypertrophy. *Clinical diagnosis:* Pulmonary emphysema with right heart failure. *Autopsy diagnosis:* Right ventricular hypertrophy.

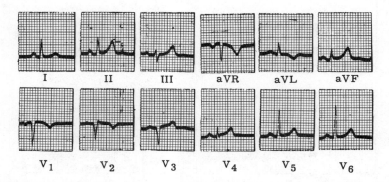

Regular sinus rhythm; P–R = 0.14 s; QRS = 0.06 s; frontal plane axis = +30 degrees; intermediate heart position. QS complexes are seen in V_{1-3} with an abrupt transition to a left ventricular epicardial complex in V_4. The T is inverted in aVL and V_{1-2}.

Interpretation: (See p 165.) Anteroseptal myocardial infarction. *Clinical and autopsy diagnosis:* Old anteroseptal infarction.

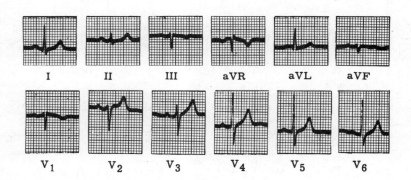

Regular sinus rhythm; P–R = 0.16 s; QRS = 0.08 s; frontal plane axis = −10 degrees; semihorizontal heart position; clockwise rotation; normal rsr′ in V_1.

Interpretation: (See p 69.) Within normal limits.

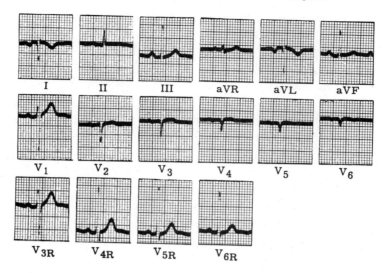

Regular sinus rhythm; P–R = 0.16 s; QRS = 0.06 s. The entire pattern of lead I is inverted. Lead aVL resembles a normal aVR. Leads V_{1-6} never reflect left ventricular epicardial potential. However, leads V_{4R-6R} do reflect the epicardial surface of the left ventricle.

Interpretation: (See p 79.) Dextrocardia (complete transposition). *Clinical diagnosis:* 30-year-old man with dextrocardia and situs inversus; no evidence of heart disease.

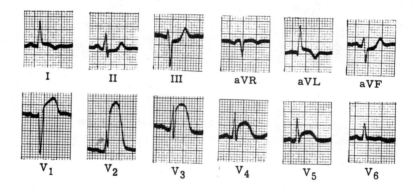

Regular sinus rhythm; P–R = 0.14 s; QRS = 0.06 s; frontal plane axis = −10 degrees; horizontal heart position. There is ST elevation with an upward convexity in leads I, aVL, and V_{2-5}. There is ST depression in leads II, III, and aVF. The T wave is inverted in leads I and aVL, and flat in V_6.

Interpretation: (See p 160.) Early anterior wall infarction. *Clinical diagnosis:* Recent (6 hours) myocardial infarction.

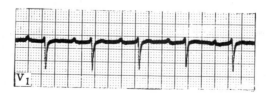

Regular sinus rhythm; P–R = 0.28 s; QRS = 0.08 s.
Interpretation: (See p 237.) First degree AV block.

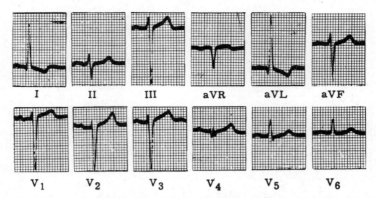

Regular sinus rhythm; P–R = 0.16 s; QRS = 0.08 s; left axis deviation (−30 degrees), ST depression and T wave inversion in lead I. The heart position is horizontal; R in aVL = 19 mm; ST depression and T wave inversion in aVL. Precordial leads are normal.

Interpretation: (See p 94.) Left ventricular hypertrophy.

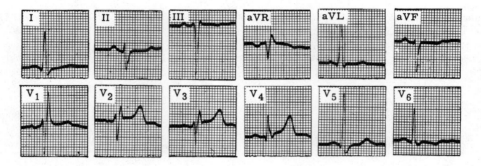

Regular sinus rhythm; P–R = 0.18 s; QRS = 0.16 s; frontal plane QRS axis = 45 degrees; low amplitude T in lead I; R in aVL = 17 mm; T of low amplitude in aVL; rSR′ complexes in V$_{1-3}$; VAT in V$_1$ = 0.1 s; wide S waves in V$_{5-6}$; inverted T in V$_6$.

Interpretation: (See p 119.) Right bundle branch block, left anterior fascicular block; the combination of the above indicates bilateral bundle branch disease; left ventricular hypertrophy. *Clinical diagnosis:* Hypertensive cardiovascular disease.

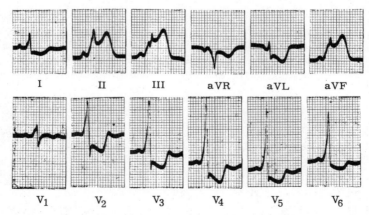

The P–R interval = 0.1 s; QRS = 0.12 s. There is slurring of the upstroke of the R in leads I, II, III, aVF, and all precordial leads. There is marked ST elevation in II, III, and aVF, with ST depression in I, aVL, and all precordial leads.

Interpretation: (See pp 169 and 272.) Recent inferior wall infarction; preexcitation (Wolff-Parkinson-White syndrome).

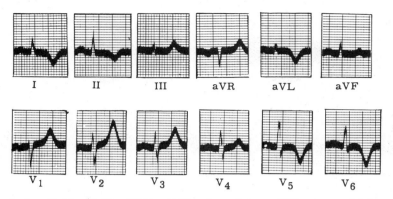

Regular sinus rhythm; P–R = 0.18 s; QRS = 0.08 s; frontal plane QRS axis = +30 degrees. The T waves are deeply and symmetrically inverted in leads I, II, aVL, and V_{5-6}. No abnormal Q waves are present.

Interpretation: (See p 180.) Abnormal ECG consistent with subendocardial infarction involving the anterior and lateral walls of the left ventricle. *Autopsy diagnosis:* Myocardial infarction involving the anterior and lateral walls. The area of infarction is not transmural but involves the inner half of the myocardium.

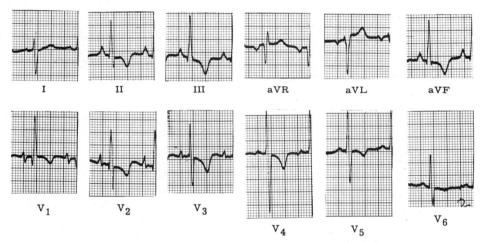

Regular sinus rhythm; P–R = 0.16 s; QRS = 0.09 s. The frontal plane QRS axis = +110 degrees. The P waves are tall and slender in II, III, and aVF and sharply diphasic in V_1. A qR complex is present in V_1. There is ST depression and T wave inversion in II, III, aVF, and V_{1-5}.

Interpretation: (See p 100.) Right atrial and right ventricular hypertrophy. *Clinical diagnosis:* Schistosomiasis mansoni with extensive pulmonary involvement and cor pulmonale in a 35-year-old man. The pulmonary artery pressure equaled the systemic pressure.

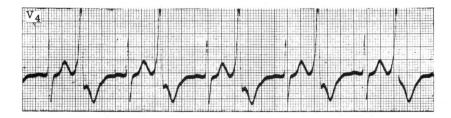

Regular sinus rhythm is present alternating with ventricular premature beats.

Interpretation: (See p 257.) Regular sinus rhythm with ventricular bigeminy.

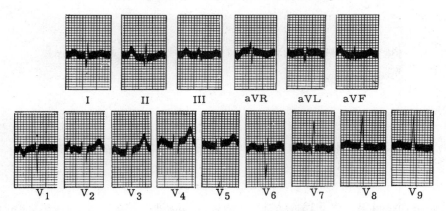

Regular sinus rhythm; P–R = 0.2 s; QRS = 0.08 s. The heart position is vertical. There are rsr' complexes in leads I, II, aVL, and aVF. Small r waves are present in V_{1-4}. rSr' complexes are present in V_{5-6}, and an rsR' complex is present in V_7. There is shallow inversion of the T in V_{7-9}.

Interpretation: (See p 152.) Abnormal ECG of nonspecific pattern. In view of the clinical findings it is consistent with the pattern of late anterior wall infarction with remaining viable muscle fibers in the epicardium.

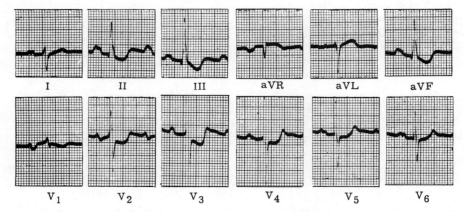

Regular sinus rhythm; P–R = 0.24 s; QRS = 0.08 s; mean frontal plane QRS axis = +100 degrees; notched P waves of the P mitrale type in leads I and II. There is ST depression with some T wave inversion in leads II and III. The heart position is vertical. There is ST depression and T wave inversion in aVF. A diphasic P with wide negative deflection is seen in V_1. A prominent r is present in V_1 and a deep S is present in V_6. There is ST depression in the precordial leads, most marked in V_{2-3}.

Interpretation: (See p 87.) Right ventricular hypertrophy; left atrial hypertrophy; first degree AV block; some of the ST–T changes could be the result of digitalis. *Clinical diagnosis:* Mitral stenosis.

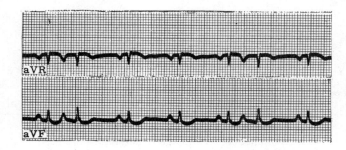

Regular sinus rhythm; rate = 75. There are premature atrial contractions. The P' waves are inverted in aVR and upright in aVF.

Interpretation: (See p 217.) Atrial premature beats arising from a high atrial focus.

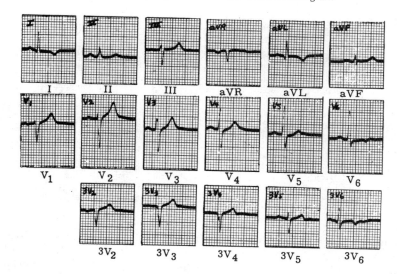

Regular sinus rhythm; P–R = 0.14 s; QRS = 0.06 s; frontal plane axis = 0 degrees; semihorizontal heart position. A small but wide q is seen in aVL. T waves are inverted in leads I, aVL, and V$_6$. Third interspace leads reveal QS complexes in the V$_{2-4}$ positions.

Interpretation: (See p 167.) High anterior and lateral myocardial infarction. *Clinical diagnosis:* Arteriosclerotic heart disease; history of myocardial infarction 1 year previously.

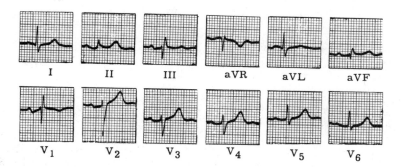

Regular sinus rhythm; P–R = 0.18 s; QRS = 0.08 s; frontal plane axis = +5 degrees; horizontal heart position. An rSR' complex is present in V$_1$; VAT in V$_1$ = 0.04 s.

Interpretation: (See p 121.) Incomplete right bundle branch block. This is not necessarily indicative of organic heart disease. The significance of this must be decided by the clinical evaluation of the patient.

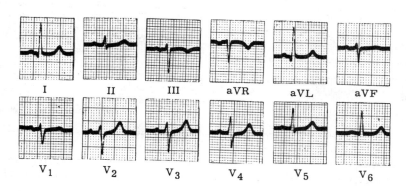

Regular sinus rhythm; P–R = 0.14 s; QRS = 0.08 s; frontal plane QRS axis = −20 degrees; horizontal heart position; voltage of R in aVL = 10.5 mm.

Interpretation: (See p 63.) Within normal limits.

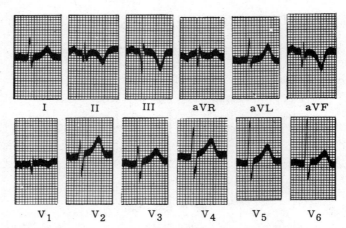

Regular sinus rhythm; P–R = 0.14 s; QRS = 0.08 s; mean frontal plane QRS axis = −20 degrees; clockwise rotation. There are abnormal Q waves with deep, symmetrically inverted T waves in leads II, III, and aVF.

Interpretation: (See p 174.) Inferior myocardial infarction, late pattern. *Clinical diagnosis:* Myocardial infarction, 4 weeks old.

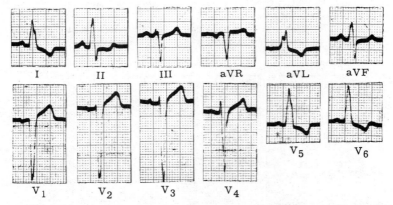

Regular sinus rhythm; P–R = 0.16 s; QRS = 0.12 s; frontal plane axis = 0 degrees. The heart position is horizontal. There are wide notched R waves in leads I, aVL, and V$_{5-6}$. VAT in aVL = 0.1 s. ST segments are depressed and the T waves inverted in these leads.

Interpretation: (See p 126.) Left bundle branch block. *Clinical diagnosis:* Hypertensive and arteriosclerotic heart disease.

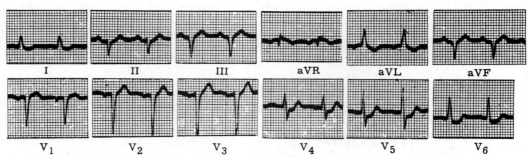

Regular sinus rhythm; P–R = 0.14 s; QRS = 0.08 s; frontal plane QRS axis = −50 degrees; ST depression in lead I. The P and T are inverted, and there is ST depression in aVL. A QS complex is present in aVF. There is ST depression in V$_{4-6}$.

Interpretation: (See p 98.) Abnormal ECG of nonspecific pattern. The QS complex in aVF can be a normal finding in a horizontal heart; yet an old inferior wall infarct cannot be excluded. The ST–T changes are not diagnostic of any specific entity. *Clinical and autopsy diagnosis:* Left ventricular hypertrophy.

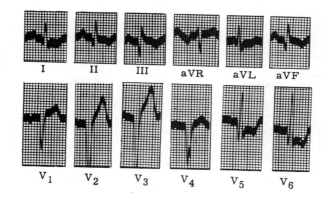

Regular sinus rhythm; P–R = 0.18 s; QRS = 0.1 s; frontal plane QRS axis = 0 degrees. There are abnormal Q waves in leads I, II, III, aVL, aVF, and V_{5-6}. QS complexes are seen in V_{1-4}. T waves are inverted in leads I, II, III, aVF, and V_{5-6}. There is ST depression in leads I, aVL, and V_{5-6}.

Interpretation: (See p 184.) Inferior wall infarction, recent; anterior wall infarction, old. *Clinical diagnosis:* Recent myocardial infarction; old myocardial infarction (by history, 10 months previously). *Autopsy diagnosis:* Old anterior wall infarction; recent posterior and inferior wall infarction; occlusion of left anterior descending and left circumflex arteries.

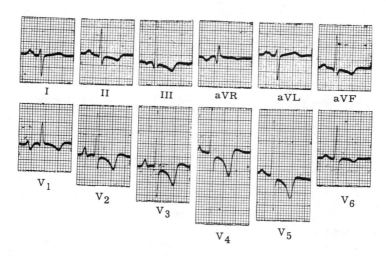

Regular sinus rhythm; P–R = 0.18 s; QRS = 0.08 s; frontal plane QRS axis = +125 degrees; notched P in lead I; ST depression and T wave inversion in leads II and III. A qR complex with ST depression and T wave inversion is seen in aVF which is a reflection of right ventricular epicardial potential. A wide diphasic P with qR complex is present in V_1. VAT in V_1 = 0.06 s. There is a deep S in V_6. The T waves are inverted in all precordial leads. There is ST depression in V_{2-5}.

Interpretation: (See p 102.) Right ventricular hypertrophy; left atrial hypertrophy. *Clinical diagnosis:* Mitral stenosis.

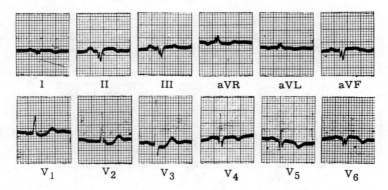

Regular sinus rhythm; P–R = 0.14 s; QRS = 0.08 s; mean frontal plane QRS axis = −100 degrees. There are notched QS complexes with inverted T waves in leads I, II, aVF, and V_6. T is also inverted in V_{4-5}. There are tall R waves with no S waves in V_{1-2}. VAT in V_1 = 0.03 s.

Interpretation: (See p 178.) Inferior, posterior, and lateral myocardial infarction. *Clinical diagnosis:* Recent myocardial infarction; no clinical evidence of right ventricular hypertrophy. *Autopsy diagnosis:* Inferior, posterior, and lateral wall infarction; normal size right ventricle; occlusion of left circumflex coronary artery.

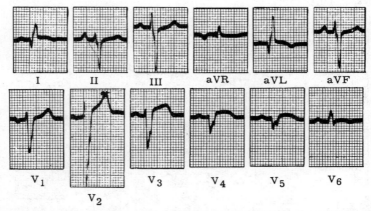

Regular sinus rhythm; P–R = 0.02 s; QRS = 0.12 s; mean frontal plane QRS axis = −60 degrees. Abnormal Q waves are seen in leads I and aVL. QS complexes are seen in V_{4-5}. There is ST elevation in leads I, aVL, and V_{2-5}. T waves are inverted in leads I, aVL, and V_6.

Interpretation: (See p 166.) Anteroapical myocardial infarction; intraventricular conduction defect (left anterior fascicular block or peri-infarction block).

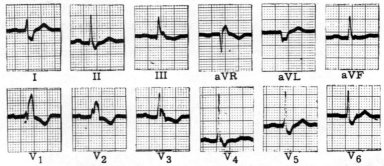

Regular sinus rhythm; P–R = 0.24 s; QRS = 0.14 s; mean frontal plane QRS axis = +90 degrees. A wide s wave is present in leads I and V_{4-6}; a wide r in aVR; an rsR′ (with a very small s) in V_1; notched and wide R in V_{2-3}; ST depression and T wave inversion in V_{1-3}; VAT in V_1 = 0.11 s.

Interpretation: (See p 195.) Possible posterior wall infarction; right bundle branch block; first degree AV block. *Clinical diagnosis:* Myocardial infarction.

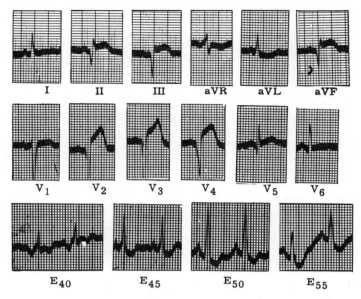

Regular sinus rhythm; P–R = 0.14 s; QRS = 0.08 s. There are abnormal Q waves in leads II, III, and aVF. QS complexes are present in V_{3-4}. There is convex ST elevation in leads II, III, aVF, and V_{4-5}. Esophageal leads over the left ventricle show ST depression but no abnormal Q waves.

Interpretation: (See p 163.) Early anterior and inferior wall infarction; no evidence of posterior wall infarction. *Clinical diagnosis:* Recent (2 days) myocardial infarction.

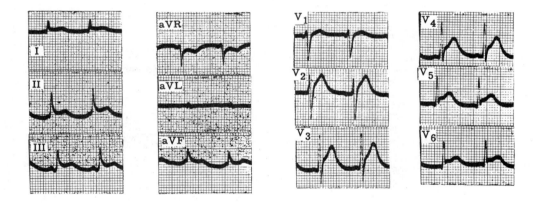

Regular sinus rhythm; P–R = 0.1 s; QRS = 0.06 s; frontal plane QRS axis = +60 degrees. There is concave ST elevation in leads I, II, III, aVF, and V_{2-6}; ST depression in aVR.

Interpretation: (See p 286.) Early pattern of pericarditis; possible preexcitation (Lown-Ganong-Levine type). *Clinical and autopsy diagnosis:* Carcinoma of the esophagus, with rupture; secondary mediastinitis and pericarditis.

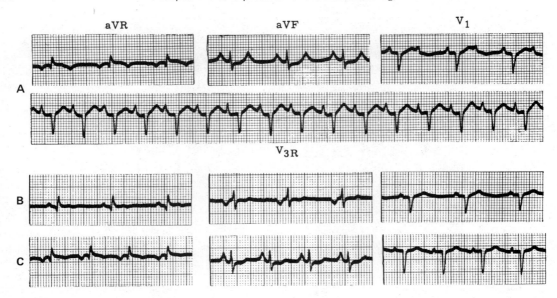

A: There is 2:1 AV conduction with an atrial rate of 142 and a ventricular rate of 71. In lead V₃ᵣ 1:1 conduction is present at a rate of 127. *B:* 1:1 conduction at a rate of 75. The P wave is upright in aVR and inverted in aVF. *C:* Sinus rhythm, rate = 100.

Interpretation: (See p 295.) *A:* Atrial tachycardia with 2:1 and 1:1 conduction owing to digitalis toxicity. *B:* Two days after (A) (digitalis discontinued); AV junctional rhythm, still indicating digitalis toxicity. *C:* Sinus rhythm reestablished 1 week after (A) and 1 week after discontinuation of digitalis.

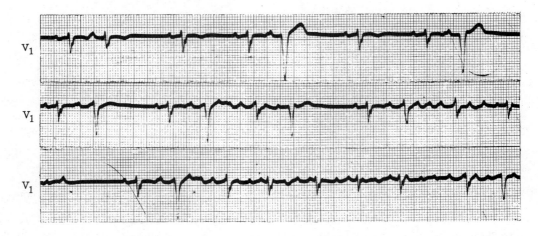

The above are portions of a continuous strip of lead V₁. Occasional regular sinus-conducted beats are seen (first, third, fourth, sixth, and seventh ventricular complexes in first strip). Frequent atrial ectopic beats are present, many with aberrant intraventricular conduction (as second, fifth, and eighth ventricular complexes in first strip). In addition, there are periods of atrial flutter-fibrillation.

Interpretation: (See p 234.) Regular sinus rhythm with atrial ectopic beats and atrial flutter-fibrillation. This illustration emphasizes the validity of the unitarian concept of the atrial arrhythmias. Each burst of atrial flutter-fibrillation is preceded by an atrial ectopic beat with a prolonged P–R interval. This permits the reentry mechanism to be activated.

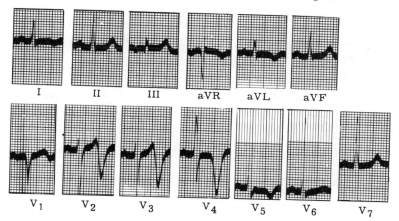

Regular sinus rhythm; P–R = 0.16 s; QRS = 0.08 s; frontal plane QRS axis = +40 degrees. There is T wave inversion in leads I and aVL; very deep, symmetrically inverted T waves in V_{2-4}. No abnormal Q waves are present. There are tall R waves in V_{5-6}. R in V_5 = 30 mm.

Interpretation: (See p 181.) Abnormal ECG consistent with subendocardial infarction of the anterior wall of the left ventricle; left ventricular hypertrophy. *Autopsy diagnosis:* Anterior wall infarction, not transmural but involving the endocardial half of the myocardium. The major area of infarction is anteroseptal.

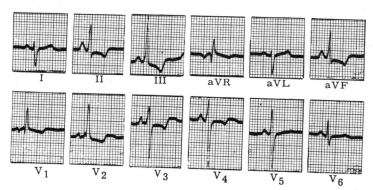

Regular sinus rhythm; P–R = 0.14 s; QRS = 0.08 s; frontal plane QRS axis = +125 degrees; ST depression and T wave inversion in leads II and III. There is ST depression and T wave inversion in aVF as a reflection of right ventricular epicardial potential. There is an rsR' complex in V_1. VAT in V_1 = 0.05 s. There is ST depression and T wave inversion in V_{1-4}.

Interpretation: (See p 120.) Incomplete right bundle branch block. In view of the clinical diagnosis of pulmonary sarcoidosis and right heart failure, this ECG is consistent with right ventricular hypertrophy.

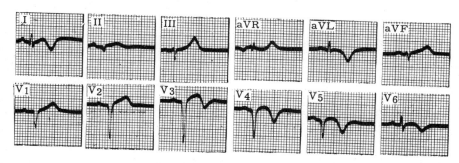

Regular sinus rhythm; P–R = 0.16 s; QRS = 0.06 s; frontal plane QRS axis = −40 degrees. There are QS complexes in V_{1-5}. T waves are inverted in leads I, aVL, and V_{3-6}.

Interpretation: (See p 182.) Anterior myocardial infarction, late pattern; left anterior fascicular block.

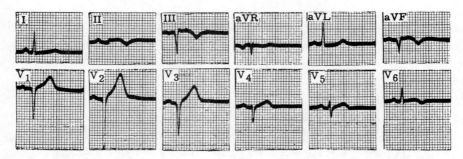

In comparison with the tracing at the bottom of p 371, a QS complex with slight ST elevation and T wave inversion is now present in aVF. The previously inverted T waves are now upright in leads I, aVL, and V$_{3-5}$.

Interpretation: (See p 183.) Recent inferior wall infarction; old anterior wall infarction.

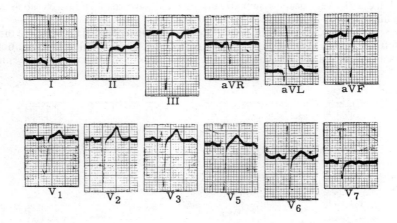

Regular sinus rhythm; P–R = 0.14 s; QRS = 0.09 s; frontal plane QRS axis = −40 degrees. ST depression with inverted T is present in leads II and III. R in aVL = 17 mm. Precordial leads show persistent S waves in V$_{5-6}$ (clockwise rotation) which are the result of the superior frontal plane axis. The T is diphasic in V$_7$.

Interpretation: (See p 96.) Left ventricular hypertrophy. *Clinical diagnosis:* Hypertensive cardiovascular disease.

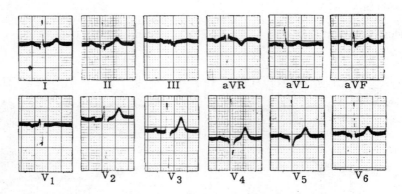

Regular sinus rhythm; P–R = 0.16 s; QRS = 0.08 s; frontal plane axis = +20 degrees.
Interpretation: (See p 65.) Within normal limits.

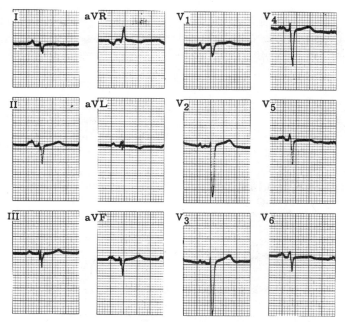

Regular sinus rhythm; the P waves are broad and notched in V_{3-6} with a wide, late negative deflection in V_1. The frontal plane QRS axis = −150 degrees with S waves in I, II, and III.

Interpretation: (See p 102.) Left atrial conduction defect which could represent left atrial hypertrophy; possible right ventricular hypertrophy. *Clinical diagnosis:* Mitral stenosis. This ECG was the initial clue to the diagnosis which was not apparent on physical examination owing to the obesity of the patient (375 lb).

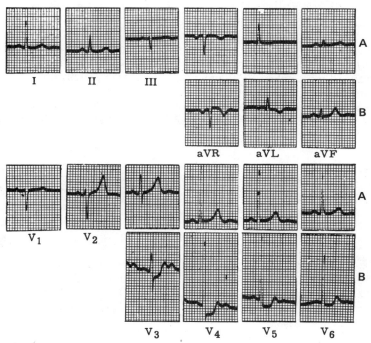

A: Regular sinus rhythm; P–R = 0.14 s; QRS = 0.06 s; frontal plane axis = +5 degrees; semihorizontal heart position. The T is flat in aVL. Precordial leads are normal. *B:* After exercise, there is horizontal ST depression in V_{3-6}; this is 4 mm in V_4; there is slight ST elevation in aVR; the T has become inverted in aVL.

Interpretation: (See p 147.) *A:* Borderline ECG; the flat T in aVL may be evidence of some lateral wall abnormality. *B:* The changes after exercise are consistent with coronary insufficiency (myocardial ischemia). *Clinical diagnosis:* Arteriosclerotic heart disease; anginal syndrome.

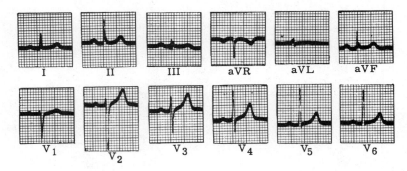

Regular sinus rhythm; P–R = 0.16 s; QRS = 0.06 s; frontal plane QRS axis = +50 degrees. *Interpretation:* (See p 67.) Within normal limits.

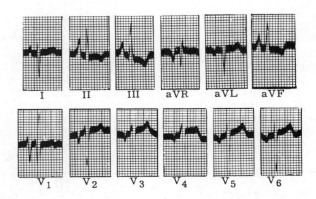

Regular sinus rhythm; P–R = 0.12 s; QRS = 0.06 s; frontal plane QRS axis = +110 degrees. There are tall, slender P waves in leads II and III; ST depression and T wave inversion in leads II and III. A tall, slender P with depressed ST and inverted T is present in aVF. A prominent diphasic P is present in V_1. An rSR′ complex is seen in V_1 and a deep S in V_6. VAT in V_1 = 0.06 s.

Interpretation: (See p 88.) Right atrial hypertrophy; incomplete right bundle branch block which is probably indicative of right ventricular hypertrophy. *Clinical diagnosis:* Pulmonary fibrosis with right heart failure.

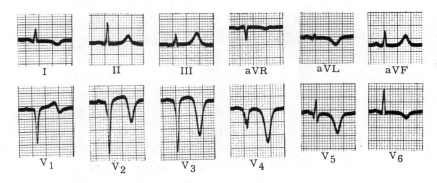

Regular sinus rhythm; P–R = 0.14 s; QRS = 0.08 s; frontal plane QRS axis = +60 degrees (semivertical heart position). There are QS complexes in V_{1-4}. There are deep, symmetrically inverted T waves in I, aVL, and V_{2-6}.

Interpretation: (See p 161.) Anterior wall infarction, late pattern (clinically 6 months old).

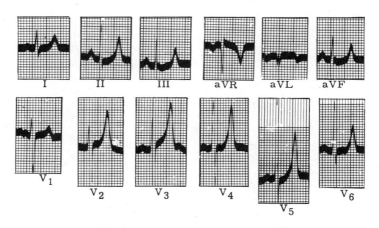

Regular sinus rhythm; P–R = 0.16 s; QRS = 0.06 s; frontal plane QRS axis = +70 degrees. The T waves are tall and slender in leads I, II, III, aVF, and V_{2-6}.

Interpretation: (See p 299.) The above record is consistent with hyperkalemia; however, such a pattern can be a normal variant.

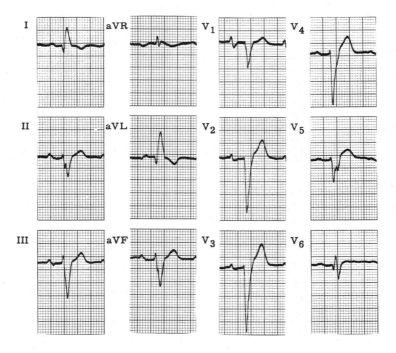

Regular sinus rhythm; P–R = 0.23 s; QRS = 0.15 s. The frontal plane QRS axis = −60 degrees. There are wide q waves in I, aVL, and V_6. The r waves in V_{1-5} are minute. There is ST depression and T wave inversion in I and aVL and ST elevation in V_{2-5}.

Interpretation: (See p 207.) Anterior and lateral myocardial infarction with peri-infarction block. *Clinical diagnosis:* Myocardial infarction, 1 year old. Large anterior ventricular aneurysm demonstrated by angiography.

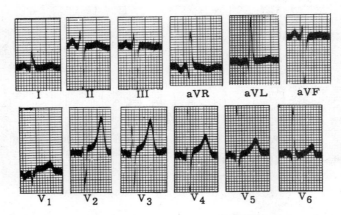

Regular sinus rhythm; P–R = 0.14 s; QRS = 0.08 s; frontal plane QRS axis = −75 degrees. The tall R wave in aVR is the result of the superior frontal plane axis. R in aVL = 16 mm. The precordial leads are normal.

Interpretation: (See p 94.) Left ventricular hypertrophy; left anterior fascicular block. *Clinical and autopsy diagnosis:* Hypertensive cardiovascular disease.

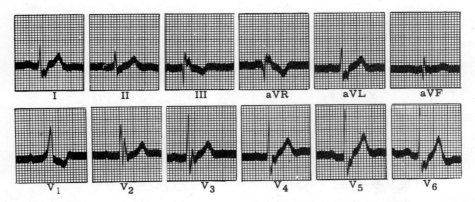

Regular sinus rhythm; P–R = 0.2 s; QRS = 0.15 s; there are wide S waves in leads I and V$_{5-6}$; a wide r in aVR; a wide, notched R in V$_1$; an RsR′ complex in V$_2$; VAT in V$_1$ = 0.09 s. The absence of an S wave in V$_1$ and the prominent initial R in V$_2$ indicate abnormally directed anterior vector forces.

Interpretation: (See p 195.) Possible posterior wall infarction; right bundle branch block. *Clinical diagnosis:* Myocardial infarction.

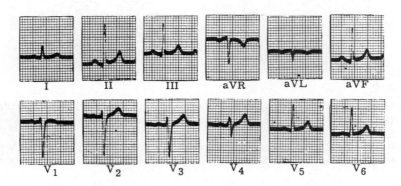

Regular sinus rhythm; P–R = 0.14 s; QRS = 0.08 s; frontal plane QRS axis = +70 degrees.
Interpretation: (See p 61.) Within normal limits.

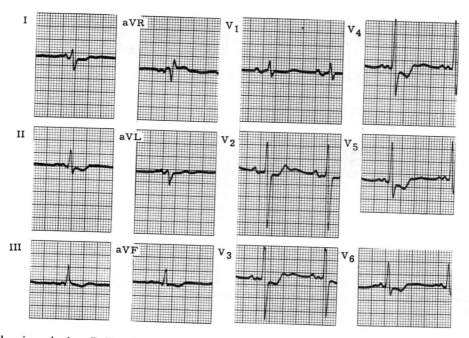

Regular sinus rhythm; P–R = 0.18 s; QRS = 0.09 s. The frontal plane QRS axis = +105 degrees. The P waves are notched in I and II with a wide, late negative deflection in V_1. The Rs ratio in V_1 = 2:1. There is ST depression in II, III, aVF, and V_{2-6}. Prominent U waves are seen in V_{4-6}.

Interpretation: (See p 102.) Right ventricular and left atrial hypertrophy. *Clinical diagnosis:* Mitral stenosis. The patient is on digitalis and quinidine therapy, which is responsible for the ST depressions and U waves.

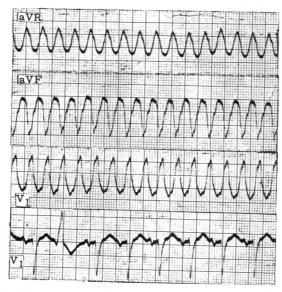

The ventricular rate is 240. The ventricular rhythm is slightly irregular. The QRS complexes are wide and slurred, upright in V_1. No definite evidence of atrial activity is seen.

Interpretation: (See p 260.) Paroxysmal ventricular tachycardia; the ectopic focus is in the left ventricle. In the bottom record, the rhythm has reverted to regular sinus with one left ventricular premature beat.

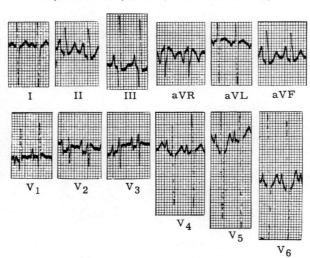

Regular sinus rhythm; rate = 177; P–R = 0.1 s; QRS = 0.06 s; frontal plane QRS axis = +105 degrees; tall P waves in leads II and III. A qR complex is seen in V_1; this initial q wave is abnormal in a 3-day-old infant.

Interpretation: (See p 104.) Right ventricular hypertrophy; probable right atrial hypertrophy; sinus tachycardia. *Clinical diagnosis:* Tetralogy of Fallot.

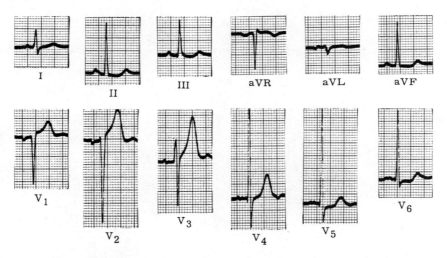

Regular sinus rhythm; P–R = 0.16 s; QRS = 0.09 s; frontal plane axis = +75 degrees; vertical heart position. The P waves are notched in all leads. $SV_1 + RV_5 = 55$ mm. There is ST depression in leads II, III, aVF, and V_{5-6}.

Interpretation: (See p 95.) Left ventricular and left atrial hypertrophy.

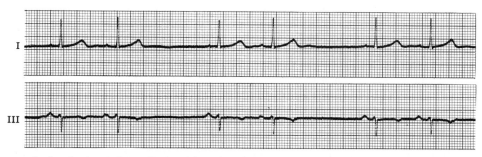

The ventricular rhythm is irregular in a bigeminal fashion. The P–P interval for conducted beats = 0.84 s. The interval between the conducted P and the nonconducted P = 0.48 s.

Interpretation: (See p 218.) The bigeminal rhythm suggests sinus rhythm alternating with atrial ectopic beats. However, all the P waves have the same morphology and the P–R intervals are constant. Atrial ectopic beats are seen superimposed upon the T wave preceding the longer pauses. The rhythm is therefore regular sinus with blocked atrial premature beats.

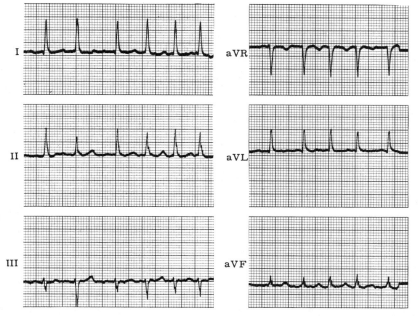

The ventricular rhythm is grossly irregular. The R–R intervals vary from 0.4–0.64 s. There is no regular atrial activity.

Interpretation: (See p 230.) Atrial fibrillation.

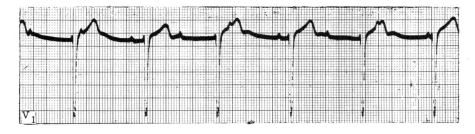

The atrial rhythm is regular at a rate of 72. The ventricular rhythm is regular at a rate of 54. There is no relation between the atrial and ventricular complexes. The QRS complexes appear normal.

Interpretation: (See p 240.) Third degree (complete) AV block; the ventricular pacemaker is close to the AV node.

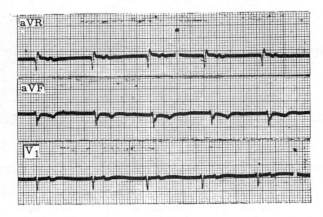

A regular ventricular rhythm is present with a rate of 70. No atrial activity precedes the QRS complexes. An atrial wave is seen following each QRS complex. The P′ is upright in aVR and inverted in aVF, indicating retrograde atrial conduction.

Interpretation: (See p 249.) AV junctional rhythm.

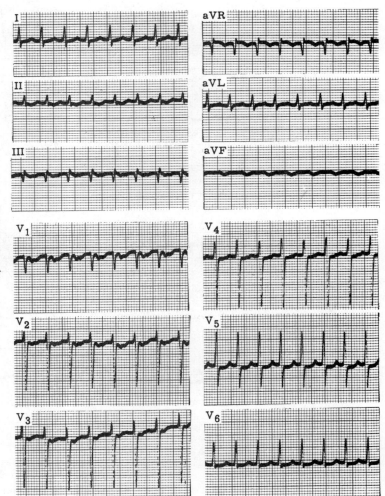

A regular ventricular rhythm is present at a rate of 188. The QRS complexes are of normal configuration. P′ waves are seen in V_{1-2}. There is minimal ST depression in precordial leads which may be the result of T_a waves.

Interpretation: (See p 250.) Paroxysmal supraventricular tachycardia.

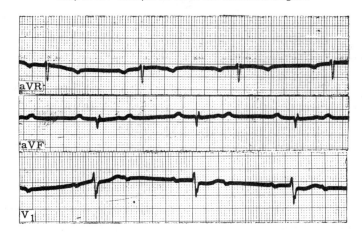

The atrial rhythm is regular at a rate of 82; the P waves are inverted in aVR and upright in aVF; the ventricular rhythm is regular at a rate of 41; there is a constant P–R interval of 0.3 s preceding each QRS complex. *Interpretation:* (See p 238.) Second degree AV block (2:1).

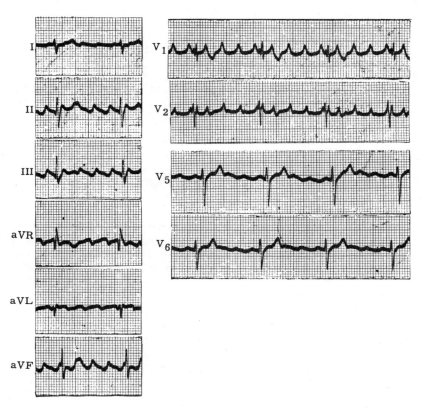

Atrial rate = 240 and regular; ventricular rate = 60 and regular; QRS = 0.08 s. The frontal plane QRS axis = +120 degrees. An rsr′ complex is seen in V₁. A deep S is present in V₆.

Interpretation: (See p 226.) Atrial tachycardia (or flutter) with 4:1 AV conduction; incomplete right bundle branch block. *Clinical diagnosis:* Mitral stenosis.

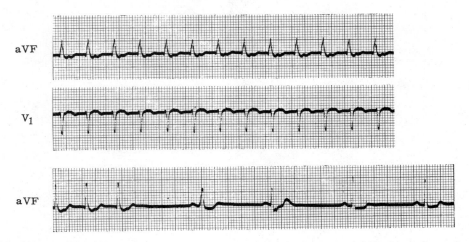

A regular ventricular rhythm is present. The rate is 150. A P wave is seen to follow each QRS complex. This could represent either a retrograde P wave from a pacemaker in the AV junction or an atrial stimulus producing ventricular activity after a P–R interval of 0.28 s. The bottom strip illustrates reversion to regular sinus rhythm with carotid pressure.

Interpretation: (See p 250.) Paroxysmal supraventricular tachycardia.

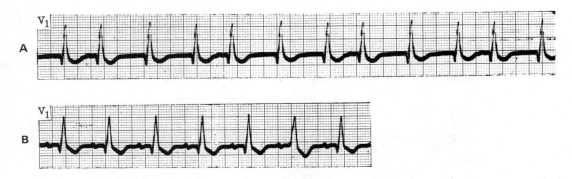

A: The basic rhythm is AV junctional at a rate of 86. An independent atrial rhythm is present at a rate of 30. On occasion (second, fifth, eighth, and eleventh complexes), the ventricle responds to the atrial stimulus. *B:* Regular sinus rhythm; rate = 86; QRS = 0.12 s; an initial deep q wave precedes the tall, wide R wave.

Interpretation: (See pp 194 and 270.) *A:* Incomplete AV dissociation. *B:* Right bundle branch block; anterior wall infarction.

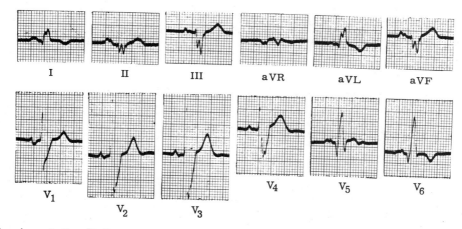

Regular sinus rhythm; P–R = 0.16 s; QRS = 0.17 s. The frontal plane QRS axis = −45 degrees. The R waves are notched and wide in leads I, aVL, and V_{5-6}. Initial q waves and inverted T waves are present in these leads.

Interpretation: (See p 196.) The initial q waves in left ventricular leads indicate that this is not an uncomplicated left bundle branch block. It is consistent with an anterolateral myocardial infarction with a marked intraventricular conduction defect (peri-infarction block). *Autopsy diagnosis:* Extensive, diffuse myocardial fibrosis due to coronary arteriolar disease in a 35-year-old man. Unfortunately, the presence or absence of a left bundle branch block was not determined by the autopsy examination.

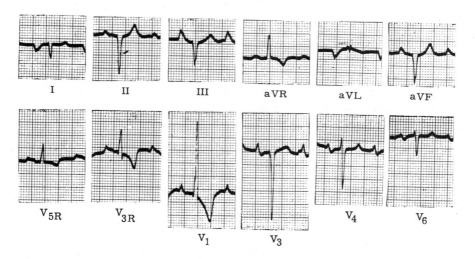

Regular sinus rhythm; P–R = 0.2 s; QRS = 0.08 s. The record is technically correct. Frontal plane QRS axis = −120 degrees (+240 degrees). The P waves are broad and large; they are inverted in I and upright in aVR. Leads aVR and aVL would appear more nearly normal if they were reversed. There are tall R waves in V_1, V_{3R}, and V_{5R}, with ST depression and T wave inversion in these leads.

Interpretation: (See pp 79 and 103.) Dextrocardia; right ventricular and right atrial hypertrophy. *Clinical diagnoses:* Situs inversus; Eisenmenger's syndrome (systolic pulmonary artery pressure = 110 mm Hg) due to an interventricular septal defect.

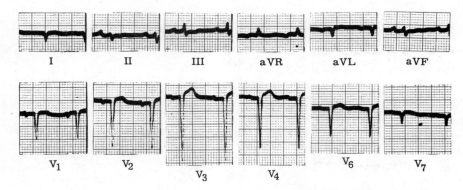

Regular sinus rhythm; P–R = 0.17 s; QRS = 0.06 s; rate = 90. QS complexes are present in leads I, aVL, and precordial leads. A prominent R is seen in aVR.

Interpretation: (See p 191.) The pattern is consistent with anterior wall infarction. However, this could represent right ventricular hypertrophy and dilatation. *Autopsy diagnosis:* Right ventricular hypertrophy and dilatation secondary to severe pulmonary emphysema; no evidence of infarction.

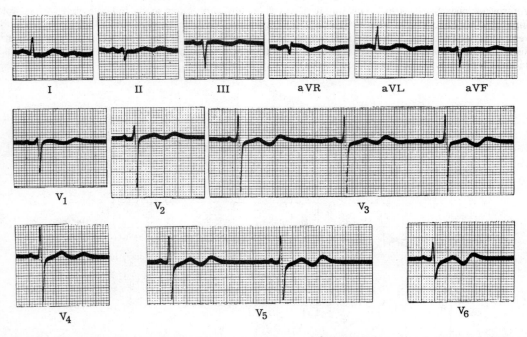

Regular sinus rhythm; P–R = 0.16 s; QRS = 0.1 s. The frontal plane QRS axis = −40 degrees. There is ST depression in leads I, aVL, and V$_{3-6}$. Prominent U waves are seen in all precordial leads. The measured Q–T interval = 0.51 s; but when corrected for a heart rate of 37, the Q–T$_c$ = 0.39 s.

Interpretation: (See p 302.) Hypokalemia. *Clinical diagnosis:* Cushing's syndrome due to adrenal hyperplasia (serum potassium = 2.5 mEq/L).

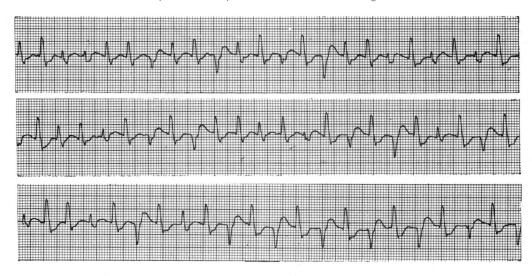

A bizarre tachycardia with a ventricular rate of 182 which is slightly irregular is present. No atrial activity can be identified. The QRS complexes are broadened and vary in configuration and polarity. There are periods of alternating direction of the QRS (right half of bottom strip).

Interpretation: (See p 283.) Ventricular tachycardia with periods of bidirectional ventricular tachycardia is a likely diagnosis. Clinically, the patient was not in digitalis toxicity.

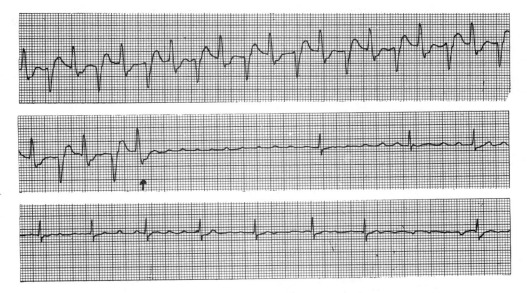

Continued record of the above patient with right carotid pressure (arrow): This results in the following changes: (1) abrupt slowing of the ventricular rate to a slow, irregular rhythm; (2) the QRS complexes become normal in duration and appearance; and (3) definite atrial activity is evident but with some fluctuation in the atrial rate and polarity. The original pattern returned when carotid pressure was released. This same phenomenon was repeated on 5 occasions, indicating that the response was not fortuitous.

Interpretation: (See p 284.) Supraventricular tachycardia with varying aberrancy of intraventricular conduction. The changing atrial rate and polarity during carotid pressure are probably the result of alterations in vagal tone. (All ECGs are lead II.)

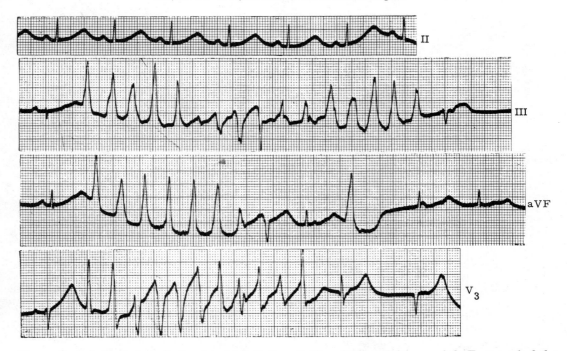

There are periods of sinus rhythm in which P–R = 0.18 s, QRS = 0.06 s, and Q–T$_c$ exceeds 0.6 s. Interspersed are periods of tachycardia with bizarre, wide, and changing QRS configuration.

Interpretation: (See p 296.) Ventricular tachycardia with borderline ventricular fibrillation. The prolonged Q–T interval during sinus rhythm should make one consider quinidine toxicity. *Clinical features:* The patient had been taking excessive doses of quinidine. Serum quinidine level was 19 mg/L (average therapeutic level, 4–8 mg/L). If this had not been appreciated, the patient could have been treated with quinidine for the ventricular arrhythmia with an almost certain fatality. He was treated with molar sodium lactate and recovered from the quinidine toxicity in 24 hours. This is an example of torsade de pointes.

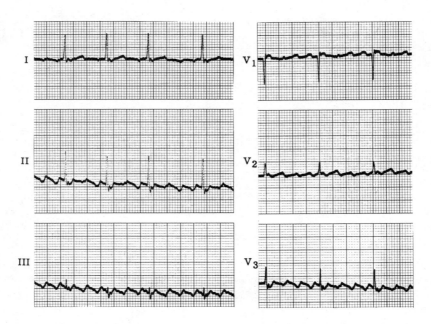

A regular atrial rhythm is present at a rate of 300. At times, there is 3:1 AV conduction with a ventricular rate of 100. At other times, there is 4:1 AV conduction with a ventricular rate of 75.

Interpretation: (See p 226.) Atrial flutter with varying 3:1 and 4:1 AV conduction.

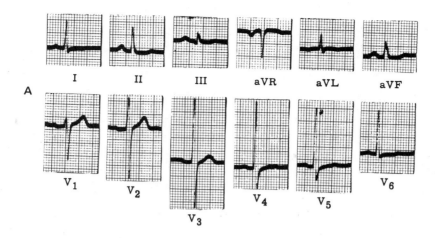

A: Regular sinus rhythm; P–R = 0.2 s; QRS = 0.08 s; the heart position is intermediate (frontal plane axis = +35 degrees). There is minimal ST depression with flattened T waves in I, aVL, and V_{4-6}.

Interpretation: Abnormal ECG indicating some abnormality of the left anterior-lateral myocardium but not diagnostic of any specific etiology. *Clinical features:* A 60-year-old man with typical angina of exertion; no evidence of previous infarction; above ECG taken when patient was asymptomatic.

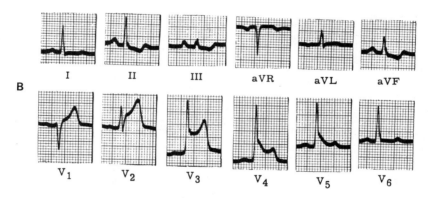

B: Nine days after (A): Marked changes have occurred since (A). There is marked ST elevation in leads V_{2-5} and ST depression in II, III, and aVF.

Interpretation: The ECG is consistent with very recent anterior wall infarction. However, it could represent the unusual variant of angina. The differential will be dependent upon clinical evaluation and serial ECGs. *Clinical features:* The above was taken at a time when the patient was experiencing anginal pain while at rest in bed. The pain lasted for 10 minutes and was promptly relieved by nitroglycerin. A repeat ECG taken after the pain had subsided was exactly the same as illustrated in (A). Serial ECGs over the next 2 months showed no change from (A). There were no clinical confirmatory signs of infarction. It must be concluded that ECG (B) represented the uncommon variant of angina (see p 145).

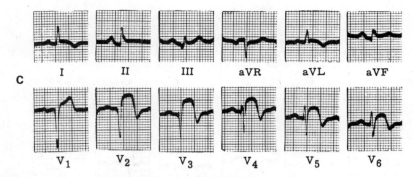

C

C: One year after (B): (See p 387.) QS complexes are now present in V_{1-3}; the ST segments are convexly elevated in I, aVL, and V_{1-6}, and the T waves are inverted in I, aVL, and V_{2-6}.

Interpretation: (See p 160.) Recent anterior wall infarction. *Clinical features:* The patient had suffered a myocardial infarct 2 days prior to the recording of the above ECG.

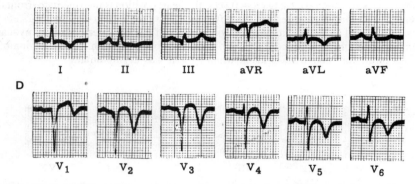

D

D: One month after (C): QS complexes present in V_{1-3}; the ST segments are now isoelectric; the T waves are deeply and symmetrically inverted in I, aVL, and V_{2-6}.

Interpretation: (See p 161.) Later pattern of anterior wall infarction. *Clinical features:* The patient had made an uneventful convalescence.

The above series of ECGs (A, B, C, D) not only illustrate the unusual variant of angina but also point out the prognostic significance of the former, ie, that myocardial infarction developed in that area of the myocardium (anterior wall) which previously showed evidence of severe myocardial ischemia.

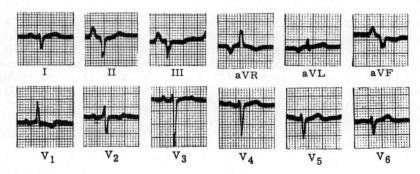

Regular sinus rhythm; P–R = 0.16 s; QRS = 0.08 s; the P waves are abnormally tall in II, III, and aVF; the QRS in the frontal plane is oriented to the right (deep S in I) and superiorly (QS complexes in II, III, and aVF) with a mean axis of −110 degrees. A tall R wave is seen in V_1.

Interpretation: (See p 191.) Right atrial and right ventricular hypertrophy. The QS complexes need not indicate inferior myocardial infarction. *Clinical and autopsy findings:* Marked right atrial and right ventricular hypertrophy and dilatation due to severe chronic lung disease. No infarction was present.

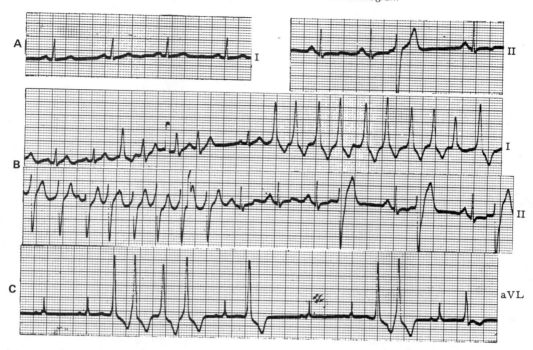

Records (A), (B), and (C) were recorded at different times during a 1-day period. Isolated ventricular ectopic beats, ventricular bigeminy, and runs of ventricular tachycardia are present.

Interpretation: (See p 258.) Ventricular arrhythmia manifested by isolated ventricular ectopic beats, ventricular bigeminy, and ventricular tachycardia. *Clinical diagnosis:* Idiopathic myocardiopathy. The patient had received no drug therapy prior to this record.

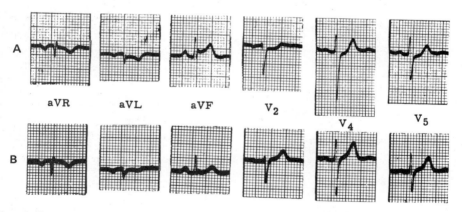

A: Taken during an episode of nocturnal chest pain. ST elevation is seen in aVF; ST depression is seen in all the other selected leads. *B:* Taken 5 minutes after above record, at which time pain has gone. The record is normal. All records taken before and for days afterward remained normal.

Interpretation: (See p 145.) There is evidence of an acute current of injury involving the inferior wall. The record in (A) could represent early inferior wall infarction. However, since the ST changes returned to normal within 5 minutes and subsequent tracings remained normal, it is indicative of acute, severe myocardial ischemia. *Clinical diagnosis:* Angina pectoris; this occurred only at rest. There was no exertional angina, and an exercise ECG was normal.

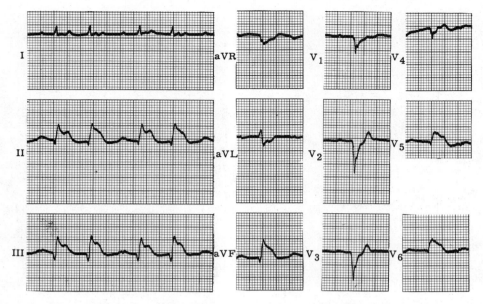

The ventricular rhythm is irregular. The P–P interval = 0.4 s. There is progressive lengthening of the P–R interval with occasional blocked ventricular response. There are wide q waves in III and aVF and QS complexes in V_{1-4}. The ST segment is markedly elevated in II, III, aVF, and V_{5-6}, and depressed in aVL and V_{1-2}.

Interpretation: Second degree AV block of the Wenckebach type, Mobitz I (see p 239); acute inferior and lateral myocardial infarction (see p 171); old anterior wall infarction (see p 160).

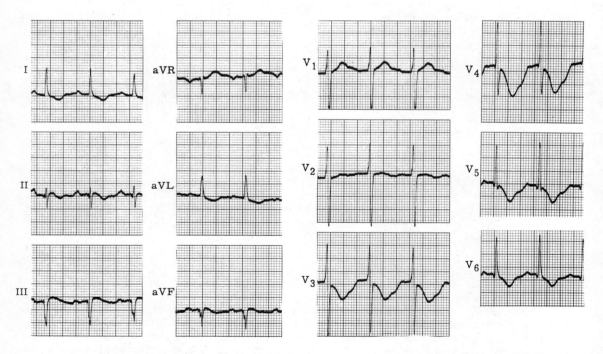

Regular sinus rhythm; rate = 90; P–R = 0.2 s; QRS = 0.08 s. A small q wave is present in lead II with QS complexes in leads III and aVF. There is ST depression and T wave inversion, most marked in leads V_{2-5}, with marked prolongation of ventricular repolarization. Q–T = 0.5 s and Q–T_c = 0.59 s.

Interpretation: (1) The marked ST–T and Q–T abnormalities are consistent with cerebral disease. (2) Probable old inferior wall infarction. *Autopsy diagnosis:* Massive intracerebral hemorrhage (see p 299) and old inferior myocardial infarction.

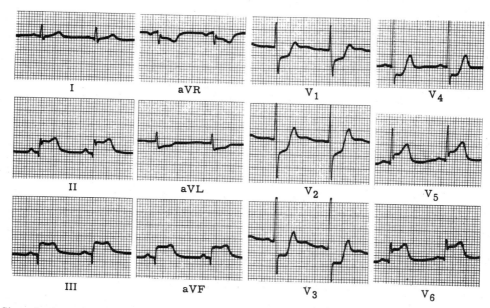

A: Sinus rhythm: rate = 75; P–R = 0.14 s; QRS = 0.08 s; frontal plane axis = +10 degrees. There are deep Q waves in leads II, III, and aVF. There is marked ST segment elevation in leads II, III, aVF, and V_{5-6} with ST segment depression in leads V_{1-4}.

Interpretation: Acute inferior-posterior-lateral myocardial infarction. The ST elevations indicate an acute current of injury involving the inferior and lateral walls, and the ST depression is due to a similar current of injury on the posterior wall.

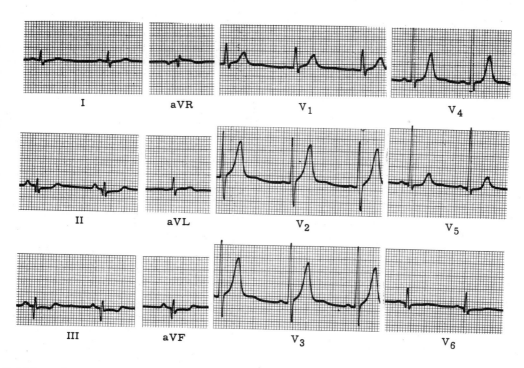

B: This tracing was recorded one week after (A). Prominent Q waves persist in II, III, aVF, and V_6. The ST segment changes have largely resolved. The R:S ratio in V_1 has increased, and the T waves are abnormally tall in V_{1-4}.

Interpretation: (See p 176.) Late pattern of inferior-posterior-lateral myocardial infarction.

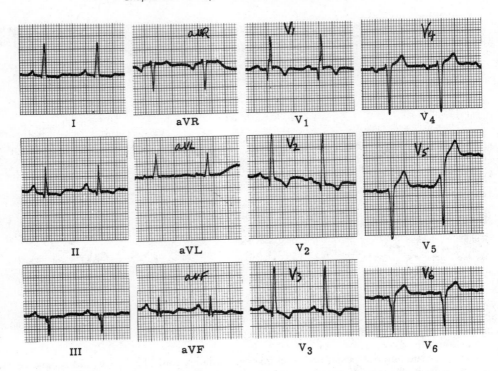

Regular sinus rhythm; rate = 75; P–R = 0.22 s; QRS = 0.08 s; frontal plane axis = +15 degrees. There are qR complexes in V_{1-3} with small r waves in V_{4-5} and a QS complex in V_6. The T waves are inverted in I, II, aVF, and V_{1-3}.

Interpretation: This tracing cannot be interpreted. Of all the precordial leads, the one labeled V_4 has a diphasic P wave that is most typical for V_1. The precordial leads have been misplaced. Leads labeled on V_{4-6} are actually V_{1-3} and leads labeled V_{1-3} are V_{4-6}. When one makes this adjustment, the diagnosis of anterior (and lateral) infarction becomes evident. This was confirmed by a properly taken ECG and illustrates a not uncommon error that occurs when all precordial leads are placed on the chest at one time (see p 9).

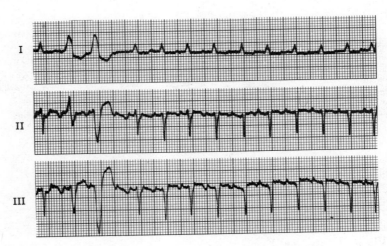

Regular ventricular rhythm, rate = 150. For most of the record a single P wave is seen preceding each QRS. In the initial portion of the record 2 ventricular ectopic beats are seen. The second is followed by a pause during which atrial activity is seen at a rate of 300. The frontal plane axis = −70 degrees.

Interpretation: Atrial flutter with 2:1 AV conduction; multiformed ventricular ectopic beats; left anterior fascicular block. In the absence of the ventricular ectopy the record could have been misinterpreted as sinus tachycardia or atrial tachycardia with 1:1 conduction (see p 227).

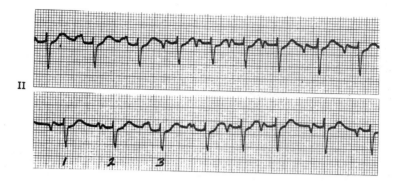

II

The ventricular rhythm is irregular. Each QRS complex is preceded by a P wave, but the P waves have varying morphology. This is a continuous recording of lead II.

Interpretation: (See p 244.) Periods of sinus rhythm (as complex 3) with first degree AV block (P–R = 0.24 s). Interspersed are periods of AV junctional rhythm (as complex 1). Other P waves (as complex 2) show a different morphology and represent fusion beats between the sinus P wave and the inverted P wave of AV junctional origin. This arrhythmia resulted from digitalis toxicity.

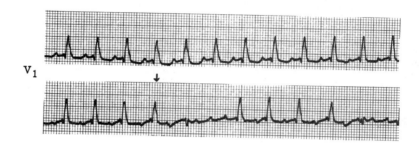

V_1

This is a continuous recording of lead V_1. The upper strip reveals a regular ventricular rhythm, rate = 135. A P wave precedes each QRS complex with a P–R interval = 0.14 s. The ventricular depolarization complexes have an rsR′ morphology.

Interpretation: (See p 228.) The upper strip could be interpreted as either sinus tachycardia or atrial tachycardia. However, one cannot exclude the possibility of atrial flutter with 2:1 AV conduction (with one of the flutter waves buried in the ventricular complex). Carotid sinus massage (at arrow on bottom strip) increases the AV block and clearly demonstrates the flutter waves at a rate of 270. In addition, a right ventricular conduction delay is present.

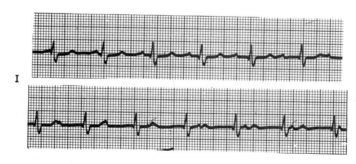

I

A regular ventricular rhythm is present, rate = 83. P waves are evident and are regular at a rate = 80 and are independent of the QRS complexes (continuous recording of lead I).

Interpretation: (See p 270.) If only a few complexes had been recorded (eg, the third, fourth, and fifth complexes in the top strip), this could have been misinterpreted as regular sinus rhythm. However, the longer strips prove complete AV dissociation, which was the result of digitalis toxicity.

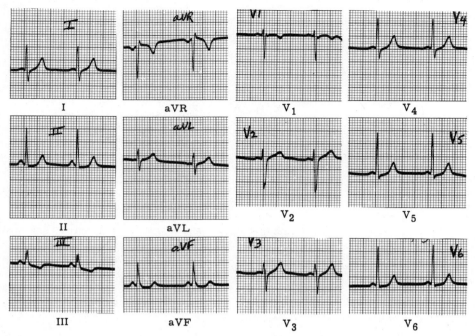

Regular sinus rhythm; rate = 75; P–R = 0.1 s, QRS = 0.08 s, frontal plane axis = +60 degrees. The QRS complexes are normal without delta waves. There is apparent ST segment depression in leads II, aVF, and V_{5-6}.

    Interpretation: (See p 275.) Lown-Ganong-Levine syndrome. The apparent ST depressions are due to atrial repolarization. The patient had episodes of paroxysmal atrial tachycardia.

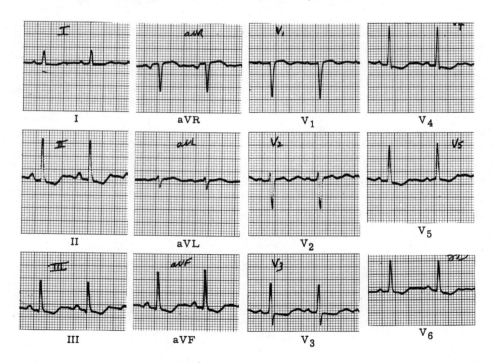

Sinus rhythm; rate = 85; P–R = 0.18 s; QRS = 0.08 s; frontal plane axis = +70 degrees. There are ST depressions in leads I, II, III, aVF, and V_{3-6}. There are prominent U waves, especially noted in V_{2-4}.

    Interpretation: (See p 302.) Nonspecific ST depressions with prolongation of ventricular repolarization. Clinically, this was the result of large doses of a phenothiazine the patient was taking without medical supervision. After discontinuation of this drug, the ECG reverted to normal.

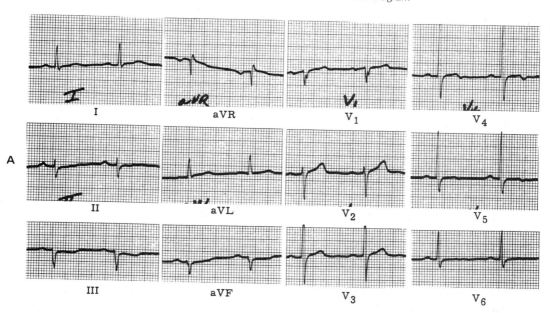

A: Sinus rhythm; rate = 65; P–R = 0.2 s; QRS = 0.08 s; frontal plane axis = −40 degrees. The T wave is diphasic in V_4 and flat in V_{5-6}.

Interpretation: Left anterior fascicular block; nonspecific lateral T wave changes. The patient had chest pain for 30 minutes prior to arrival in the emergency room but was pain-free at the time of the recording. He was admitted to the coronary care unit.

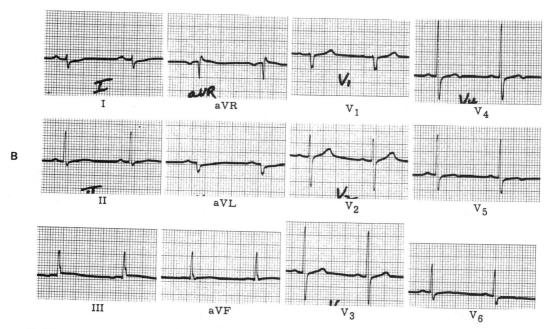

B: This tracing was taken 12 hours after (A). He had just had a recurrent bout of chest pain relieved by nitroglycerin. The major change has been a significant shift of the frontal plane QRS axis from −40 degrees (A) to +90 degrees (B). This immediately suggested an acute right ventricular overload probably secondary to pulmonary embolization. However, on more careful inspection it becomes apparent that leads aVL and aVF are reversed. This modifies the standard leads as follows: Lead I records LL-RA (II of [A]), lead II records LA-RA (I of [A]), and lead III records LA-LL (−III or mirror image of [A]). This was confirmed by a repeat, properly taken ECG.

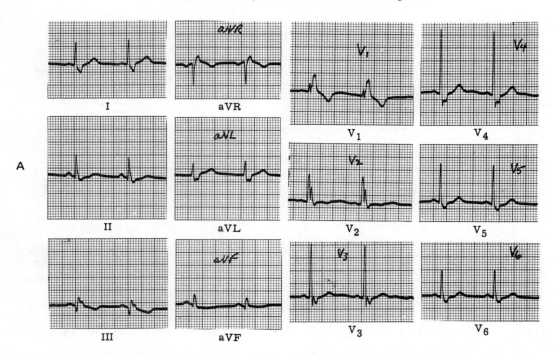

A: Sinus rhythm; rate = 75; P–R = 0.16 s; QRS = 0.14 s. There are wide S waves in leads I and V_{4-6} and a wide, tall R' wave in V_1.

Interpretation: (See p 115.) Right bundle branch block. *Clinical diagnosis:* Coronary artery disease with crescendo angina.

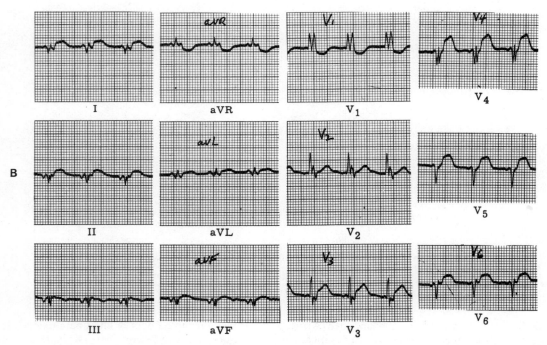

B: This tracing was recorded 1 week after (A). The following changes have occurred: (1) The P waves are now inverted in leads II and aVF and are upright in aVR; (2) P–R = 0.08 s; (3) new Q waves are present in I, aVF, and V_{4-6} with ST segment elevation in these leads; and (4) heart rate = 105.

Interpretation: (See pp 178 and 250.) AV junctional tachycardia; recent anterolateral and inferior (apical) myocardial infarction.

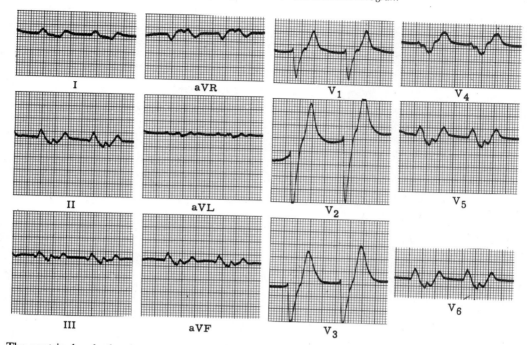

The ventricular rhythm is regular, rate = 80. No P waves are evident. The QRS interval = 0.2 s. The T waves are upright and relatively tall in all precordial leads.

Interpretation: (See p 300.) Hyperkalemia (serum potassium = 9.1 mEq/L). The absent P waves need not represent an AV junctional focus, but could be the result of sinoventricular rhythm. The above was the result of inadvertent use of potassium in a patient receiving spironolactone therapy.

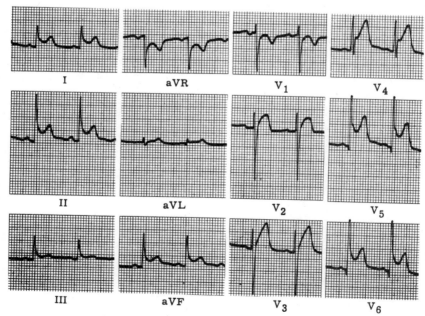

Sinus rhythm; rate = 95; P–R = 0.16 s; QRS = 0.08 s. There is concave ST segment elevation in leads I, II, III, aVF, and V$_{2-6}$. The ST segment is isoelectric in aVL and depressed in aVR and V$_1$.

Interpretation: (See p 285.) Acute pericarditis. The mean ST vector in the frontal plane is +60 degrees, resulting in an isoelectric ST segment in aVL, elevated ST segments in I, II, III, and aVF, and a depressed ST segment in aVR (cavity complex). The ST segment elevation in leads I and V$_{2-6}$ indicate an ST vector oriented anteriorly and leftward, resulting in ST depression in V$_1$ (cavity complex). *Clinical and autopsy diagnosis:* Acute purulent pericarditis secondary to staphylococcal aortic valve endocarditis with an aortic root abscess.

First Appendix:
Review of the Normal Electrocardiogram & Common Abnormalities

This appendix is offered as a simplified review of the normal ECG and the more common abnormalities recognized in clinical practice. Electrophysiologic explanations, clinical significance, and complex problems are purposely not included. This section is intended only as a review for the beginner; the reader should refer to the text for a more complete understanding of electrocardiography.

ment must be corrected for heart rate (Q–Tc). Use nomogram on p 27.

ST segment: The measurement from the end of the QRS complex to the beginning of the T wave. Usually isoelectric. May accept up to 1 mm elevation or 0.5 mm depression.

THE NORMAL ADULT ELECTROCARDIOGRAM

An ECG is a representation of the electrical forces of depolarization and repolarization of the heart. The conventional 12-lead ECG records these electrical forces along 12 different lead axes. Leads I, II, III, aVR, aVL, and aVF record events in the frontal plane. Leads V_{1-6} record events in the horizontal plane.

WAVES, COMPLEXES, & INTERVALS OF THE ELECTROCARDIOGRAM

P wave: The result of depolarization of right and left atria.

Ta (or Pt) wave: The result of atrial repolarization. This is usually not evident in the normal ECG.

QRS complex: The result of depolarization of right and left ventricles.

T wave: The result of ventricular repolarization.

U wave: Probably the result of normal late repolarization of ventricular Purkinje fibers.

P–R interval: The measurement from the beginning of the P wave to the beginning of the q wave (or R wave if q is not present). Normally 0.12–0.20 s.

QRS interval: The measurement from the beginning of the q wave to the end of the S wave. Up to 0.10 s.

Q–T interval: The measurement from the beginning of the q wave to the end of the T wave. Measure-

EVENTS OF THE ELECTROCARDIOGRAM

P wave: Upright in leads I, II, aVF, V_{2-6}; inverted in aVR; may be upright, diphasic, or inverted in III, aVL, and V_1.

Q waves:

1. A small q wave is commonly seen in leads I, II, aVF, and V_{4-6}. It is under 0.03 s in duration and is less than 25% of the height of the R wave in the same QRS complex. Q waves of varying size are normal in lead aVR.

2. A larger Q wave (ie, 0.04 s or more in duration or greater than 25% of the R) may be seen in lead III alone. Draw no conclusion from this finding alone. Abnormal Q waves must be present in aVF, in addition to III, for diagnostic significance.

3. Similarly, a larger Q wave in aVL may be normal. Draw no conclusion from this finding alone. Abnormal Q waves must be present in lead I or precordial leads for diagnostic significance.

4. A QS complex (entirely negative) is often a normal finding in V_1 and occasionally in V_2.

R wave: The R wave is the dominant (largest) wave in leads I and V_{4-6}. It is the dominant wave in leads I, II, and aVF in a vertical heart position and in leads I and aVL in a horizontal heart position. The r is small in V_1 and becomes progressively larger in leads V_{2-6}.

S wave: The S wave is the dominant wave in leads V_{1-3}. It becomes progressively smaller from V_{3-6}. S waves may be seen in leads I and II and are always smaller than the R wave in the respective lead. The S is the dominant wave in leads III and aVF in a horizontal heart position and in lead aVL in a vertical heart position. It is the dominant wave in aVR.

T wave: Upright in leads I, II, aVF, and V_{2-6} and

inverted in aVR. It may be upright, diphasic, or inverted in III, aVL, and V_1.

U wave: Often is not evident. When present, it is a small upright deflection of lower amplitude than the T wave in the same lead. It is usually best seen in leads V_{2-4}.

VARIATIONS OF THE ELECTROCARDIOGRAM

Because of many biologic variables, 100% of a selected normal population will not meet all the criteria given above. Approximately 2% will fall out of the average "normal" range and could be considered "abnormal" if this is not appreciated.

Infants: The ECG of a normal infant is typical of right ventricular hypertrophy using adult standards.

Children and young adults (up to about age 30): The ECG may have T inversion in leads V_{1-3}.

ST elevation: Elevation of ST segment greater than 1 mm with or without late T inversion in many leads (I, II, aVL, aVF, V_{3-6}). This is more commonly seen in young black adults.

ST depression: Depression of ST segment greater than 0.5 mm with or without T wave flattening or inversion may be seen in many leads in association with hyperventilation, anxiety, and 30–60 minutes after a high-carbohydrate meal.

Dextrocardia: In dextrocardia, a congenital anomaly, the alterations in the ECG are simply the result of the reversal of the polarity of the right-left lead axis (lead I). Therefore, lead I is the mirror image of the normal, and leads II-III and aVR-aVL are reversed. The precordial leads must be recorded over the right side of the chest.

Interchange of right and left arm electrodes in a normal person will produce the typical electrocardiographic findings of dextrocardia in frontal plane leads. However, precordial leads will be normal.

MEASUREMENT OF ELECTRICAL FORCES

The frontal plane axis is a measurement of the mean electrical forces in the frontal plane of the body (see p 29). Although it is most commonly used to express the mean frontal plane QRS axis, similar measurements are made for the P and T axes.

Mean P axis: The range of normal is 0 to +90 degrees. Therefore, the P is upright in leads I, II, and aVF and inverted in aVR. It may be upright, diphasic, or inverted in III and aVL. If the P axis is less than +30 degrees, the P will be inverted in lead III. If the P axis is greater than +60 degrees, the P will be inverted in aVL.

Mean QRS axis: The wide range of normal for all age groups is −30 to +110 degrees. The range in

individuals over the age of about 40 is −30 to +90 degrees. An axis greater than +90 degrees is right axis deviation. An axis above −30 degrees is a superior (or left) axis deviation. Either one implies an abnormal state.

Mean T axis: The range of normal is 0 to +90 degrees (similar to P).

QRS–T angle in frontal plane: The value of this angular measurement between the mean QRS axis and the mean T axis is normally less than 50 degrees.

ANALYSIS OF THE ELECTROCARDIOGRAM

Knowing the meaning of the various waves, complexes, and intervals and the range of normal for each, one is now prepared to analyze an ECG in the following manner.

Determine Heart Rate

A. Ventricular Rate: Measure the distance between one or more R waves and correct for rate per minute. One can use tables or scales (see inside back cover) to simplify this determination.

B. Atrial Rate: Will be the same as the ventricular rate if sinus rhythm is present. If the rhythm is not normal sinus and regular atrial activity is evident, measure the P–P interval and determine the atrial rate per minute.

Determine Rhythm

A. Sinus Rhythm: Regular and equal atrial and ventricular rates; P waves are normal; the P–R interval is normal.

1. Sinus bradycardia–Sinus rhythm, rate less than 60.

2. Sinus tachycardia–Sinus rhythm, rate greater than 100.

3. Sinus arrhythmia–Sinus rhythm with cyclic variations in rate usually related to respiration. The rate increases with inspiration and slows with expiration.

B. AV Block:

1. First degree–Sinus rhythm, P–R interval greater than 0.21 s.

2. Second degree–At regular or irregular intervals, a P wave is not followed by a QRS complex, ie, there is a dropped beat. The P–P interval is constant.

a. Mobitz I (Wenckebach)–Cyclically there is progressive lengthening of the P–R interval from beat to beat until a P wave is not followed by a QRS.

b. Mobitz II–In a regular sequence (eg, 2:1, 3:1) or in an irregular sequence (eg, 3:2, 4:3, etc), a P wave is not followed by a QRS. The P–R interval for the conducted beats is constant.

3. Third degree–Complete dissociation between atrial and ventricular rhythms. The atrial rhythm may be normal sinus or any atrial arrhythmia, but in either event the atrial impulse does not capture the ventricle.

Ventricular depolarization (the QRS) is initiated by a secondary pacemaker either in the AV junction, resulting in a regular ventricular rhythm, rate = 50–60±, with normal-appearing QRS complexes, or in the ventricle (idioventricular), resulting in a regular rhythm, rate = 30–40±, with wide, slurred, or notched QRS complexes.

C. Atrial Arrhythmias:

1. SA block–Periods in which there is disappearance of P waves and total absence of electrical activity for many seconds. Sinus rhythm then usually resumes or a second pacemaker in the AV junction (junctional escape beats) or in the ventricle (ventricular escape beats) induces ventricular depolarization. The QRS complexes will be normal in appearance with junctional escape beats.

2. Atrial premature (ectopic) beats–A P wave occurs prematurely (ie, at an interval shorter than the basic P–P interval) and is followed by a normal-appearing QRS–T complex. A pause which is different from the normal R–R interval follows this beat. The P–R interval of the premature beat may be the same as, longer than, or shorter than the P–R interval of the sinus-conducted beats.

a. High atrial focus–The direction of the P is normal, ie, the P is upright in I and aVF.

b. Low atrial focus–The P wave is inverted in II, III, and aVF. The P–R interval is usually shorter than that of the sinus beat. These beats are indistinguishable from those arising in the AV junction.

c. Blocked atrial beats–A premature P wave occurs shortly after the preceding QRS, in which instance the AV node is still refractory from the previously conducted beat and therefore blocks conduction into the ventricles.

d. Wandering atrial pacemaker–The ventricular rhythm may be regular or irregular. Each QRS is preceded by a P wave of varying configuration and changing P–R intervals.

3. Atrial tachycardia–There is regular atrial activity (ie, a constant P–P interval, and the atrial rate is 160–220±). The P wave axis may be normal, indicating a high atrial focus, or the P may be inverted in II, III, and aVF, indicating a low atrial (or AV junctional) focus.

a. Atrial tachycardia with 1:1 conduction–Each P wave is followed by a QRS complex.

b. Atrial tachycardia with AV block–Most commonly, 2:1 AV block is present with a resulting ventricular rate one-half the atrial rate. Less commonly, other ratios of AV block occur (ie, 3:1, 4:1, 3:2, etc).

c. Chaotic (multifocal) atrial tachycardia–A tachycardia characterized by a ventricular rate of 120 or greater. A P wave precedes each QRS complex, the P waves vary in configuration and direction, the P–R intervals vary, and the ventricular rhythm may be irregular because of the changing P–R interval and the presence of blocked atrial beats.

4. Atrial flutter–There is evidence of regular atrial activity (ie, a constant P–P interval) and an atrial rate of 260–320±. The P waves have a "sawtooth" configuration and usually appear to be inverted in II, III, and aVF. AV block is present, most commonly 2:1 or 4:1, producing a slower and regular ventricular rhythm. On occasion, the degree of AV block may be variable (ie, 2:1, 3:1, 4:1, etc), producing an irregular ventricular response.

5. Atrial fibrillation–There is no regular atrial activity. Instead, there are a multitude of deflections seen in the base line of the ECG. The ventricular rhythm is grossly irregular.

Atrial fibrillation with regular ventricular rhythm is indicative of complete AV dissociation. Normal-appearing QRS complexes are indicative of an independent AV junctional rhythm. The ventricular rate is usually in the 50–100 range. In contrast, if the QRS complexes are wide, slurred, or notched, an idioventricular rhythm is present and the ventricular rate is usually less than 50.

D. AV Junctional Rhythms:

1. Junctional ectopic beats–Indistinguishable from low atrial ectopic beats (see above).

2. Junctional rhythm–A regular atrial rhythm with 1:1 AV conduction at a rate of 50–100. The P waves are inverted in II, III, and aVF. The P–R interval is usually short but may be normal, or the P wave may follow the QRS complex. On occasion, the P wave is "buried" in the QRS complex and not visible.

3. Junctional tachycardia–Similar to junctional rhythm, but the rate is 120–200.

E. Ventricular Rhythms:

1. Ventricular premature (ectopic) beats–In the presence of sinus rhythm, a ventricular premature beat is evidenced by a wide, notched, or slurred QRS which is not preceded by a P wave and occurs prematurely in relation to the R–R interval.

a. Unifocal–All the QRS complexes of the ventricular premature beats have the same appearance in a single lead.

b. Multifocal–The QRS complexes of the ventricular ectopic beats vary in configuration and direction in a single lead.

c. More "dangerous"–A ventricular premature beat which occurs on the peak or downstroke of the preceding T wave.

2. Ventricular tachycardia–A run of 3 or more consecutive ventricular ectopic beats. The ventricular rate is usually in the 140–200 range and may be slightly irregular. Usually no P waves are seen. On occasion, one may identify completely independent, regular P waves of sinus origin.

3. Idioventricular rhythm–A regular or slightly irregular ventricular rhythm at a rate of 30–40. Independent sinus rhythm or any atrial mechanism may coexist.

4. Accelerated idioventricular rhythm–The same as idioventricular rhythm except the ventricular rate = 60–120.

5. Ventricular fibrillation–A rapid, irregular wavy electrocardiographic recording. ***This is cardiac arrest.***

6. Ventricular asystole–Absence of ventricular complexes for seconds to minutes. *This is cardiac arrest.*

F. Aberrancy of Intraventricular Conduction in Atrial Arrhythmias: This is one of the most difficult areas in interpretation. Differential diagnosis between such arrhythmias and ventricular arrhythmias may be impossible without the use of clinical measures (eg, response to vagal maneuvers) or intracardiac or esophageal electrocardiography.

1. Atrial ectopic beats with aberrancy–In the presence of sinus rhythm, a premature P consistently precedes the QRS complex, which is wide, slurred, and notched and morphologically resembles a ventricular ectopic beat. Most commonly this beat has an rSr′ configuration in V_1.

2. Aberrancy in the presence of atrial fibrillation–Sporadic QRS complexes resembling ventricular ectopic beats will be seen. Although not absolute, an rSr′ morphology in V_1 and the appearance of such a beat after a short R–R interval preceded by a long R–R interval favor aberrancy over ventricular ectopy.

3. Atrial tachyarrhythmias (tachycardia, flutter, or fibrillation) with aberrancy–A major problem in differentiation from ventricular tachycardia. It is often necessary to perform intra-atrial or esophageal ECGs or bundle of His recordings to make a definitive diagnosis.

G. Preexcitation Syndromes:

1. Wolff-Parkinson-White (WPW) syndrome–The ECG is characterized by (1) a short P–R interval, usually 0.1 s or less, with a normal P wave axis, and (2) initial slurring of the upstroke of the R wave (delta wave) or of the downstroke of a Q wave. This prolongs the QRS interval and is often associated with ST depression and T wave inversion.

2. Lown-Ganong-Levine (LGL) syndrome–The ECG is characterized by a short P–R interval, 0.1 s or less, a normal P axis, and normal QRS–T complexes.

ABNORMAL PATTERNS OF THE ELECTROCARDIOGRAM

RECOGNITION OF HYPERTROPHY

Left Atrial Hypertrophy

Broad, upright, and notched P waves are evident in many frontal plane leads and V_{4-6}. Of major importance is a diphasic P in V_1 in which the terminal portion of the P is negative (at least 1 mm) and broad (at least 0.04 s).

Right Atrial Hypertrophy

Tall (over 2.5 mm) and peaked P waves in II, III, and aVF.

Left Ventricular Hypertrophy
  A. Voltage criteria (valid only over age 35):
    1. RI + SIII > 26 mm.
    2. RaVL > 11 mm.
    3. RV_5 or RV_6 > 26 mm.
    4. SV_1 + RV (or RV) > 35 mm.
  B. ST depression and T wave inversion in those leads with high QRS voltage.
  C. Frontal plane QRS axis superior to −30 degrees; this may be present but is not essential diagnostically.
  D. Slight to moderate prolongation of QRS interval (0.1–0.12 s) may be seen.

Right Ventricular Hypertrophy
  A. Right axis deviation: Mean frontal plane QRS axis greater than +110 degrees in infants and young children; greater than +90 degrees in adults over about age 40.
  B. Tall R wave in V_1 (and V_2): RV_1 greater than 5 mm and R:S ratio in V_1 greater than 1. This is most commonly seen in children or young adults with congenital or acquired heart diseases which result in right ventricular hypertrophy.
  C. ST depression and inverted T waves in V_{1-3}.
  D. In contrast to B above, right ventricular hypertrophy acquired late in life (eg, cor pulmonale in adults over about age 60) is commonly characterized by small or absent r waves in V_{1-3}, and the ECG mimics anterior myocardial infarction.
  E. The association of criteria for left or right atrial hypertrophy aids in the recognition of right ventricular hypertrophy.

Biventricular Hypertrophy
  Uncommonly recognized by ECG.
  A. Voltage criteria for left ventricular hypertrophy with ST depression and T wave inversion in leads V_{5-6}, plus
  B. A frontal plane QRS axis of +90 degrees or greater.

INTRAVENTRICULAR CONDUCTION DEFECTS

Bundle Branch Block
  A. Right bundle branch block (RBBB):
    1. QRS interval = 0.12 s or greater (complete RBBB); 0.1–0.12 s = incomplete RBBB.
    2. Wide, slurred S waves in leads I, V_{5-6}.
    3. Wide, slurred R′ waves in leads V_{1-2} (occasionally V_3).
    4. ST depression and T wave inversion in V_{1-2} (V_3).
  B. Left bundle branch block (LBBB):
    1. QRS interval = 0.12 s or greater (complete LBBB); 0.1–0.12 s = incomplete LBBB.

2. No q wave in leads I, V_{5-6}.
3. QRS complexes wide, notched, or slurred.
4. QRS upright in leads I, V_{5-6}.
5. ST depression and T wave inversion in leads I, V_{5-6}.

Peripheral Left Ventricular Conduction Defects

A. Left anterior fascicular block:
1. Frontal plane QRS axis greater than -30 degrees.
2. Dominant R wave in lead I.
3. R:S ratio in lead II is less than 1.
B. Left posterior fascicular block:
1. Frontal plane QRS axis greater than $+110$ degrees.
2. Must exclude right ventricular hypertrophy and lateral wall infarction by clinical evaluation.

Bilateral Bundle Branch Block

A. RBBB + left anterior fascicular block:
1. All the criteria given for RBBB, plus
2. Frontal plane QRS axis greater than -30 degrees.
B. RBBB + left posterior fascicular block:
1. All the criteria given for RBBB, plus
2. Frontal plane QRS axis greater than $+110$ degrees, plus
3. Absence of clinical evidence of right ventricular hypertrophy or lateral wall infarction.
C. RBBB plus first degree AV block.*
D. LBBB plus first degree AV block.*
E. Alternating RBBB and LBBB in single or serial records.

Trifascicular Block

A. RBBB, plus
B. Left anterior (or posterior) fascicular block.
C. First degree AV block.*

MYOCARDIAL ISCHEMIA

Myocardial ischemia, which is expressed clinically as angina, is associated with transient and reversible ST segment changes. More commonly, this involves the subendocardial region of the myocardium and is manifested by one of the following criteria: (1) ST segment depression of 1 mm or more in one or more leads. (2) The ST segment depression must be horizontal or downward sloping and have a duration of at least 0.08 s. (3) It is essential to differentiate the above from normal J point depression. The latter may begin 1–3 mm below the isoelectric line, but the ST segment is directed sharply in an upward direction. (4) The above criteria are also used to define a positive exercise ECG.

*This will often require His bundle recordings to prove the block is distal to the His bundle.

A less common electrocardiographic finding in myocardial ischemia is marked ST segment elevation in association with spontaneous angina or exercise testing. Up to 10 mm ST segment elevation may be seen. This disappears within minutes when the pain or exercise ceases. Ventricular arrhythmias often accompany the above.

Transient T wave inversions may be seen during periods of myocardial ischemia. However, in the evaluation of an exercise ECG, T wave changes alone, in the absence of above-described ST segment criteria, do not warrant the interpretation of a positive exercise test.

MYOCARDIAL INFARCTION

The typical sequence of events in the ECG as a result of acute transmural myocardial infarction are the following:

(1) ST segment elevation: This is the earliest sign of myocardial infarction and persists for a few days up to 2 weeks.

(2) Large ("giant," "hyperacute") upright T waves may be seen in those leads which show the ST elevation. This finding is usually gone within 24 hours.

(3) Over the course of 1–3 days, the T wave becomes inverted. This is usually maximal within 1–2 weeks, by which time the T wave is deeply and symmetrically inverted.

(4) Within 1–3 days, abnormal Q waves develop and are indicative of transmural infarction. The abnormal Q wave is defined by the following criteria:

(a) Q duration = 0.04 s or more.
(b) Q:R ratio = 25% or greater.
(c) A QS complex may be considered as equivalent to a Q wave.

Note: The above criteria, if present only in lead III, aVL, or V_1, is not diagnostic of infarction.

The localization of the site of myocardial infarction is made by applying the above criteria to specific leads:

Location of Infarction	Leads
Anterior	V_{2-4}
Inferior	aVF
Lateral	I, V_6
Posterior*	Tall R, upright T, V_{1-2}

*None of the leads of the conventional 12-lead ECG directly reflect the posterior wall of the left ventricle. A lead directly over an area of posterior wall infarction, such as an esophageal lead, would record the abnormal Q wave and ST–T changes. Leads directly opposite the posterior wall (ie, anterior leads V_{1-2}) will record a mirror image of the infarct pattern. There will be abnormally tall R waves (R:S ratio greater than 1 in V_1) and tall, upright T waves in V_{1-2}. In the early stage of infarction, the ST segment will be depressed in V_{1-2} (ie, the reciprocal of ST elevation on the posterior wall).

Later Sequence of Events

Over the course of months following an acute episode of transmural myocardial infarction, the above-described T waves gradually become upright. In a smaller percentage of such patients, the abnormal Q wave eventually disappears. Therefore, it is not uncommon (about 10%) to see a normal ECG months to years after a well-documented episode of transmural myocardial infarction.

SUBENDOCARDIAL MYOCARDIAL INFARCTION

It had been generally accepted that an abnormal Q wave is not seen in subendocardial infarction and that the only changes in the ECG consist of ST depression and T wave inversion. However, several autopsy studies have shown that subendocardial (nontransmural) infarction can produce abnormal Q waves and that transmural infarction need not be associated with an abnormal Q wave. Therefore, the electrocardiographic differentiation between transmural and nontransmural infarction is grossly inaccurate.

VENTRICULAR ANEURYSM

As stated above, ST segment elevation is an early sign of transmural myocardial infarction and is usually gone within 2 weeks. Persistence of this ST segment elevation for months to years following the acute event is indicative of a ventricular aneurysm. The absence of this finding does not exclude such a possibility.

DIFFERENTIAL DIAGNOSIS OF INFARCTION

Clinical conditions other than myocardial infarction result in ECGs which mimic myocardial infarction. Common examples are the following:

(1) **Left ventricular hypertrophy:** In 10–20% of patients with left ventricular hypertrophy (and autopsy documentation of the absence of infarction), there will be very small r waves or QS complexes in V_{1-3} simulating anterior wall infarction. The presence of voltage criteria for left ventricular hypertrophy will obviously favor the latter diagnosis but will not exclude the additional possibility of anterior infarction. Clinical evaluation and serial ECGs are needed to make this differentiation.

(2) **Pulmonary disease and cor pulmonale:** It is very common to see very small r waves or QS complexes in V_{1-3} which mimic anterior myocardial infarction. The presence of right axis deviation, P waves meeting criteria for right atrial hypertrophy, and low voltage of all complexes are features which favor the diagnosis of pulmonary disease. Less commonly, patients with severe pulmonary disease (and autopsy documentation of the absence of infarction) will show abnormal Q waves in aVF simulating inferior wall infarction, or abnormal Q waves in lead I simulating lateral wall infarction. Pulmonary emphysema often produces a superior (left) axis deviation greater than -30 degrees. This is not due to a lesion in the left anterior fascicle.

(3) **Left bundle branch block:** Very small r waves or QS complexes are commonly present in V_{1-3}. There is often ST elevation in these leads. These findings are merely those of the LBBB alone. In most instances, in the presence of a typical LBBB, using the criteria given for such, it is impossible to make the electrocardiographic diagnosis of myocardial infarction.

(4) **WPW syndrome:** The delta wave in the ECG may be positive or negative. When negative, it records a slurred, wide Q wave. Such is common in leads II, III, and aVF. Once the ECG is recognized to be a WPW, no other electrocardiographic diagnosis should be made from that single record.

(5) **Right ventricular hypertrophy versus posterior myocardial infarction:** Both of these clinical states have abnormally prominent anterior QRS forces, ie, tall R waves in V_1 (R:S ratio > 1) and V_2. In right ventricular hypertrophy, the T wave is inverted and the ST segment depressed in V_{1-2}. In posterior myocardial infarction, the T wave is upright and often abnormally tall in these leads. P waves consistent with left or right atrial hypertrophy favor the probability of right ventricular hypertrophy. Right axis deviation may be present in either condition.

PERICARDITIS

(1) Initially there is ST segment elevation in all leads except aVR, aVL (in a vertical heart position), V_1, and V_2.

(2) Over the course of days, the ST segment returns to the isoelectric line and the T wave becomes inverted.

(3) Atrial arrhythmias are common.

(4) There are no changes in the QRS complex and no disturbance of AV or intraventricular conduction.

(5) The above-described ST–T changes do not occur in uremic pericarditis.

PERICARDIAL EFFUSION

In addition to the change associated with pericarditis, if such is present clinically, pericardial effusion will result in the following:

(1) Low voltage.

(2) Electrical alternans: This finding is not pathognomonic nor a very frequent finding but, when present, is most commonly associated with pericardial effusion. However, other myocardial diseases may also produce an electrical alternans.

Note: Electrical alternans, in association with supraventricular tachycardia, has no clinical significance.

MYOCARDITIS

A wide variety of electrocardiographic abnormalities may result from myocarditis, including the following:

(1) Those associated with pericarditis.

(2) AV or intraventricular conduction defects.

(3) Ventricular hypertrophy (usually left ventricular hypertrophy).

(4) Ventricular arrhythmias.

DRUG EFFECTS

Digitalis

A. **Effect:** The following are electrocardiographic changes which indicate that the patient is taking digitalis. They are not signs of toxicity nor do they correlate with the degree of clinical efficacy.
   1. ST segment depression, often having a "scooped" appearance.
   2. Slowing of the ventricular rate, especially in the presence of atrial fibrillation.
   3. Shortening of Q–T interval.

B. **Toxicity:** The following are signs of digitalis toxicity:
   1. Marked sinus bradycardia, rate under 50.
   2. First degree AV block, P–R greater than 0.24 s.
   3. Second–third degree AV block.
   4. Atrial tachycardia, most commonly with 2:1 AV conduction.
   5. Ventricular ectopic beats; bigeminy.
   6. Ventricular tachycardia.

Quinidine

A. **Effect:** The following effects on the ECG may or may not represent toxicity. Clinical evaluation is necessary to make this decision.
   1. ST depression and T wave flattening.
   2. Prolongation of ventricular repolarization with prominent U waves.

B. **Toxicity:** The following are definite electrocardiographic signs of quinidine toxicity:
   1. Prolongation of QRS interval: A 50% increase above the pretreatment interval.

2. AV block.
3. AV dissociation.
4. Ventricular ectopic beats.
5. Ventricular tachycardia.

Other Drugs

Other drugs such as procainamide, the phenothiazines, and tricyclic antidepressants have similar "quinidine-like" effects on the ECG.

ELECTROLYTE ABNORMALITIES

Hyperkalemia

With increasing levels of serum potassium, the following changes are seen:

A. Tall, slender, peaked T waves.

B. AV conduction defects.

C. Disappearance of P waves.

D. Widening of QRS interval.

E. Ventricular tachycardia, fibrillation.

Hypokalemia

With decreasing levels of serum potassium, the following changes are seen:

A. ST depression and lowering of T waves.

B. Prolongation of ventricular repolarization with large, upright U waves, best seen in leads V_{2-4}. This finding is identical to that produced by quinidine.

Hypercalcemia

Marked shortening of Q–T interval is seen. The ST segment, as a distinct isoelectric period, is eliminated as the T wave begins immediately at the end of the QRS.

Hypocalcemia

Prolongation of Q–T interval is seen owing to lengthening of the ST segment.

PROLONGED VENTRICULAR REPOLARIZATION

Prolongation of ventricular repolarization can result from Q–T prolongation alone (with or without ST prolongation) or the presence of an abnormal U wave that merges with or is separate from the T wave. The more common clinical causes are as follows:

(1) Myocardial ischemia.

(2) Drugs: Quinidine, procainamide, tricyclic antidepressants, phenothiazines.

(3) Hypokalemia and probably hypomagnesemia.

(4) Hypocalcemia (specifically prolongs the ST segment).

(5) Congenital syndromes.

(6) Central nervous system disease.

(7) Prolonged ventricular depolarization.

PROMINENT ANTERIOR QRS FORCES

This is defined by an R:S ratio in V_1 greater than 1. The common causes are as follows:

(1) Normal in infants and children.

(2) Cardiac displacement: Congenital or acquired.

(3) Incorrect lead placement.

(4) Right ventricular hypertrophy.

(5) Right bundle branch block.

(6) Posterior myocardial infarction.

(7) Preexcitation: Type A WPW.

(8) Left anterior conduction delay.

(9) Error in the indifferent electrode of the unipolar lead system.

Second Appendix:
Abnormalities & Differential Diagnosis of the Adult Twelve-Lead Electrocardiogram

The following is offered as a guide to the evaluation of electrocardiographic abnormalities. It is not intended as a complete diagnostic index since the diagnosis must always depend upon evaluation of the complete tracing in the light of the clinical findings. Even though many electrocardiographic tracings are considered "diagnostic," experience has shown that this is not always the case. The ECG is a laboratory test, and as such must be integrated with the clinical situation.

Many patients are made unnecessary cardiac invalids solely on the basis of an "abnormal" or "diagnostic" ECG. This appendix is intended to be used only as an aid in suggesting possible explanations of abnormal complexes. It is hoped that the reader will refer to the text for a more detailed explanation and, finally, correlate the clinical picture with the ECG before arriving at a final diagnosis.

P WAVE ABNORMALITIES

I. Abnormalities of P wave configuration and magnitude.

① Broad, notched P waves in leads I, aVL, and V_{4-6}. Diphasic P wave with broad negative deflection in lead V_1.

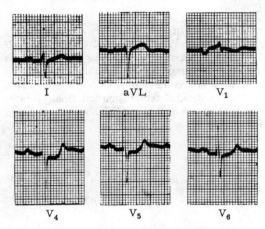

Left atrial hypertrophy (see p 87)

② Tall, peaked P waves in leads II, III, and aVF. Tall or diphasic peaked wave in lead V_1.

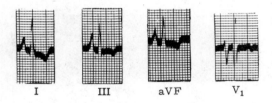

Right atrial hypertrophy (see p 88)

II. Abnormalities of direction of P wave.

① Inverted P wave in lead I. Upright P wave in lead aVR.

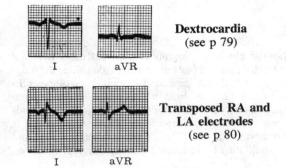

Dextrocardia
(see p 79)

Transposed RA and LA electrodes
(see p 80)

② Inverted P waves in lead aVF (also II and III); upright P waves in aVR.

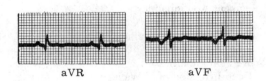

Ectopic atrial focus low in atrium or in AV junction (see p 217)

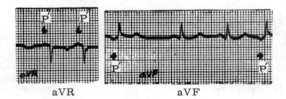

Low AV junctional rhythm (see p 247)

QRS COMPLEX ABNORMALITIES

I. Abnormal "mean" frontal plane direction with normal QRS duration.

(1) QRS upright in lead I. QRS diphasic; S > R in lead II. (Left [or superior] axis deviation [left anterior fascicular block].)

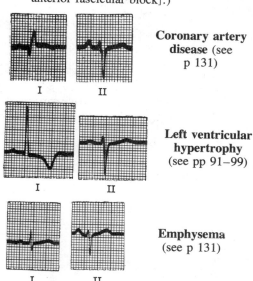

Coronary artery disease (see p 131)

Left ventricular hypertrophy (see pp 91–99)

Emphysema (see p 131)

Note: The above patterns may be seen in other myocardial diseases also.

(2) QRS upright, diphasic, or inverted in lead aVF. QRS diphasic; S > R in lead I. (Right axis deviation.)

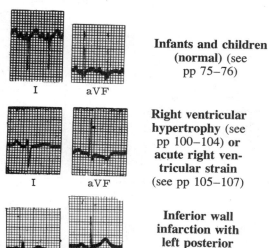

Infants and children (normal) (see pp 75–76)

Right ventricular hypertrophy (see pp 100–104) **or acute right ventricular strain** (see pp 105–107)

Inferior wall infarction with left posterior fascicular block (see pp 204–207)

II. Abnormal QRS duration (> 0.12 s).

(1) Wide S in leads I and V$_{4-6}$. Wide R' in lead V$_1$.

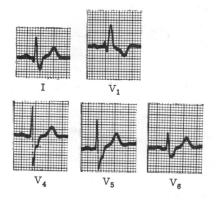

Right bundle branch block (see pp 114–122)

(2) Wide, notched RR' or RSR' in leads I and V$_{4-6}$, with absent q.

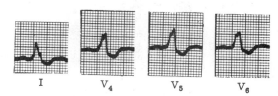

Left bundle branch block (see pp 123–131)

(3) Wide QRS complexes in all leads.

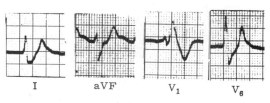

Hyperkalemia (see p 299–301)

Q WAVE ABNORMALITIES
(0.04 s or more in duration, or > 25% of R)

(1) Abnormal Q waves in leads II, III, and aVF.

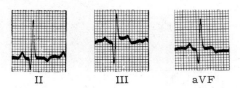

II   III   aVF

Inferior infarction (see pp 169–174)

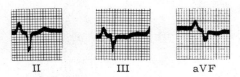

II   III   aVF

Pulmonary emphysema or right ventricular hypertrophy (see p 191–192)

(2) Abnormal Q waves in leads I, aVL, and V$_{4-6}$.

I   aVL

V$_4$ V$_5$ V$_6$

Anterior infarction (see pp 155–168)

(3) Abnormal Q waves in leads V$_{3R}$-V$_1$, V$_{1-2}$, V$_{1-3}$, or V$_{1-4}$.

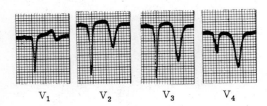

V$_1$ V$_2$ V$_3$ V$_4$

Anteroseptal infarction (see p 165)

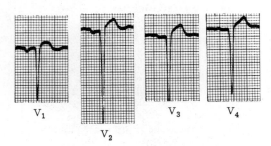

V$_1$ V$_2$ V$_3$ V$_4$

Left ventricular hypertrophy
(see p 190)

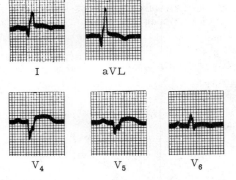

V$_1$ V$_2$ V$_4$

Left bundle branch block
(see pp 123–131)

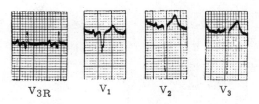

V$_{3R}$ V$_1$ V$_2$ V$_3$

Right ventricular hypertrophy
(see pp 102, 191, and 192)

QS COMPLEX ABNORMALITIES

(1) QS complex in leads V_{1-2}, V_{1-3}, or V_{1-4}.

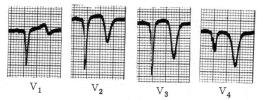

V_1 V_2 V_3 V_4

Anteroseptal infarction (see p 165)

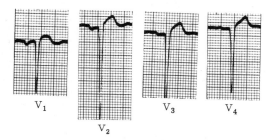

V_1 V_2 V_3 V_4

Left ventricular hypertrophy (see p 190)

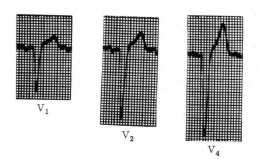

V_1 V_2 V_4

Left bundle branch block (see p 124)

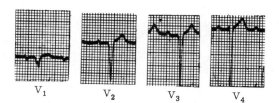

V_1 V_2 V_3 V_4

Right ventricular hypertrophy
(see pp 191–192)

(2) QS complex in leads I and $V_{1-3(4)}$.

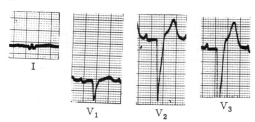

I V_1 V_2 V_3

Anterior infarction (see pp 155–168)

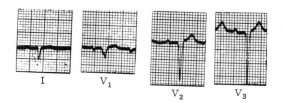

I V_1 V_2 V_3

Emphysema; right ventricular hypertrophy
(see pp 191–192)

(3) QS complex in leads II, III, and aVF.

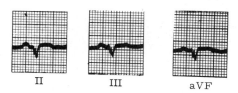

II   III   aVF

Inferior infarction (see pp 169–174)

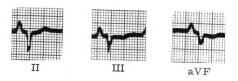

II   III   aVF

**Emphysema or right ventricular
hypertrophy** (see p 192)

ABNORMALITIES OF R WAVE MAGNITUDE

(1) R wave > 13 mm in aVL, or > 27 mm in V_5 or V_6, or > 35 mm in V_5 (or V_6) plus S in V_1.

(2) R wave > S in V_1.

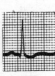

aVL

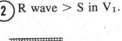

V_1

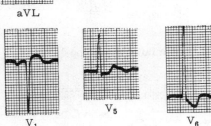

V_1 V_5 V_6

Left ventricular hypertrophy (with exceptions) (see p 91)

Right ventricular hypertrophy (especially if right axis deviation is present) (see p 100)

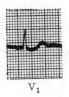

V_1

Posterior infarction (see pp 175–177)

(3) R wave > S in V_1 or V_2.

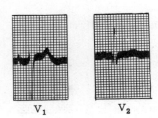

V_1 V_2

Dextroversion (see p 78)

S WAVE ABNORMALITIES
(See QRS complex, QS complex, and R wave.)

ST SEGMENT ABNORMALITIES

I. Elevation of ST segment. (Elevation of ST segment 1 mm or more.)*

1 Elevation of ST segment in all leads except aVR and V_1, and in aVL in a vertical heart.

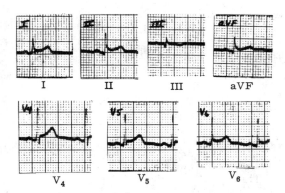

Pericarditis (see pp 285–287)

2 Elevation of ST segment in II, III, and aVF.

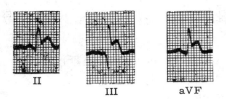

Inferior infarction (see p 173)

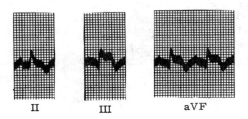

Ventricular aneurysm (see p 188)

3 Elevation of ST segment in I, aVL, and V_{4-6}.*

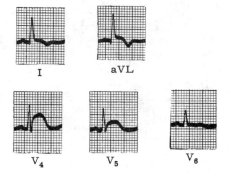

Anterior infarction (see pp 155–168)

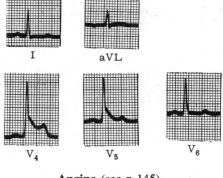

Angina (see p 145)

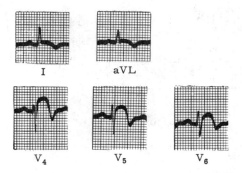

Ventricular aneurysm (see p 188)

II. Depression of ST segment.*

(1) Oblique or horizontal depression of ST in any lead except aVR and aVL with vertical heart.

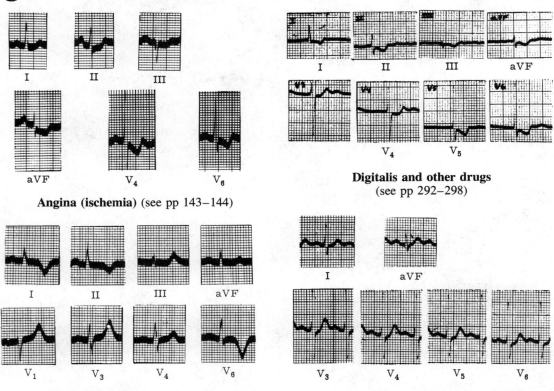

Angina (ischemia) (see pp 143–144)

Digitalis and other drugs
(see pp 292–298)

Subendocardial infarction (see pp 180–181)

Anxiety or tobacco (see p 83)

(2) Oblique or horizontal depression of ST segment in leads V₁, V₂, and V₃.

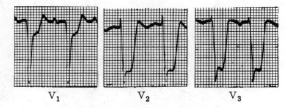

Ischemia (see p 143)

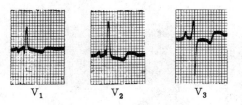

Right bundle branch block
(see pp 114–122)
(But need other [QRS and T] criteria
for diagnosis.)

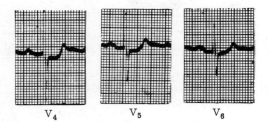

Right ventricular hypertrophy
(see pp 100–106)

*0.5 mm or more: in any lead except aVR and aVL
with vertical heart. An associated QRS complex or
T wave abnormality is usually required before a
definitive electrocardiographic diagnosis is justified. "Scooped" depression of the ST segment in
any lead except aVR and aVL with vertical heart
favors a diagnosis of digitalis effect (see p 292).

II. Depression of ST segment. (Cont'd.)

(3) Oblique or horizontal depression of ST segment in leads I, aVL, and V_{4-6}.

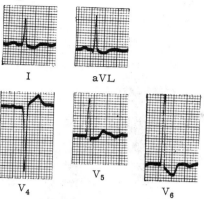

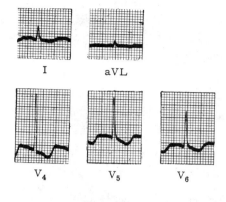

Left ventricular hypertrophy
(see pp 91–99)

Ischemia (see p 143)

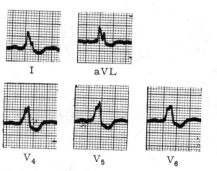

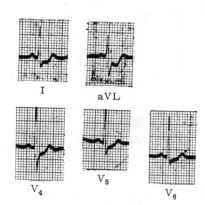

Left bundle branch block (see pp 123–131)
(But need other [QRS and T] criteria
for diagnosis.)

**Reciprocal of ST elevation with inferior
infarction** (see p 173)

(4) Oblique or horizontal depression of ST segment in leads II, III, and aVF.

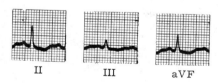

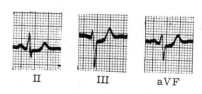

Ischemia (see p 143)

**Reciprocal of ST elevation with anterior
infarction** (see p 160)

T WAVE ABNORMALITIES

I. Deep inversion of T wave.

(1) Symmetric in any lead except aVR and aVL in vertical heart.

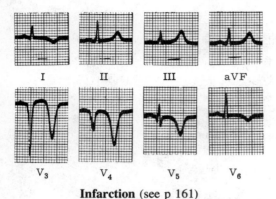

Infarction (see p 161)

Ischemia (see p 147)

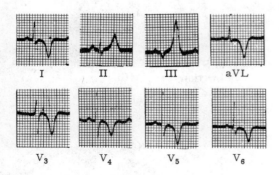

Pericarditis (see p 287)

(2) Symmetric inversion of T waves in leads I, aVL, and V_{4-6}.

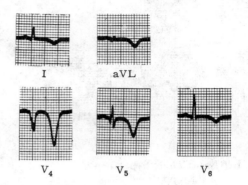

Anterior infarction (see pp 155–168)

(3) Symmetric in leads II, III, and aVF.

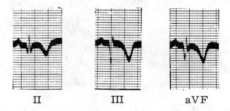

Inferior infarction
(Diagnosis more certain if associated with abnormal Q waves; see pp 169–174.)

II. T wave flat to inverted.

(1) Asymmetric in any lead except aVR and aVL in vertical heart. Usually not diagnostic unless associated with QRS–ST abnormalities. Possibilities same as for ST depression.

III. Upright T wave.

(1) Tall, peaked, and slender upright T waves in all leads except aVR and aVL in vertical heart.

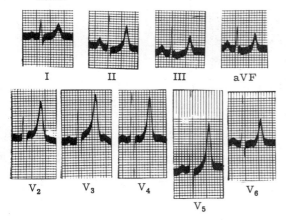

I II III aVF

V₂ V₃ V₄ V₅ V₆

Hyperkalemia (see pp 299–301)

(2) Tall, symmetric T waves in leads V₁₋₄.

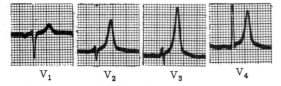

V₁ V₂ V₃ V₄

Posterior infarction (see pp 170 and 177)

U WAVE ABNORMALITIES

Upright U wave, taller than T in same lead, especially in V₂₋₄.

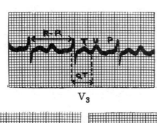

V₃

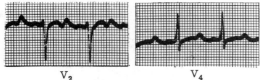

V₂ V₄

Hypokalemia (see pp 302–303)

ABNORMAL INTERVALS*

I. P–R interval, > 0.21 s in any lead.

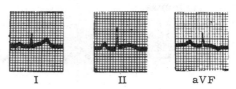

I II aVF

First degree AV block (see p 237)

II. Prolonged S–T interval in any lead.

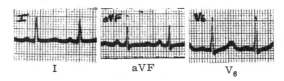

I aVF V₆

Hypocalcemia (see pp 304–305)
(Also seen in liver disease.)

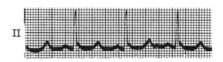

II

Hypothermia (see p 291)

III. Q–T꜀ interval, > 0.42–0.43 s in any lead.

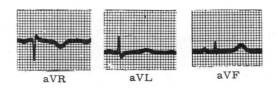

aVR aVL aVF

Multiple causes: any type of myocardial disease, quinidine effect or toxicity, hypocalcemia, hypothermia (see pp 288, 291, 296, and 304)

*QRS interval: See QRS complex.

ARRHYTHMIAS

I. Sinus arrhythmias.

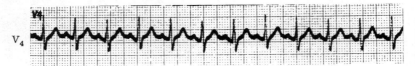

Sinus tachycardia; rate 100–160 (see p 213)

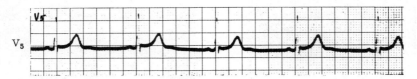

Sinus bradycardia; rate < 60 (see p 213)

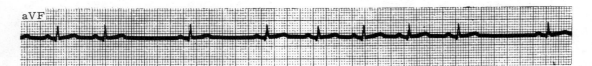

Sinus arrhythmia (see p 214)

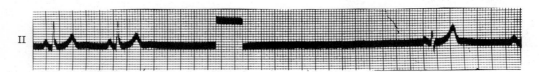

Sinus arrest (see p 215)

II. Atrial arrhythmias.

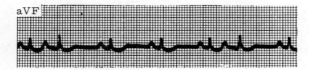

Premature beats (see pp 214, 217, and 218)

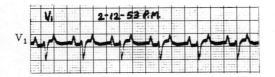

Tachycardia with AV block
(see pp 294–295)

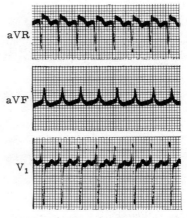

Tachycardia with 1:1 AV conduction
(see p 222)

II. Atrial arrhythmias. (Cont'd.)

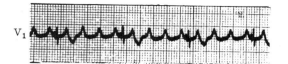

Atrial flutter (see pp 225–229)   **Atrial fibrillation** (see pp 229–233)

III. AV blocks and AV junctional arrhythmias.

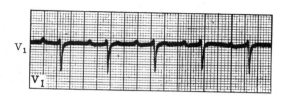
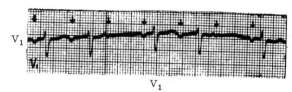

First degree AV block (see pp 235–237)

Second degree AV block, Wenckebach type
(see p 239)

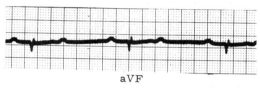
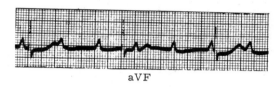

Second degree AV block, constant
(see pp 238)

Third degree AV block (see pp 240–243)

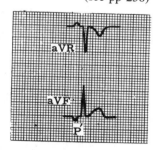
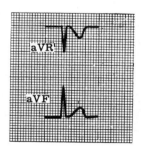
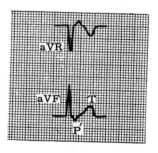

High AV junctional focus.
Note upright P′ in aVR and
inverted P′ in aVF pre-
ceding the QRS complex.

AV junctional focus. P′
buried in QRS complex.

Low AV junctional focus.
Note upright P′ in aVR and
inverted P′ in aVF following
the QRS complex.

Premature beats (see pp 244–248)

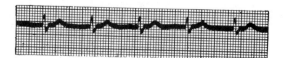
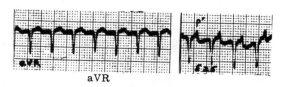

AV junctional rhythm (see p 249)   **AV junctional tachycardia** (see p 250)

IV. Ventricular arrhythmias.

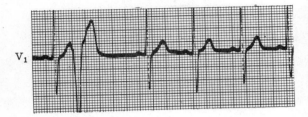

Premature beats (see pp 251–259)

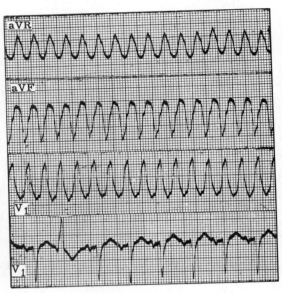

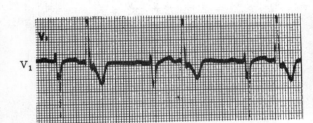

Bigeminy (see p 257)

Tachycardia (see pp 259–265)

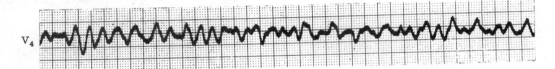

Fibrillation (see pp 265–267)

V. Pararrhythmias.

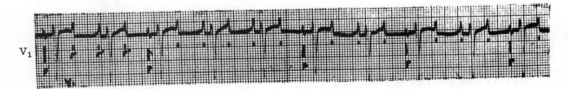

Parasystole (see pp 268–270)

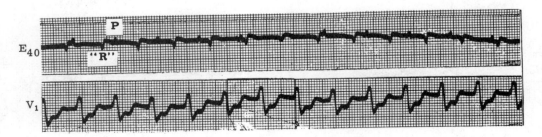

AV dissociation (see pp 270–271)

VI. Preexcitation.

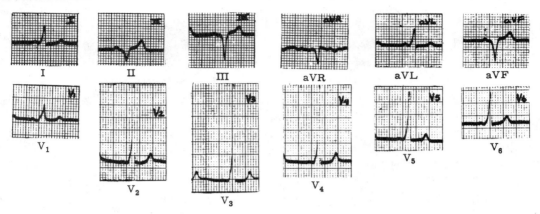

Wolff-Parkinson-White syndrome (see pp 276–278)

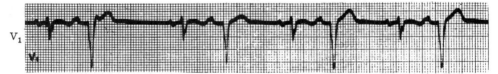

Isolated preexcitation beats (see p 278)

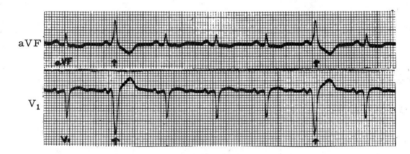

Aberrant intraventricular conduction with atrial premature beats (see p 281)

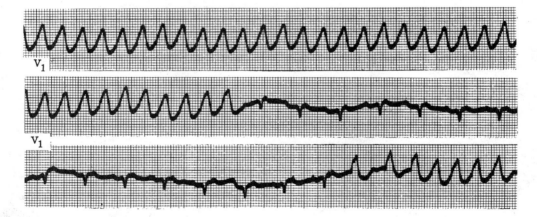

Aberrant intraventricular conduction with atrial tachycardia (see pp 282–284)

Third Appendix:
Application of Statistics to the Electrocardiogram

It is necessary for a physician, student, or nurse involved in evaluation of an ECG to have an understanding of the following commonly used statistical terms.

$$\text{Sensitivity} = \frac{\text{True positives}}{\text{True positives} + \text{False negatives}}$$

ie, the percentage of individuals with a specific diagnosis recognized by the electrocardiographic criteria.

$$\text{Specificity} = \frac{\text{True negatives}}{\text{True negatives} + \text{False positives}}$$

ie, the percentage of normal individuals who do not meet the electrocardiographic criteria for a specific abnormality.

$$\text{False positives} = \frac{\text{False positives}}{\text{False positives} + \text{True negatives}}$$

ie, 1 minus specificity.

$$\text{False negatives} = \frac{\text{False negatives}}{\text{True positives} + \text{False negatives}}$$

ie, 1 minus sensitivity.

$$\text{Accuracy for positive prediction} =$$
$$\frac{\text{True positives}}{\text{True positives} + \text{False positives}}$$

$$\text{Accuracy for negative prediction} =$$
$$\frac{\text{True negatives}}{\text{True negatives} + \text{False negatives}}$$

Another important concept is expressed by Bayes' theorem, which states that the probability that certain electrocardiographic criteria are indicative of a specific disease entity depends not only on the sensitivity and specificity of such criteria but also on the prior probability of that individual having such a disease as assessed by other nonelectrocardiographic criteria. Expressed mathematically, the correct electrocardiographic probability equals the product of the prior probability times the test sensitivity divided by the sum of this product plus the product of 1 minus the prior probability and 1 minus the test specificity (ie, false positives).

Example 1: Let us assume that certain electrocardiographic criteria for left ventricular hypertrophy have a sensitivity of 95% and a specificity of 95% (false positives = 5%). Such criteria seem excellent. They are now applied to a survey of a general population of 100,000 individuals in whom the estimated prior probability of left ventricular hypertrophy (by nonelectrocardiographic, epidemiologic criteria) is 10%. Therefore, 95% (sensitivity) of the 10,000 abnormal cases = 9500; 5% (false positives) of the 90,000 normal cases = 4500. The total abnormal ECGs = 14,000. However, the positive predictive accuracy = 4500/14,000, or 68%!

The same criteria is used to evaluate a group of 100 patients with critical aortic stenosis. The prior probability of left ventricular hypertrophy by nonelectrocardiographic criteria is at least 95%. Therefore, 95% (sensitivity) of 95 patients (90.25) plus 5% (false positives) of 5 patients (0.25 patients) gives a total recognition rate of 90.5. In this instance, the positive predictive accuracy = 90.25/90.5, or over 99%.

Therefore, it is obvious that prior probability is a major factor in predictive accuracy even though sensitivity and specificity remain constant.

Example 2: A 50-year-old man complains of atypical anginal pain. Based on available data (eg, Framingham study), the prior probability of coronary artery disease is 60%. An exercise electrocardiographic test is performed which is said to have a sensitivity of 75% and a specificity of 85%, and the test is interpreted as positive (ie, consistent with myocardial ischemia). Based on Bayes' theorem, the positive predictive accuracy of the exercise test is 0.88.

Given a 30-year-old woman with similar complaints of chest pain, the prior probability of coronary artery disease is under 10%. Using the same sensitivity and specificity of an exercise test, the positive predictive accuracy is 0.35! This is a less accurate means of reaching decisions than tossing a coin.

REFERENCES: BOOKS

Cassels DE, Ziegler RF: *Electrocardiography in Infants and Children*. Grune & Stratton, 1966.

Chou T, Helm RA: *Clinical Vectorcardiography*, 2nd ed. Grune & Stratton, 1974.

Cranefield PF: *The Conduction of the Cardiac Impulse*. Futura (New York), 1975.

Grant RP: *Clinical Electrocardiography*. McGraw-Hill, 1957.

Hoffman BF, Cranefield PF: *Electrophysiology of the Heart*. Blakiston-McGraw, 1960.

Katz LN, Pick A: *Clinical Electrocardiography*. Part 1. *The Arrhythmias*. Lea & Febiger, 1956.

Kossman CE: *Advances in Electrocardiography*. Grune & Stratton, 1958.

Lepeschkin E: *Modern Electrocardiography*. Vol 1. Williams & Wilkins, 1951.

Massie E, Walsh TJ: *Clinical Vectorcardiography and Electrocardiography*. Year Book, 1960.

Narula OS: *Cardiac Arrhythmias: Electrophysiology, Diagnosis and Management*. Williams & Wilkins, 1979.

Pick A, Langendorf R: *Interpretation of Complex Arrhythmias*. Lea & Febiger, 1979.

Prinzmetal M et al: *The Auricular Arrhythmias*. Thomas, 1952.

Schamroth L: *The Disorders of Cardiac Rhythm*, 2nd ed. 2 vols. Mosby, 1980.

Scherf D, Schott A: *Extrasystoles and Allied Arrhythmias*, 2nd ed. Heinemann, 1973.

Simonson E: *Differentiation Between Normal and Abnormal in Electrocardiography*. Mosby, 1961.

Sodi-Pallares D, Calder RM: *New Bases of Electrocardiography*. Mosby, 1956.

REFERENCES: ARTICLES

THE NORMAL ELECTROCARDIOGRAM

Alimurung BN: The influence of early repolarization variant on the exercise ECG: A correlation with coronary arteriograms. *Am Heart J* 1980;**99**:739.

Bethesda Conference Report: Optimal electrocardiography. *Am J Cardiol* 1978;**41**:113.

Blackburn HW Jr, Simonson E: The total QRS duration. *Am Heart J* 1957;**53**:699.

Brody JI, Golden LH, Tobin JL: A review of 3369 electrocardiograms in young male hospitalized patients. *Am Heart J* 1957;**53**:821.

Buxton TM, Hsu I, Barter RH: Fetal electrocardiography. *JAMA* 1963;**185**:441.

Cohen JC et al: The heart of a dancer: Noninvasive cardiac evaluation of professional ballet dancers. *Am J Cardiol* 1980;**45**:959.

Einthoven W: The telecardiogram. [Translated by HW Blackburn, Jr.] *Am Heart J* 1957;**53**:602.

Einthoven W, Fahr G, de Waart A: On the direction and manifest size of the variations of potential in the human heart and on the influence of the position of the heart on the form of the electrocardiogram. [Translated by HE Hoff and P Sekeli.] *Am Heart J* 1950;**40**:163.

Gardberg M, Rosen IL: The effects of nonpathologic factors on the electrocardiogram. *Am Heart J* 1957;**53**:494, 711.

Hariman RJ et al: Method for recording electrical activity of the sinoatrial node and automatic atrial foci during cardiac catheterization in human subjects. *Am J Cardiol* 1980;**45**:775.

Hoffman BF: Fine structure of internodal pathways. *Am J Cardiol* 1979;**44**:385.

James TH: The connecting pathways between the sinus node and A-V node and between the right and left atrium in the human heart. *Am Heart J* 1963;**66**:498.

Johnston FD: Reflection on electrocardiography. (Editorial.) *Circulation* 1957;**15**:801.

Kennamer R et al: Studies on the mechanism of ventricular activity. 5. Intramural depolarization potentials in the normal heart with a consideration of currents of injury in coronary heart disease. *Am J Heart* 1953;**46**:379.

Kossman CE: The normal electrocardiogram. *Circulation* 1953;**8**:920.

Lamb LE: The effects of respiration on the electrocardiogram in relation to differences in right and left ventricular stroke volume. *Am Heart J* 1957;**54**:342.

Lepeschkin EL, Surawicz B: The measurement of the QT interval of the electrocardiogram. *Circulation* 1952;**6**:378.

Osborne JA, Dower GI: False RVH pattern due to Wilson's central terminal error. *Am Heart J* 1957;**54**:722.

Palati IJ, Ikaheimo MJ: Runner's heart. *Primary Cardiol* (April) 1981;**7**:73.

Prinzmetal M et al: Studies on the nature of the repolarization process. 19. Studies on the mechanism of ventricular activity. *Am Heart J* 1957;**53**:100.

Raskoff WJ, Goldman S, Cohn K: The "athletic heart": Prevalence and physiological significance of left ventricular enlargement in distance runners. *JAMA* 1976;**236**:158.

Rosen KM: Clinical cardiac electrophysiology. (Key references.) *Circulation* 1980;**61**:1262.

Scher AM: The sequence of ventricular excitation. *Am J Cardiol* 1964;**14**:294.

Stern S, Eisenberg S: The effect of propranolol on the ECG of normal subjects. *Am Heart J* 1969;**77**:192.

Symposium on cardiology in aviation: Electrocardiographic findings in 67,375 asymptomatic subjects. *Am J Cardiol* 1960;**6**:76–200.

Symposium on the U wave of the electrocardiogram. *Circulation* 1957;**15**:68.

Tranchesi J et al: Atrial repolarization: Its importance in clinical electrocardiography. *Circulation* 1960;**22**:635.

Uhley HN, Rivkin L: Peripheral distribution of the canine A-V conduction system: Observations on gross morphology. *Am J Cardiol* 1960;**5**:688.

Van Dam RT, Durrer D: The T wave and ventricular repolarization. *Am J Cardiol* 1964;**14**:294.

Wasserburger RN, Corliss RJ: Value of oral potassium salts in differentiation of functional and organic T wave changes. *Am J Cardiol* 1962;**10**:673.

Wolferth CC: Clinical electrocardiography: Offspring of science or empiricism? *Circulation* 1957;**16**:321.

HYPERTROPHY

DiBianco R et al: Left atrial overload: A hemodynamic, echocardiographic, electrocardiographic and vectorcardiographic study. *Am Heart J* 1979;**98**:478.

Liu C, DeCristofaro D: Sensitivity and specificity of electrocardiographic evaluation of LVH in 364 unselected autopsy cases. *Am Heart J* 1968;**76**:596.

Milnor WR: Electrocardiogram and vectorcardiogram in right ventricular hypertrophy and right bundle branch block. *Circulation* 1957;**16**:348.

Romhilt DW et al: A critical appraisal of the electrocardiographic criteria for the diagnosis of left ventricular hypertrophy. *Circulation* 1969;**40**:185.

Scott RC: The correlation between the electrocardiographic patterns of ventricular hypertrophy and the anatomic findings. *Circulation* 1960;**21**:256.

Sokolow M, Lyon TP: The ventricular complex in left ventricular hypertrophy as obtained by unipolar precordial and limb leads. *Am Heart J* 1949;**37**:161.

Sokolow M, Lyon TP: The ventricular complex in right ventricular hypertrophy as obtained by unipolar precordial and limb leads. *Am Heart J* 1949;**38**:273.

Walker IC Jr, Helm RA, Scott RC: Right ventricular hypertrophy. *Circulation* 1955;**11**:215, 223.

INTRAVENTRICULAR CONDUCTION DEFECTS

Banta HD, Greenfield JC Jr, Estes EH Jr: Left axis deviation. *Am J Cardiol* 1964;**14**:330.

Braunwald E, Morrow AG: Sequence of ventricular contraction in human bundle branch block. *Am J Med* 1957;**23**:205.

Damato AN, Gallagher JJ, Lau SH: Application of His bundle recordings in diagnosing conduction disorders. *Prog Cardiovasc Dis* 1972;**14**:601.

Damato AN, Lau SH: Clinical value of the electrogram of the conduction system. *Prog Cardiovasc Dis* 1970;**13**:119.

Damato AN et al: Study of atrioventricular conduction in man using electrode catheter recordings of His bundle activity. *Circulation* 1969;**39**:287.

Damato AN et al: A study of heart block in man using His bundle recordings. *Circulation* 1969;**39**:297.

Denes P et al: A characteristic precordial repolarization abnormality with intermittent left bundle branch block. *Ann Intern Med* 1978;**89**:55.

Dodge HT, Grant RP: Mechanisms of QRS complex prolongation in man: Right ventricular conduction defects. *Am J Med* 1956;**21**:534.

Dreifus LS et al: Atrioventricular block. *Am J Cardiol* 1971;**28**:371.

Eliot RS, Millhon WA, Millhon J: The clinical significance of uncomplicated marked left axis deviation in men without known disease. *Am J Cardiol* 1963;**12**:767.

El-Sherif N et al: Normalization of bundle branch block patterns by distal His bundle pacing. *Circulation* 1978;**57**:473.

Fisher ML et al: Left anterior fascicular block: Electrocardiographic criteria for its recognition in the presence of inferior myocardial infarction. *Am J Cardiol* 1979;**44**:645.

Grant RP, Dodge HT: Mechanisms of QRS complex prolongation in man: Left ventricular conduction disturbances. *Am J Med* 1956;**20**:834.

Hoffman I et al: Anterior conduction delay: A possible cause for prominent anterior QRS forces. *J Electrocardiol* 1976;**9**:15.

James TN, Sherf L: Specialized tissues and preferential conduction in the atria of the heart. *Am J Cardiol* 1971;**28**:414.

Kennamer R, Prinzmetal M: Studies on the mechanism of ventricular activity. 10. Depolarization of the ventricle with bundle branch block. *Am Heart J* 1954;**47**:769.

Langendorf R, Cohen H, Gozo EG: Observations on second degree A-V block. *Am J Cardiol* 1972;**29**:111.

Pryor R: Fascicular blocks and the bilateral bundle branch block syndrome. *Am Heart J* 1972;**83**:441.

Pryor R, Blount SG Jr: The clinical significance of true left axis deviation. *Am Heart J* 1966;**72**:391.

Ranganathan N et al: His bundle electrogram in bundle branch block. *Circulation* 1972;**45**:282.

Reiffel JA, Bigger JT Jr: Pure anterior conduction delay: A variant "fascicular" defect. *J Electrocardiol* 1978;**11**:315.

Rosenbaum MB: The hemiblocks: Diagnostic criteria and clinical significance. *Mod Concepts Cardiovasc Dis* 1970;**39**:141.

Rosenbaum MB, Elizari MV, Lazzari JO: The hemiblocks. Oldsmar, Florida, Tampa Tracings, 1970.

Scott RC: Left bundle branch block: A clinical assessment. *Am Heart J* 1965;**70**:813.

Tuna IC, Tuna N: Clinical significance of acquired left axis deviation. *Pract Cardiol* 1980;**6**:81.

Uhley HN, Rivkin L: Electrocardiographic patterns following interruption of the main and peripheral branches of the canine bundle of His. *Am J Cardiol* 1961;**7**:810 and 1964;**13**:41.

Watt TB, Pruitt RD: Character, cause, and consequence of combined left axis deviation and right bundle branch block in human electrocardiograms. *Am Heart J* 1969;**77**:460.

Wyndham CR et al: Epicardial activation in human left anterior fascicular block. *Am J Cardiol* 1979;**44**:638.

MYOCARDIAL ISCHEMIA & INFARCTION

Bellet S, Deliyiannis S, Eliakim M: The electrocardiogram during exercise as recorded by radioelectrocardiography. *Am J Cardiol* 1961;**8**:385 and *Circulation* 1962;**25**:5, 686.

Bodenheimer MM, Helfant RH: Problems in the evaluation of Q waves. *Pract Cardiol* 1979;**5**:50.

Bruce RA, Kusumi F, Hosmer D: Maximal oxygen intake and nomographic assessment of functional aerobic impairment in cardiovascular disease. *Am Heart J* 1973;**85**:546.

Gardin JM: Pseudoischemic "false positive" S–T segment changes induced by hyperventilation in patients with mitral valve prolapse. *Am J Cardiol* 1980;**45**:952.

Gazes PC: False-positive exercise test in the presence of the Wolff-Parkinson-White syndrome. *Am Heart J* 1969;**78**:13.

Georgopoulos AJ et al: Effect of exercise on electrocardiograms of patients with low serum potassium. *Circulation* 1961;**23**:567.

Goldschlager N, Cake D, Cohn K: Exercise induced ventricular arrhythmias in patients with coronary artery disease and their relationships to angiographic findings. *Am J Cardiol* 1973;**31**:434.

Goldschlager N, Selzer A, Cohn K: Treadmill stress tests as indicators of presence and severity of coronary artery disease. *Ann Intern Med* 1976;**85**:277.

Grant RP: Peri-infarction block. *Prog Cardiovasc Dis* 1959;**2**:237.

Hollenberg M et al: Treadmill score quantifies electrocardiographic response to exercise and improves test accuracy and reproducibility. *Circulation* 1980;**61**:276.

Ideker RE: Q waves and transmural infarcts. (Abstract.) *Am J Cardiol* 1981;**47 (2-part 2)**:464.

Lahiri A et al: Exercise-induced S–T segment elevation in variant angina. *Am J Cardiol* 1980;**45**:887.

Lepeschkin E: Exercise tests in the diagnosis of coronary artery disease. *Circulation* 1960;**22**:986.

Lopez EA et al: Q-wave abnormalities in chronic obstructive pulmonary disease and myocardial infarction. *J Electrocardiol* 1980;**13**:173.

Massumi RA et al: Studies on the mechanism of ventricular activity. 16. Activation of the human ventricle. *Am J Med* 1955;**19**:832.

McNeer JF et al: The role of the exercise test in the evaluation of patients for ischemic heart disease. *Circulation* 1978;**57**:64.

Myers GB, Klein HA, Hiratzka T: Correlation of electrocardiographic and pathologic findings in anteroposterior infarction. *Am Heart J* 1949;**37**:205.

Myers GB, Klein HA, Hiratzka T: Correlation of electrocardiographic and pathologic findings in large anterolateral infarcts. *Am Heart J* 1948;**36**:838.

Myers GB, Klein HA, Hiratzka T: Correlation of electrocardiographic and pathologic findings in posterior infarction. *Am Heart J* 1949;**38**:547.

Myers GB, Klein HA, Hiratzka T: Correlation of electrocardiographic and pathologic findings in posterolateral infarction. *Am Heart J* 1949;**38**:837.

Myers GB, Klein HA, Stofer BE: Correlation of electrocardiographic and pathologic findings in anteroseptal infarction. *Am Heart J* 1948;**36**:535.

Myers GB, Klein HA, Stofer BE: Correlation of electrocardiographic and pathologic findings in lateral infarction. *Am Heart J* 1949;**37**:374.

Pearce ML, Chapman MG: The evaluation of Q aVF by the initial sagittal QRS vectors in 70 autopsied cases. *Am Heart J* 1957;**53**:782.

Pipberger HV, Lopez EA: "Silent" subendocardial infarcts: Fact or fiction. *Am Heart J* 1980;**100**:597.

Platt ML, Peter T, Mendel WJ: Evaluation of ST–T segment abnormalities in the ECG. *Pract Cardiol* 1979;**5**:37.

Prinzmetal M et al: Angina pectoris: Clinical and experimental difference between ischemia with ST elevation and ischemia with ST depression. *Am J Cardiol* 1961;**7**:412.

Prinzmetal M et al: A variant of angina pectoris. *Am J Med* 1959;**27**:375.

Pruitt RD, Dennis EW, Kinard SA: The difficult ECG diagnosis of myocardial infarction. *Prog Cardiovasc Dis* 1963;**6**:85.

Raunio H et al: Changes in the QRS complex and ST segment in transmural and subendocardial myocardial infarctions: A clinicopathologic study. *Am Heart J* 1979;**98**:176.

Ruben IL, Gross H: Abnormal Q waves in ECG in absence of infarction. *Pract Cardiol* 1979;**5**:52.

Scherf D: The electrocardiographic exercise test. *J Electrocardiol* 1968;**1**:141.

Schuster EH et al: Nontransmural vs. transmural myocardial infarction. (Abstract.) *Am J Cardiol* 1981;**47** (**2-part 2**):459.

Sheffield LT: Clinical exercise stress testing. (Key references.) *Circulation* 1980;**61**:1053.

Simonson E: Electrocardiographic stress tolerance tests. *Prog Cardiovasc Dis* 1970;**13**:269.

Simonson E: Use of the ECG in exercise tests. *Am Heart J* 1963;**66**:552.

Spodick DH: Transmural vs. nontransmural infarction. *Circulation* 1980;**62**:447.

Strasberg B et al: Treadmill exercise testing in the Wolff-Parkinson-White syndrome. *Am J Cardiol* 1980;**45**:742.

Watanabe K, Bhargava V, Froelicher V: Computer analysis of the exercise ECG: A review. *Prog Cardiovasc Dis* 1980;**22**:423.

ARRHYTHMIAS

Aronson RS, Keung EC: Electrophysiologic mechanism of cardiac arrhythmias. *Cardiovasc Rev Rep* 1980;**1**:403.

Basu D, Scheinman M: Sustained accelerated idioventricular rhythm. *Am Heart J* 1975;**89**:227.

Berlinerblau R, Feder W: Chaotic atrial rhythm. *J Electrocardiol* 1972;**5**:135.

Castellanos A Jr, Castillo CA, Agha AS: Contribution of His bundle recordings to the understanding of clinical arrhythmias. *Am J Cardiol* 1971;**28**:499.

Castellanos A Jr et al: The electrocardiogram in patients with pacemakers. *Prog Cardiovasc Dis* 1970;**13**:190.

Chardack WM: Heart block treated with implantable pacemaker. *Prog Cardiovasc Dis* 1964;**6**:507.

Chatterjee K et al: ECG changes subsequent to artificial ventricular depolarization. *Br Heart J* 1969;**31**:770.

Cobb FR et al: Successful surgical resection of the bundle of Kent in a patient with W-P-W syndrome. *Circulation* 1968;**38**:1018.

Cohn K: Arrhythmias in exercise testing. *Pract Cardiol* 1978;**4**:153.

Culler MR, Boone JA, Gazes RC: Fibrillatory wave size as a clue to etiological diagnosis. *Am Heart J* 1963;**66**:435.

Dreifus LS et al: Control of recurrent tachycardia of W-P-W syndrome by surgical ligature of the A-V bundle. *Circulation* 1968;**38**:1030.

Dreifus LS et al: Ventricular fibrillation: A possible mechanism of sudden death in patients with W-P-W. *Circulation* 1971;**43**:520.

Fisch C, Knoebel SB: Junctional rhythms. *Prog Cardiovasc Dis* 1970;**13**:141.

Fisher JD: Role of electrophysiologic testing in the diagnosis and treatment of patients with known and suspected bradycardias and tachycardias. *Prog Cardiovasc Dis* 1981;**24**:25.

Fox TT: Further remarks on the syndrome of aberrant A-V conduction (Wolff-Parkinson-White). *Am Heart J* 1969;**22**:711.

Gallagher JJ et al: The preexcitation syndromes. *Prog Cardiovasc Dis* 1978;**20**:285.

Goldreyer BN, Bigger JT: Site of reentry in paroxysmal supraventricular tachycardia in man. *Circulation* 1971;**43**:15.

Han J: The concepts of reentrant activity responsible for ectopic rhythms. *Am J Cardiol* 1971;**28**:253.

Hoffman BF: The genesis of cardiac arrhythmias. *Prog Cardiovasc Dis* 1966;**8**:319.

James TN: The Wolff-Parkinson-White syndrome. *Prog Cardiovasc Dis* 1970;**13**:159.

Josephson ME et al: Sustained ventricular tachycardia: Role of the 12-lead ECG in localizing site of origin. *Circulation* 1981;**64**:257.

Kastor JA et al: Clinical electrophysiology of ventricular tachycardia. *N Engl J Med* 1981;**304**:1004.

Kennelly BM, Lloyd E, Rose AG: ECG recognition of extent of acute myocardial infarction in ventricular extrasystoles. *Arch Intern Med* 1980;**140**:970.

Kleiger R, Lown B: Cardioversion and digitalis. *Circulation* 1966;**33**:878.

Krikler DM, Curry PV: Torsade de pointes, an atypical ventricular tachycardia. *Br Heart J* 1976;**38**:117.

Lange WR, Kennedy HL: The ECG recognition of AV junctional rhythms. *Pract Cardiol* 1979;**5**:49.

Langendorf R, Pick A: Atrioventricular block, type II (Mobitz): Its nature and clinical significance. *Circulation* 1968;**38**:819.

Lichtenberg SB, Schwartz MJ, Case RB: Value of premature ventricular contraction morphology in the detection of myocardial infarction. *J Electrocardiol* 1980;**13**:167.

Lipman BS: Aberrancy, ectopy and re-entry in the ECG. *Pract Cardiol* 1978;**4**:107.

Lown B, Amarasingham R, Newman J: New method for terminating cardiac arrhythmias: Use of synchronized capacitor discharge. *JAMA* 1962;**182**:548.

Lown B, Levine S: The carotid sinus. *Circulation* 1961;**23**:766.

Marriott HJL: Interactions between atria and ventricle during interference dissociation and complete A-V block. *Am Heart J* 1957;**53**:884.

Marriott HJL, Fogg E: Constant monitoring for cardiac dysrhythmias and blocks. *Mod Concepts Cardiovasc Dis* 1970;**39**:103.

Marriott HJL, Sandler IA: Criteria, old and new, for differentiating between ectopic beats and aberrant ventricular conduction in the presence of atrial fibrillation. *Prog Cardiovasc Dis* 1966;**9**:18.

Miller R, Sharrett RH: Interference dissociation. *Circulation* 1957;**16**:803.

Moore EN, Knoebel SB, Spear JF: Concealed conduction. *Am J Cardiol* 1971;**28**:406.

Nathan DA et al: Long-term correction of complete heart block: Clinical and physiologic studies of a new type of implantable synchronous pacer. *Prog Cardiovasc Dis* 1966;**6**:538.

Nelson WP: Atrioventricular dissociation. *Resident Staff Physician* (Feb) 1981;**27**:48 and (March) 1981;**27**:96.

Pick A: A-V dissociation. *Am Heart J* 1963;**66**:147.

Pick A, Dominguez P: Nonparoxysmal A-V nodal tachycardia. *Circulation* 1957;**16**:1022.

Pick A, Langendorf R, Katz LN: Advances in the electrocardiographic diagnosis of cardiac arrhythmias. *Med Clin North Am* 1957;**41**:269.

Rosen KM: Dual AV nodal pathways and AV nodal reentrant paroxysmal tachycardia. *Am Heart J* 1981;**101**:691.

Rosenbaum MB, Lepeschkin EL: The effect of ventricular systole on auricular rhythm in auriculoventricular block. *Circulation* 1955;**11**:240.

Rubenstein JJ et al: Clinical spectrum of the sick sinus syndrome. *Circulation* 1972;**46**:5.

Runge TM et al: Extremely rapid arrhythmias and regular tachycardias in paroxysms in patients with and without accelerated A-V conduction. *Am J Med Sci* 1957;**234**:170.

Rytand DA: The circus movement (entrapped circuit wave) hypothesis and atrial flutter. *Ann Intern Med* 1966;**65**:125.

Scherf D: The atrial arrhythmias. *N Engl J Med* 1955;**252**:928.

Singer DH, Ten Eick E: Aberrancy: Electrophysiologic aspects. *Am J Cardiol* 1971;**28**:381.

Surawicz B: Role of electrolytes in etiology and management of cardiac arrhythmias. *Prog Cardiovasc Dis* 1966;**8**:364.

Sutton R, Davies M: The conduction system in acute myocardial infarction complicated by heart block. *Circulation* 1968;**38**:987.

Tye K et al: R on T or R on P phenomenon: Relation to the genesis of ventricular tachycardia. *Am J Cardiol* 1979;**44**:632.

Vassalle M: Automaticity and automatic rhythms. *Am J Cardiol* 1971;**28**:245.

Vera Z, Mason DT: Reentry vs. automaticity. *Am Heart J* 1981;**101**:329.

Watanabe Y: Reassessment of parasystole. *Am Heart J* 1971;**81**:451.

Watson RM, Josephson ME: Atrial flutter. 1. Electrophysiologic substrates and modes of initiation and termination. *Am J Cardiol* 1980;**45**:732.

Wolff L, Parkinson J, White PD: Bundle branch block with short PR interval in healthy people prone to paroxysmal tachycardia. *Am Heart J* 1930;**5**:685.

DRUGS, ELECTROLYTES, MISCELLANEOUS

Abildskov JA et al: The electrocardiogram and the central nervous system. *Prog Cardiovasc Dis* 1970;**13**:210.

Alexander CS: Cardiotoxic effects of phenothiazine and related drugs. *Circulation* 1968;**38**:1014.

Bellet S: The electrocardiogram in electrolyte imbalance. *Arch Intern Med* 1955;**96**:618.

Bigger JT, Basset AL, Hoffman BF: Electrophysiological effects of diphenylhydantoin on canine Purkinje fibers. *Circ Res* 1968;**22**:221.

Bruce MA, Spodick DH: Atypical ECG in acute pericarditis. *J Electrocardiol* 1980;**13**:61.

Clements SD Jr, Hurst JW: Diagnostic value of ECG abnormalities observed in subjects accidentally exposed to cold. *Am J Cardiol* 1972;**29**:729.

Cropp GJ, Manning GW: Electrocardiographic changes simulating myocardial ischemia and infarction associated with spontaneous intracerebral hemorrhage. *Circulation* 1960;**22**:25.

Curtiss EI, Heibel RH, Shaver JA: Autonomic maneuvers in hereditary QT interval prolongation. *Am Heart J* 1978;**95**:420.

Goldman MJ: Common errors in the interpretation of the ECG. *Pract Cardiol* 1979;**5**:140.

Lary D, Goldschlager N: ECG changes during hyperventilation. *Am Heart J* 1974;**87**:383.

Morgan JR, Rogers AK, Forker AD: Congenital absence of the left pericardium. *Ann Intern Med* 1971;**74**:370.

Mullican WS, Fisch C: Postextrasystolic alternans of the U waves due to hypokalemia. *Am Heart J* 1964;**68**:383.

Pick A: Digitalis and the electrocardiogram. *Circulation* 1957;**15**:603.

Pryor R: The long QT syndrome. *Primary Cardiol* (Feb) 1981;**7**:53.

Ryan C, Suddeth B: ECG recognition of pacemaker malfunction. *Pract Cardiol* 1978;**4**:142.

Schwartz PJ: The long Q–T syndrome. *Am Heart J* 1975;**89**:378.

Smith W, Gallagher JJ: QT prolongation syndromes. *Pract Cardiol* 1979;**5**:118.

Spodick DH: The ECG in acute pericarditis. *Am J Cardiol* 1974;**33**:470.

Surawicz B et al: Quantitative analysis of the electrocardiographic pattern of hypopotassemia. *Circulation* 1957;**16**:750.

Villamil A et al: Electrocardiographic changes in artificial hibernation. *Am Heart J* 1957;**53**:365.

SPATIAL VECTORCARDIOGRAPHY

Brinberg L: The ventricular gradient in space. *Am J Med* 1957;**23**:212.

Cosma J, Levy B, Pipberger HV: The spatial ventricular gradient during alterations in the ventricular activation pathway. *Am Heart J* 1966;**71**:84.

Draper HW et al: The corrected orthogonal electrocardiogram and vectorcardiogram in 510 normal men. *Circulation* 1964;**30**:853.

Eddleman EE Jr, Pipberger HV: Computer analysis of orthogonal ECG and VCG in 1002 patients with MI. *Am Heart J* 1971;**81**:608.

Frank E: An accurate, clinically practical system for spatial vectorcardiography. *Circulation* 1956;**13**:737.

Frank E: General theory of heart vector projection. *Circ Res* 1954;**2**:258.

Frank E: The image surface of a homogeneous torso. *Am Heart J* 1954;**47**:757.

Goldman MJ, Ferrari L: A simplified, inexpensive bedside technique for recording corrected orthogonal scalar electrocardiograms. *Am J Med Sci* 1963;**246**:212.

Goldman MJ, Pipberger HV: Analysis of the orthogonal ECG and VCG in ventricular conduction defects with and without myocardial infarction. *Circulation* 1969;**39**:243.

Helm RA: An accurate lead system for spatial vectorcardiography. *Am Heart J* 1957;**53**:415.

Helm RA: Vectorcardiographic notation. *Circulation* 1956;**13**:581.

Hoffman I: Clinical vectorcardiography in adults. (2 parts.) *Am Heart J* 1980;**100**:239, 373.

Ishikawa K, Berson AS, Pipberger HV: ECG changes due to cardiac enlargement. *Am Heart J* 1971;**81**:635.

Ishikawa K, Eddleman EE, Pipberger HV: Electrocardiograms in pulmonary emphysema mimicking myocardial infarction. *Med Ann DC* 1970;**39**:20.

Ishikawa K, Kini PM, Pipberger HV: P wave analysis in 2464 orthogonal ECGs. *Circulation* 1973;**48**:565.

Johnston FD: The clinical value of vectorcardiography. *Circulation* 1961;**23**:297.

Kerr A, Adicoff A, Klingeman JD: Computer analysis of the orthogonal ECG in pulmonary emphysema. *Am J Cardiol* 1970;**25**:34.

Kini PM, Eddleman EE, Pipberger HV: ECG differentiation between LVH and anterior MI. *Circulation* 1970;**42**:875.

Kini PM, Pipberger HV: Criteria for ECG differentiation of RVH from true posterior myocardial infarction. *Am J Cardiol* 1974;**33**:608.

Kornbluth AW, Allenstein BJ: The normal direct spatial vectorcardiogram. *Am Heart J* 1957;**54**:396.

McCaughan D, Littmann D, Pipberger HV: Computer analysis of the orthogonal ECG and VCG in 939 cases with hypertensive cardiovascular disease. *Am Heart J* 1973;**85**:467.

Milnor WR, Talbot SA, Newman EV: A study of relationship between unipolar leads and spatial vectorcardiograms, using the panoramic vectorcardiograph. *Circulation* 1953;**7**:545.

Nemati M et al: The orthogonal ECG in normal women. *Am Heart J* 1978;**95**:12.

Pipberger HV: Correlation and clinical information in the standard 12 lead ECG and in a corrected orthogonal 3 lead VCG. *Am Heart J* 1961;**61**:35.

Pipberger HV: Current status and persistent problems of electrode placement and lead systems for vectorcardiography and electrocardiography. *Prog Cardiovasc Dis* 1959;**2**:248.

Pipberger HV: The normal orthogonal electrocardiogram and vectorcardiogram. *Circulation* 1958;**17**:1102.

Pipberger HV et al: Clinical application of a second generation of an ECG computer program. *Am J Cardiol* 1975;**35**:597.

Pipberger HV et al: Correlations of the orthogonal electrocardiogram and vectorcardiogram with constitutional variables in 518 normal men. *Circulation* 1967;**35**:536.

Simonson E et al: Diagnostic accuracy of the vectorcardiogram and electrocardiogram. *Am J Cardiol* 1966;**17**:829.

Walston A, Pipberger HV: Computer analysis of orthogonal ECG and VCG in mitral stenosis. *Circulation* 1974;**59**:472.

Yankopoulos NA, Haisty WK, Pipberger HV: Computer analysis of the orthogonal electrocardiogram and vectorcardiogram in 257 patients with aortic valve disease. *Am J Cardiol* 1977;**40**:707.

Index

NORMAL RANGES & VARIATIONS IN THE ADULT
TWELVE-LEAD ELECTROCARDIOGRAM

A true understanding of the normal range and the normal variation of the ECG depends upon a basic understanding of both normal and abnormal cardiac electrophysiology. It must be remembered that many of the configurations tabulated below may represent cardiac abnormalities when interpreted in the context of the entire tracing and in the light of the clinical history and physical examination. Therefore, the information contained in the following table is intended to be used only as a rough preliminary guide to the interpretation of ambiguous and borderline tracings.

Lead	P	Q	R	S	T	ST
I	Upright deflection	Small. < 0.04 s and < 25% of R.	Dominant. Largest deflection of the QRS complex.	< R, or none	Upright deflection	Usually isoelectric; may vary from +1 to −0.5 mm.
II	Upright deflection	Small or none	Dominant	< R, or none	Upright deflection	Usually isoelectric; may vary from +1 to −0.5 mm.
III	Upright, flat, diphasic, or inverted, depending on frontal plane axis (Table 6−1).	Small or none, depending on frontal plane axis (Table 6−1); or large (0.04−0.05 s or > 25% of R).	None to dominant, depending on frontal plane axis (Table 6−1).	None to dominant, depending on frontal plane axis (Table 6−1).	Upright, flat, diphasic, or inverted, depending on frontal plane axis (Table 6−1).	Usually isoelectric; may vary from +1 to −0.5 mm.
aVR	Inverted deflection	Small, none, or large	Small or none, depending on frontal plane axis (Table 6−1).	Dominant (may be QS)	Inverted deflection	Usually isoelectric; may vary from +1 to −0.5 mm.
aVL	Upright, flat, diphasic, or inverted, depending on frontal plane axis (Table 6−1).	Small, none, or large, depending on frontal plane axis (Table 6−1).	Small, none, or dominant, depending on frontal plane axis (Table 6−1).	None to dominant, depending on frontal plane axis (Table 6−1).	Upright, flat, diphasic, or inverted, depending on frontal plane axis (Table 6−1).	Usually isoelectric; may vary from +1 to −0.5 mm.
aVF	Upright deflection	Small or none	Small, none, or dominant, depending on frontal plane axis (Table 6−1).	None to dominant, depending on frontal plane axis (Table 6−1).	Upright, flat, diphasic, or inverted, depending on frontal plane axis (Table 6−1).	Usually isoelectric; may vary from +1 to −0.5 mm.
V_1	Inverted, flat, upright, or diphasic	None (may be QS)	< S, or none (QS); small r′ may be present (Fig 5−9).	Dominant (may be QS)	Upright, flat, diphasic, or inverted*	0 to +3 mm
V_2	Upright; less commonly, diphasic or inverted.	None (may be QS)	< S, or none (QS); small r′ may be present (Fig 5−9).	Dominant (may be QS)	Upright; less commonly, flat, diphasic, or inverted.*	0 to +3 mm
V_3	Upright	Small or none	R <, >, or = S	S >, <, or = R	Upright*	0 to +3 mm
V_4	Upright	Small or none	R > S	S < R	Upright*	Usually isoelectric; may vary from +1 to −0.5 mm.
V_5	Upright	Small	Dominant (< 26 mm)	S < SV_4	Upright	
V_6	Upright	Small	Dominant (< 26 mm)	S < SV_5	Upright	

*Inverted in infants, children, and occasionally in young adults (Figs 7−2, 7−3, 7−11, and 7−12).